Internet of Things enabled Machine Learning for Biomedical Applications

The text begins by highlighting the benefits of the Internet of Things–enabled machine learning in the healthcare sector, examines the diagnosis of diseases using machine learning algorithms, and analyzes security and privacy issues in the healthcare systems using the Internet of Things. The text elaborates on image processing implementation for medical images to detect and classify diseases based on magnetic resonance imaging and ultrasound images.

This book:

- Covers the procedure to recognize emotions using image processing and the Internet of Things–enabled machine learning.
- Highlights security and privacy issues in the healthcare system using the Internet of Things.
- Discusses classification and implementation techniques of image segmentation.
- Explains different algorithms of machine learning for image processing in a comprehensive manner.
- Provides computational intelligence on the Internet of Things for future biomedical applications, including lung cancer.

It is primarily written for graduate students and academic researchers in the fields of electrical engineering, electronics and communications engineering, computer science and engineering, and biomedical engineering.

Internet of Things enabled Machine Learning for Biomedical Applications

Edited by
Neha Goel and Ravindra Kumar Yadav

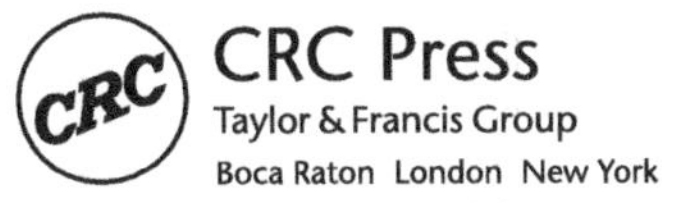

CRC Press
Taylor & Francis Group
Boca Raton London New York

CRC Press is an imprint of the
Taylor & Francis Group, an **informa** business

Designed cover image: Neha Goel

First edition published 2025
by CRC Press
2385 NW Executive Center Drive, Suite 320, Boca Raton FL 33431

and by CRC Press
4 Park Square, Milton Park, Abingdon, Oxon, OX14 4RN

CRC Press is an imprint of Taylor & Francis Group, LLC

ISBN: 978-1-032-55082-4 (hbk)
ISBN: 978-1-032-78392-5 (pbk)
ISBN: 978-1-003-48764-7 (ebk)

DOI: 10.1201/9781003487647

Typeset in Sabon
by KnowledgeWorks Global Ltd.

Contents

List of contributors ix
Editors' biographies xv

1 ML and IoT coupled biomedical applications in healthcare: Smart growth and upcoming challenges 1

VASANTH R., PARANTHAMAN M., AND SIVAPRAKASH P.

2 Recent advances in ubiquitous sustainable healthcare systems 23

SHWETHA BALIGA AND PUSHKAR R. KULKARNI

3 IoT-enabled healthcare system using machine learning 41

P. JOTHI THILAGA, K. VIGNESH SARAVANAN, S. KAVI PRIYA, AND K. VIJAYALAKSHMI

4 An efficient architecture for classification of super-resolution enhanced human chromosome images 58

D. MENAKA AND K. S. SUBHASHINI

5 Applications of machine learning to the impact of IoT in biomedical applications 77

SHWETHA BALIGA, RAKSHITA BASARAKOD, KALATHMIKA G., NANDANA P. PILLAI, JAYASHREE SHIVAKUMAR, AND PREETI YADAV

6 Ovarian cancer detection using IoT-based intelligent assistant and blockchain technology 97

MOHSEN GHORBIAN AND SAEID GHORBIAN

7 Blood oxygen level and pulse rate measurement using hemodialysis using IoT and computational intelligence 116

N. VIGNESHWARI, C. SIVAMANI, S. SELVI, AND G. REVATHY

8   Dental shade matching using machine learning models   131

SHISHIRA R., S. DEEPTHI NAYAK, M. N. SUMA, AND GEETISHREE MISHRA

9   Brain tumor detection for recognizing critical brain damage in patients using computer vision   145

VIVEK VEERAIAH, PARTH SHARMA, KUMUD SAXENA, NIRAJ KUMAR SAHU, KHUSHBOO SHARMA, JAY KUMAR PANDEY, R. K. YADAV, AND MRITUNJAY RAI

10   Smart therapist: The mental health detector   167

ARUNABHA DUTT, NIZAR BANU P. K., AKARSHI BANSAL, AND KRISHNA BANSAL

11   Medical image analysis based on deep learning approach and Internet of Medical Things (IoMT) for early diagnosis of retinal disease   188

S. KARKUZHALI, THENDAL P., AND SENTHILKUMAR S.

12   Intelligent e-learning platform consolidating Web of Things and ChatGPT   202

NEHA KATIYAR, MAYANK DEEP KHARE, JATIN KUMAR, AYUSH SHARMA, SACHIN RAWAT, AND JYOTI SRIVASTAV

13   Issues and challenges in security and privacy with e-Healthcare: A thorough literature analysis   222

MANIKANDAN A., SANJAY T., GAUTHAM MENON, ASWIN R., PARTHIV BIJUMON BHASKAR, MAHADEV GOVIND R., AND RAMPRASAD OG

14   Harnessing the power of distributed cloud and edge computing for advanced healthcare systems   248

SAMPATH BOOPATHI

15   Securing cloud-based IoT: Exploring the significance of lightweight cryptography for enhanced security   273

GAIKWAD VIDYA S., NILESH P. SABLE, DISHA S. WANKHEDE, VAISHALI MISHRA, MADHURI P. KARNIK, NITIN AMBHORE, AND AKSHAY MANIKJADE

16   Security and privacy in the Internet of Medical Things (IoMT)-based healthcare: Ensuring trust and safety   295

DEEPALI VASHISTHA, DHAIRYA MEHTA, PRANAV VASHISTHA, PRANJAL MAIRAL, MALARAM KUMHAR, AND JITENDRA BHATIA

17 A comprehensive study of the problem and challenges
associated with machine learning-enabled IoT
in biomedical applications   320

SANDEEP BHATIA, BASETTY MALLIKARJUN, NEHA GOEL,
AMIT KUMAR GOEL, BHARAT BHUSHAN NAIB,
AND SONIYA VERMA

18 A machine learning-enabled Internet of Things
model for cloud-based biomedical applications   341

PALANIVEL KUPPUSAMY, NANDHU PALANIVEL,
AND SURESH JOSEPH K

19 Machine learning-enabled IoT for biomedical
applications: Problem and challenges   367

HASHMAT USMANI AND RENU RANI

20 IoT-driven machine learning mechanisms
for healthcare applications   379

GOPALAKRISHNAN KARUPPAIAH, KARTHIKEYAN VELAYUTHAPANDIAN,
AND SRIDHAR RAJ SANKARA VADIVEL

Index   407

Contributors

Manikandan A.
Amrita School of Engineering
Amrita Vishwa Vidyapeetham
Kollam, Kerala, India

Nitin Ambhore
Vishwakarma Institute of Information
　Technology
Pune, Maharashtra, India

Ramachandran Balasubramanian
SRM Institute of Science and
　Technology
Chennai, Tamil Nadu, India

Shwetha Baliga
RV College of Engineering
Bengaluru, Karnataka, India

Akarshi Bansal
CHRIST (Deemed to be University)
Bangalore, Karnataka, India

Krishna Bansal
CHRIST (Deemed to be University)
Bangalore, Karnataka, India

Rakshita Basarakod
RV College of Engineering
Bangalore, Karnataka, India

Parthiv Bijumon Bhaskar
Amrita School of Engineering

Amrita Vishwa Vidyapeetham
Kollam, Kerala, India

Jitendra Bhatia
Institute of Technology
Nirma University
Ahmedabad, Gujarat, India

Sandeep Bhatia
School of Computing Science
　and Engineering
Galgotias University
Greater Noida, Uttar Pradesh,
　India

Sampath Boopathi
Muthayammal Engineering
　College
Namakkal, Tamil Nadu, India

Sachin Chaudhary
School of Computer Science and
　Applications
IIMT University
Meerut, Uttar Pradesh, India

Arunabha Dutt
CHRIST (Deemed to be University)
Bangalore, Karnataka, India

Kalathmika G.
RV College of Engineering
Bangalore, Karnataka, India

Mohsen Ghorbian
Islamic Azad University
Qom, Iran

Saeid Ghorbian
Islamic Azad University
Ahar, Iran

Amit Kumar Goel
School of Engineering and
Technology
Apeejay Stya University
Gurugram, Haryana, India

Neha Goel
Raj Kumar Goel Institute of
Technology
Ghaziabad, Uttar Pradesh, India

Suresh Joseph K
Pondicherry University
Puducherry, India

S. Karkuzhali
Mepco Schlenk Engineering College
Sivakasi, Tamil Nadu, India

Madhuri P. Karnik
Vishwakarma Institute of
Information Technology
Pune, Maharashtra, India

Gopalakrishnan Karuppaiah
Mepco Schlenk Engineering
College
Sivakasi, Tamil Nadu, India

Neha Katiyar
Bennett University
Greater Noida, Uttar Pradesh, India

Mayank Deep Khare
Noida Institute of Engineering
and Technology
Greater Noida, Uttar Pradesh, India

Pushkar R. Kulkarni
RV College of Engineering
Bengaluru, Karnataka, India

Bhupendra Kumar
School of Computer Science
and Applications
IIMT University,
Meerut, Uttar Pradesh, India

Jatin Kumar
Noida Institute of Engineering
and Technology
Greater Noida, Uttar Pradesh,
India

Malaram Kumhar
Institute of Technology
Nirma University
Ahmedabad, Gujarat, India

Palanivel Kuppusamy
Pondicherry University
Puducherry, India

Paranthaman M.
Kongunadu College of Engineering
and Technology
Thottiam, Namakkal, India

Pranjal Mairal
Institute of Technology
Nirma University
Ahmedabad, Gujarat,
India

Basetty Mallikarjun
Institute of Aeronautical
Engineering
Dundigal, Telangana, India

Akshay Manikjade
Vishwakarma Institute of
Information Technology
Pune, Maharashtra, India

Dhairya Mehta
Institute of Technology
Nirma University
Ahmedabad, Gujarat, India

D. Menaka
Sri Venkateswara College
of Engineering
Sriperumbudur, India

Gautham Menon
Amrita School of Engineering
Amrita Vishwa Vidyapeetham
Kollam, Kerala, India

Geetishree Mishra
B.M.S. College of Engineering
Bangalore, Karnataka, India

Vaishali Mishra
Vishwakarma Institute of
Information Technology
Pune, Maharashtra, India

Bharat Bhushan Naib
School of Computer Science
Galgotia University
Greater Noida, India

S. Deepthi Nayak
B.M.S. College of Engineering
Bangalore, Karnataka, India

Ramprasad OG
Conservatory Ln
Aurora, IL

Sivaprakash P.
Rathinam College of Arts and
Science
Echanari, Coimbatore, India

Nizar Banu P.K.
CHRIST (Deemed to be University)
Bangalore, Karnataka, India

Nandhu Palanivel
Indian Institute of Science Education
& Research
Thiruvananthapuram, Kerala, India

Jay Kumar Pandey
Department of Electronics and
Communication Engineering
Shri Ramswaroop Memorial
University
Barabanki, Uttar Pradesh, India

Rajneesh Panwar
School of Computer Science and
Applications
IIMT University
Meerut, Uttar Pradesh, India

Nandana P. Pillai
RV College of Engineering
Bangalore, Karnataka, India

S. Kavi Priya
Mepco Schlenk Engineering
College
Sivakasi, Tamil Nadu, India

Thendal P.
Mepco Schlenk Engineering
College
Sivakasi, Tamil Nadu, India

Aswin R.
Amrita School of Engineering
Amrita Vishwa Vidyapeetham
Kollam, Kerala, India

Mahadev Govind R.
Amrita School of Engineering
Amrita Vishwa Vidyapeetham
Kollam, Kerala, India

Shishira R.
B.M.S College of Engineering
Bangalore, Karnataka, India

Vasanth R.
Rathinam College of Arts and
Science
Echanari, Coimbatore, India

Mritunjay Rai
Shri Ramswaroop Memorial
University
Barabanki, UP, India

Subash Rajendran
SRM Institute of Science and
Technology
Chennai, Tamil Nadu, India

Renu Rani
Raj Kumar Goel Institute of
Technology
Dr. APJ Abdul Kalam Technical
University
Lucknow, Uttar Pradesh, India

Sachin Rawat
Noida Institute of Engineering and
Technology
Greater Noida, Uttar Pradesh, India

G. Revathy
SASTRA DEEMED UNIVERSITY
Kumbakonam, Tamil Nadu, India

Gaikwad Vidya S.
Vishwakarma Institute of
Information Technology
Pune, Maharashtra, India

Senthilkumar S.
Ayya Nadar Janaki Ammal
College
Sivakasi, Tamil Nadu, India

Nilesh P. Sable
Vishwakarma Institute of
Information Technology
Pune, Maharashtra, India

Niraj Kumar Sahu
Department of Information
Technology
Shri Shankaracharya Institute of
Professional Management and
Technology
Raipur, Chhattisgarh, India

K. Vignesh Saravanan
Ramco Institute of Technology
Rajapalayam, Tamil Nadu, India

Kumud Saxena
Department of Computer Science
& Engineering
Noida Institute of Engineering and
Technology
Greater Noida, Uttar Pradesh, India

S. Selvi
Builders Engineering College,
Nathakadaiyur
Tirrupur, Tamil Nadu, India

Ayush Sharma
Noida Institute of Engineering and
Technology
Greater Noida, Uttar Pradesh,
India

Kewal Krishan Sharma
School of Computer Science and
Applications
IIMT University
Meerut, Uttar Pradesh, India

Khushboo Sharma
Department of Electrical
Engineering
Vivekananda Global University
Jaipur, India

Neetu Sharma
Galgotias University
Greater Noida, Uttar Pradesh, India

Parth Sharma
Symbiosis Law School Nagpur
Symbiosis International (Deemed
    University)
Pune, Maharashtra, India

Vikas Sharma
School of Computer Science
    and Applications
IIMT University
Meerut, Uttar Pradesh, India

Jayashree Shivakumar
RV College of Engineering
Bangalore, Karnataka, India

C. Sivamani
Kalaignar Karunanidhi Institute
    of Technology
Coimbatore, Tamil Nadu,
    India

Jyoti Srivastava
Madan Mohan Malviya University
    of Technology
Greater Noida, Uttar Pradesh,
    India

K. S. Subhashini
Sri Venkateswara College of
    Engineering
Sriperumbudur, India

M. N. Suma
B.M.S College of Engineering
Bangalore, Karnataka, India

Sanjay T.
JPMorgan Chase & Co.
Bengaluru, Karnataka, India

P. Jothi Thilaga
Ramco Institute of Technology
Rajapalayam, Tamil Nadu,
    India

Hashmat Usmani
Raj Kumar Goel Institute
    of Technology
Dr. APJ Abdul Kalam Technical
    University
Lucknow, Uttar Pradesh,
    India

Sridhar Raj Sankara Vadivel
Mepco Schlenk Engineering College
Sivakasi, Tamil Nadu, India

Vivek Veeraiah
Adichunchanagiri University
Mandya, Karnataka, India

N. Vigneshwari
Kalaignar Karunanidhi Institute of
    Technology
Coimbatore, Tamil Nadu, India

K. Vijayalakshmi
Ramco Institute of Technology
Rajapalayam, Tamil Nadu,
    India

Tarun Kumar Vashishth
School of Computer Science and
    Applications
IIMT University
Meerut, Uttar Pradesh, India

Deepali Vashistha
Institute of Technology
Nirma University
Ahmedabad, Gujarat, India

Pranav Vashistha
Institute of Technology
Nirma University
Ahmedabad, Gujarat, India

Karthikeyan Velayuthapandian
Mepco Schlenk Engineering College
Sivakasi, Tamil Nadu, India

Soniya Verma
School of Liberal Arts
Pimpri Chinchwad University
Pune, Maharashtra, India

Disha S. Wankhede
Vishwakarma Institute of
  Information Technology
Pune, Maharashtra, India

Preeti Yadav
RV College of Engineering
Bangalore, Karnataka, India

Ravindra Kumar Yadav
Raj Kumar Goel Institute of Technology
Dr. APJ Abdul Kalam Technical
  University
Lucknow, Uttar Pradesh, India

Editors' Biographies

Dr. Neha Goel is working as **Professor** in the Department of Electronics & Communication Engineering, RKGIT, Ghaziabad, India. She **has Ph.D. degree** from SRM University, Chennai, in 2019. She has 18 years of rich experience in **teaching and research and development activities**. Her area of interest is VLSI design, CMOS design, Internet of Things, and machine learning. She has guided several **B.Tech and M.Tech** Projects and has published **45 papers** in various national/ international journals and conferences. She has received many grants and has published **Four patents**. She has also attended various workshops and seminars in various fields.

Dr. Ravindra Kumar Yadav is Professor and Head of the Department of Electronics & Communication Engineering, RKGIT, Ghaziabad, India. He has B.E., M.E., and Ph.D. degrees in the field of Electronics & Communication Engineering. He has 26 years of rich experience in teaching, research and development activities, administration and managing, and establishing higher educational institutions. He has guided several B. Tech. and M.Tech. projects and is also guiding Ph.D. students from IIT Dhanbad as a co-guide. He has 90 papers to his credit, published in international/national journals, conferences, and symposiums. Prof. Yadav is **reviewer** for several national/international journals of high repute. He has chaired/participated in technical sessions at multiple international and national conferences/seminars held throughout the country.

Chapter 1

ML and IoT coupled biomedical applications in healthcare

Smart growth and upcoming challenges

Vasanth R., Paranthaman M., and Sivaprakash P.

1.1 INTRODUCTION

1.1.1 Internet of Things (IoT)

IoT is the idea of tethering everyday physical items, devices, and even living creatures to the internet. These devices' connection enables them to gather, exchange, and respond to data, building a seamless network of interconnected "things." The primary objectives of IoT are to boost productivity, enhance decision-making, and allow one-of-a-kind services that can significantly improve many facets of our daily life [1]. The following are the key elements of IoT: (i) *Things/devices:* IoT is built on the actual objects or machinery that is connected to sensors, actuators, and communication interfaces. These may also include everyday gadgets like smartphones and smart watches, as well as sophisticated home and office furnishings, industrial machinery, environmental sensors, and other items. (ii) *Connections:* Smooth communication is made possible by a range of connection options found in the IoT ecosystem. Devices connect with one another and with centralised systems using a variety of protocols, including Wi-Fi, Bluetooth, Zigbee, cellular networks, and low-power wide-area networks (LPWAN). (iii) *Data processing:* IoT is a network of networked devices that produces vast volumes of data. For this data to produce useful insights, a crucial analysis and transformation procedure is necessary. Data processing is necessary for this, during which the data is reviewed and useful insights are generated. Data processing may be done using edge computing as well as cloud computing. Edge computing processes data locally, either on the device or nearby, reducing latency and conserving bandwidth. (iv) *Storage:* The data gathered by IoT devices must be stored for later analysis and historical reference. Cloud-based storage alternatives are frequently employed to fill this demand. The IoT's massive amounts of data may be safely stored on a scalable and accessible platform called cloud storage. (v) *User interface:* To enable user interaction and control over connected devices, user interfaces are often employed in IoT applications. These user interfaces are designed to offer a seamless and straightforward experience. They might show up as voice assistants, web portals, or mobile apps,

DOI: 10.1201/9781003487647-1

among other things. These interfaces enable simple and efficient administration over the networked environment by allowing users to effortlessly manage and monitor their IoT devices. Overall, the automated and broad use of IoT improves the quality of service (QoS), leading to a more effective, sustainable, and environment-friendly system [2].

1.1.2 Healthcare and IoT

IoT and healthcare are intertwining more and more, with the IoT technology offering the healthcare industry a plethora of benefits and potentially game-changing opportunities. IoT has the power to completely alter patient outcomes, boost operational efficiency, and alter how healthcare is provided. IoT is having a significant impact on healthcare in a number of important areas, including remote patient monitoring, telemedicine and virtual consultations, medication management, smart medical equipment, healthcare asset tracking, health and wellness monitoring, data-driven decision-making, disease management, and prevention [3]. Although there are many advantages of IoT in healthcare, there are also problems that must be fixed. Data security and patient privacy are crucial because healthcare data is sensitive and requires strong protection. Frictionless data exchange may be limited by issues with compatibility across different IoT platforms and devices. When using IoT technology, the healthcare industry has ongoing challenges that include controlling the likelihood of data breaches and preserving regulatory compliance. IoT has the potential to transform healthcare by delivering more patient-centric, effective, and individualised services. There has to be more research, development, and collaboration between technology businesses and healthcare professionals if IoT is to truly deliver on its promise of improving healthcare outcomes [4].

1.1.3 IoT health and big data

The large amount of data generated by IoT devices and sensors in the healthcare industry is referred to as "big data" in the context of IoT. The integration of IoT technology with healthcare applications creates both opportunities and challenges for managing, assessing, and utilising this data to enhance patient care and healthcare services. Big data is transforming the healthcare industry in a number of ways, including data collecting, real-time monitoring, predictive analytics, personalised treatment, population health management, and research and development. Big data in IoT health has the potential to completely transform the healthcare industry since it allows for tailored medicine, real-time insights, and faster medical research [4]. To fully benefit from this revolutionary technology and enhance patient care and healthcare outcomes, it is crucial to address difficulties with data security, interoperability, and ethical considerations. By effectively resolving these issues, we can unlock the full potential of big data in IoT health and usher in a new era of medical advancements. Patients nowadays are a part of an extensive sensor network that continually gathers and records environmental, physical, physiological, and behavioural data. This tendency is highlighted even more by the development of progressive therapeutic splendid devices with increased reminiscence and handing out influence [1]. Better particle swarm optimisation techniques are used by these super sensors to distribute medications accurately to various organs, locate medications, and do other tasks. These sensors produce a huge amount of linked, diverse data that is sometimes referred to as "big data." This data was historically transported to a centralised server for feature mining and examination due to network restrictions during data transmission and a lack of real-time processing power and resources for analysis [5].

1.1.4 IoT health machine learning (ML) for big data

Smart systems are increasingly using deep learning and ML approaches. These complex systems are composed of a number of connected components, each of which serves a specific purpose. It is crucial to break down intelligent systems into their fundamental parts, such as computer networks, computer vision, natural language processing (NLP), reinforcement learning, and general reasoning, in order to comprehend them. Over the past few decades, intensive research has been conducted to enhance the capabilities of each of these parts, each of which performs a specific role. Due to the variety and depth of these fields, we won't go into extensive detail on any of them. We will instead concentrate on the important architectural and algorithmic frameworks that have been utilised often in recent case studies. These fundamental methods have been crucial in helping intelligent systems complete challenging tasks and make wise decisions, benefiting various fields of study and industries [5].

Algorithms for ML may be roughly divided into supervised and unsupervised techniques. The model is given unlabelled data in unsupervised procedures with the aim of discovering important patterns and hidden structures using the clustering process. Popular unsupervised algorithms include K-means, fuzzy C-means, expectation–maximisation algorithm, and hidden Markov model. Regression and classification are, on the other hand, subcategories of supervised models. In classification, the model is taught to properly categorise incoming data into recognisable groups by utilising labelled data during training. Popular classifiers include K-nearest neighbour (KNN), random forest, C4.5 model, naive Bayes, support vector machine (SVM), neural networks, and deep belief networks [6]. Convolutional neural networks (CNNs) have transformed image- and video-related tasks. Since they employ pooling and convolutional layers to automatically extract essential information, they are very effective for a range of vision problems, including picture classification, object localisation, object identification, semantic segmentation, and instance segmentation. VGG, Inception, and ResNet are CNN architectures that perform admirably when solving these issues. In circumstances where temporal considerations are important, recurrent neural networks (RNNs), such as long short-term memory (LSTM) or gated recurrent unit (GRU), can be stacked on top of CNNs to learn time-related patterns. CNN designs frequently include a feed-forward neural network or a basic classifier like KNN in their final classification layers. Only after training, when they may be merged with other features and fed to other classifiers or ensembles as needed, can the convolutional layers be used as feature extractors. Regression, on the other hand, focuses on predicting numbers in the continuous domain. Support vector regression (SVR), suitably structured neural networks, and linear regression are often employed techniques for this purpose. Overall, ML techniques, including supervised and unsupervised methods, as well as specialist architectures like CNNs and RNNs, have completely changed a number of sectors and are still advancing the discipline [7].

1.2 IoT CHANNEL

1.2.1 Collection of data and sensing

Through the automation of formerly manual processes, IoT aims to improve the quality of human existence. This translates to complete patient monitoring and treatment with improved responsiveness and accuracy in the setting of healthcare. Wearables and implants are now feasible in the healthcare industry because of the development of portable microcontrollers and microprocessors like Arduino and Raspberry Pi, as well as the effective, fairly costly, yet precise sensors and communication modules like Zigbee. Wearables are gadgets that may be worn as accessories and come in a range of shapes, sizes, and designs. Smart watches, fitness trackers, wristbands, and smart rings are some of the more well-known examples. Along with other features, they enable users to measure and keep track of important health indicators, including heart rate, blood pressure, amount of activity, calories burned, and sleep patterns. Contrarily, implants are objects that are designed to be inserted into or beneath the skin. Spiral neurons, hearing restoration, glucose monitoring, and cardiac pacemakers are just a few of their specialties. In contrast to wearables, implants frequently have more narrowly targeted goals that aim to restore an organ's natural function. By automatically releasing insulin from a built-in insulin tank as needed, a glucose-monitoring implant, for instance, may regulate blood glucose levels. This is accomplished by routinely monitoring blood glucose levels [8]. The overview of IoT channel is shown in Figure 1.1.

1.2.2 Data preparation and storage

It is common practice to keep the collected data on local memory within the device for early analysis and pre-processing because the real-time transmission of data from wearables and implants might be costly. However, the aforementioned sophisticated ML models, such as CNNs and RNNs, typically need a lot of processing power and working memory, making them unsuitable for

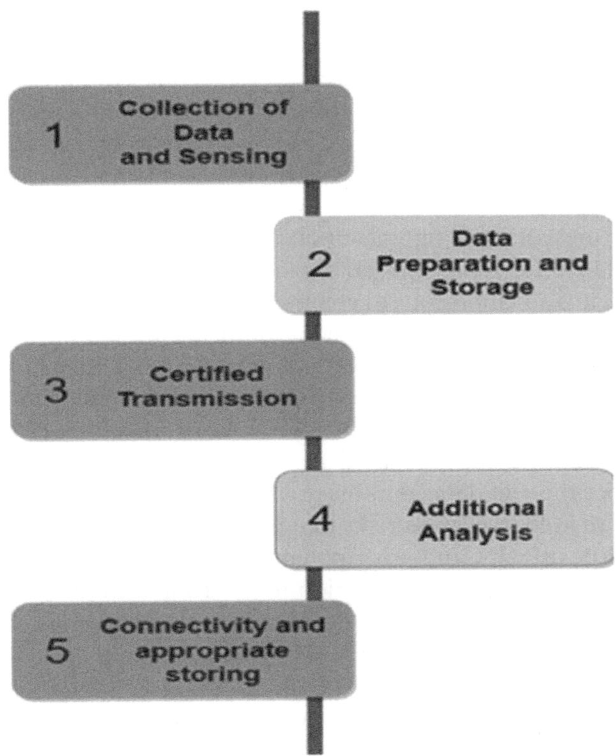

Figure 1.1 Overview of IoT channel.

wearables and implants that have limited resources. To get over this limitation, lighter neural network models are employed to give efficient computations while still giving appropriate performance. These lightweight models may cause a slight loss of accuracy, but continual design improvements make them ever more effective. The use of trained variants of pruned or reduced neural networks, such SqueezeNet, MobileNet, and EfficientNet, is best suited for such devices. These models enable thorough data stream analysis and can even handle video streams captured by small cameras built into some implants. By utilising these less resource-intensive neural network models, wearables and implants may assess locally stored data in real time without straining their limited resources. This approach strikes a balance between efficiency and accuracy, allowing ML to be used even in low-resource devices, enhancing their functionality and perhaps having a favourable impact on healthcare and other applications [9].

1.2.3 Certified transmission

The devices' own pre-processing models allow for asynchronous, passive data delivery to centralised servers. These algorithms search for patterns in the flowing data and pinpoint them. If no anomalies are discovered, the data may be retained and sent later or in accordance with a predetermined schedule when the network is less congested. However, if the models detect, suspect, or anticipate any issues with the data, they can quickly submit the pertinent information for more research. They are unable to do in-depth studies on the integrated processor and battery because they have a limited amount of computational power, even with the aid of pre-processing models, especially in the absence of data from other patients. As a result, sending the whole data set to the server presents two significant challenges. Firstly, a sizeable amount of highly correlated data from several sensors adds to the total amount of data. To solve this, it is advantageous to compress the data before transmission. This may be done by locating and removing outliers, noise, and redundant data using lightweight local models. The remaining data may then be merged, compressed, and divided into manageable chunks before being transferred to the central server when the network demand is at its lowest. Swarm intelligence concepts may be studied and used to improve data transmission methods. Secondly, since the sent data contains private patient data, secure transfer techniques must be used to prevent risks like data breaches, eavesdropping, denial-of-service (DoS) attacks, and other potential risks brought on by inadequately designed networks and communication tools. To guarantee patient confidentiality even in the event of network breaches, the data must be encrypted. Therefore, stringent security standards and procedures are consistently put into place to guarantee the safety of patient data at all costs. By resolving these problems, healthcare systems may effectively integrate IoT technology, wearables, and implants to monitor patients, enhance diagnoses, and improve general healthcare services while prioritising data privacy and security [10].

1.2.4 Additional analysis

The key benefit of central computing servers is that they have access to a lot of resources and processing power, which allows them to do comprehensive analysis and identify patterns in the data. By integrating and fusing their data, as well as data from more than one patient, these servers' ML algorithms may access data from several patients at once. This method allows for the identification of patterns and correlations at a higher semantic level by using a broader lens. Due to their expanded processing capabilities, central server analytical frameworks may include history data from patients' past medical visits, data from several service providers and sensors, demographic data, and other supplemental data [11]. By merging these many data sources, the central servers may get a more complete and all-encompassing view, enabling a more in-depth and precise analysis. By collecting and aggregating data from diverse people and sources, it is possible to improve diagnoses, gain a deeper understanding of population-level health trends and patterns, and make better healthcare decisions. These big studies' collective data help progress medical research, which ultimately leads to better patient care and more effective healthcare services. In the healthcare sector, the interpretability of the results from deep learning and ML technologies is crucial. Due to their complex internal workings, these models can occasionally be perceived as "black boxes," making it challenging for doctors and clinicians to understand the reasoning behind their decisions, despite the fact that they can do fairly well when processing complex data. Interpretability is crucial in the healthcare sector since doctors and clinicians need to trust and comprehend the judgements and decisions made by these models. When the model's predictions are incorrect or have unintended repercussions, it is critical to understand the reasoning and factors that motivated such decisions. The deep learning models' intricate design makes it difficult to establish easy interpretability. However, scientists are working hard to create techniques that will allow them to extract the most popular routes in these models and produce rules from neural networks. With additional information about these models' decision-making processes, medical practitioners will be able to better comprehend and apply them. When dealing with image and video processing tasks, attention models are a helpful technique to increase interpretability. Thanks to attention approaches, deep learning models may focus on certain regions of an image or a video that are crucial for reaching a particular result. By displaying these attention maps, we can more clearly see the areas that the model focuses on when arriving at its conclusions. This visualisation helps validate the model's reasoning and provides insightful information about how it decides. Since interpretability is a crucial aspect of AI applications in healthcare, researchers are always trying to develop methods that balance between the complexity of deep learning models and their explainability. By improving the readability and transparency of AI models, we can progress their usage in healthcare for improved patient care and results. This will promote trust and make it possible for healthcare personnel and AI systems to work together successfully [12].

1.2.5 Connectivity and appropriate storing

Controlling and managing data in a centralised framework while ensuring interoperability across different systems may be challenging. It could be more difficult to exchange and use the data among several servers and apps if all the data were just poured into one database. To achieve semantic interoperability, standardised norms, data formats, and interfaces must be created and followed by all essential frameworks and services. By doing this, it is ensured that the data's meaning is clear and that different computer systems may easily communicate, understand, and use it. An important concept in IoT is semantic interoperability. Each piece of data should have meta-information that provides context for the values it relates to, allowing data from various sources to be linked together. This enables autonomous reasoning and inference to transform unstructured data into knowledge that can be utilised to generate new insights and make informed decisions [13]. Two essential methods for developing semantic interoperability are the Resource Description Framework (RDF) and the Web Ontology Language (OWL). RDF provides a flexible method for describing resources and their linkages, whereas OWL permits the creation of ontologies to define and categorise ideas in a domain. These techniques complement one another and are crucial for structuring and querying data because they function together. Using SPARQL, a query language developed for RDF, data is accessed and modified from several web sources, enabling data integration and knowledge discovery. Semantic interoperability is a broad and intricate subject with several standards and approaches. The IoT and other linked settings require effective data transfer and integration, even if attaining full interoperability across several systems and data sources is challenging [11].

1.3 SEVERAL IoT APPLICATIONS IN THE HEALTHCARE INDUSTRY

IoT applications in healthcare encompass a wide range of tools, platforms, and technologies that collect and share data to improve patient outcomes, healthcare management, and medical services. They provide an overview of many significant IoT applications in the healthcare industry, highlighting their benefits, disadvantages, and potential impacts on the healthcare ecosystem. IoT-enabled wearables, sensors, and medical apparatus are used to remotely monitor patients' vital signs and health issues. RPM makes it simpler to continually monitor a patient's vital indicators, such as heart rate, blood pressure, glucose levels, and more. This real-time data sharing allows healthcare personnel to watch patients from a distance, identify warning signs before they become serious, and intervene quickly when necessary. RPM improves the level of care for patients with chronic illnesses, boosts patient involvement, and lowers the rate of readmissions to hospitals [14].

In reaction to real-time patient data, a new class of intelligent medical devices, including pacemakers, inhalers, and insulin pumps, may autonomously change a patient's treatment plan. With the aid of this technological advancement, patients may have better control over their chronic illnesses, and there is a lower likelihood of human error while filling prescriptions. The fusion of IoT technology and smart medical equipment enables the adoption of personalised treatment plans that are tailored to the unique needs of each patient. The IoT features of these smart devices enable more specialised, efficient, and patient-centred healthcare.

No matter where they are physically situated, interactions between patients and healthcare professionals have never been simpler, thanks to the emergence of IoT-driven telemedicine solutions. These systems use videoconferencing and data-sharing capabilities to provide remote diagnosis and treatment, which removes geographical boundaries and significantly improves access to healthcare services. By delivering medical expertise to patients who may have few local options, telemedicine plays a critical role in improving healthcare accessibility, especially in rural or underdeveloped areas. By moving non-urgent patients to virtual consultations, telemedicine also helps hospitals reduce their workload and focus more efficiently on critical and emergency circumstances. With this strategy, telemedicine powered by the IoT helps create a healthcare system that is more efficient, patient-centred, and accessible [15].

IoT-driven pharmaceutical management systems help patients adhere to suggested prescription regimens. Smart pill dispensers and medication reminders alert patients or caretakers when it is time to take a drug, reducing the probability that a dosage will be missed and increasing the medication adherence. These technologies can also notify medical workers when a patient is complying, enabling prompt interventions and changes to treatment plans.

The predictive healthcare analytics solutions enable early treatments, enabling medical professionals to identify and address health issues before they worsen. Early intervention enables healthcare practitioners to customise therapy to meet the unique needs of each patient, thereby enhancing patient satisfaction and health outcomes [10].

A new age has begun with the introduction of IoT, which has inspired innovation and transformation in the healthcare sector. IoT applications have improved a variety of things, including patient outcomes, operational efficiency, and accessibility to healthcare services. However, it is crucial to overcome issues with data security, interoperability, and privacy in order to properly exploit IoT in healthcare. As a result of ongoing technology advancements, IoT is anticipated to play a larger role in healthcare, producing a more connected and patient-focused healthcare environment. By embracing IoT technology and making headway on associated challenges, the healthcare sector may continue to grow and offer top-notch care to patients throughout the world [11].

1.4 IoT HEALTHCARE ML CHALLENGES

In this part, we concentrate on outlining the main constraints and difficulties that ML in the context of IoT healthcare presents. Figure 1.2 illustrates the relationship between IoT, ML, and personal healthcare (PH). Numerous studies show the many ways that ML is used in the fields of PH and IoT. The graphic shows how IoT creates enormous volumes of data that are later used to train ML algorithms. These ML algorithms produce useful solutions for PH, including illness detection, analysis of patient behaviour, and recommendations for assistive care. ML- and IoT-based supported PH services already have had a significant impact on people's lives because of how quickly technology is evolving. These innovative techniques have the potential to considerably enhance healthcare results. But as they proceed, they encounter challenging issues that must be overcome [13].

The use of ML-based PH services enables us to employ a predictive analytic method that benefits patients who have been released from the hospital but may need to be readmitted, according to a study. Predictive analysis tries to build a risk categorisation model that can detect which patients are at higher

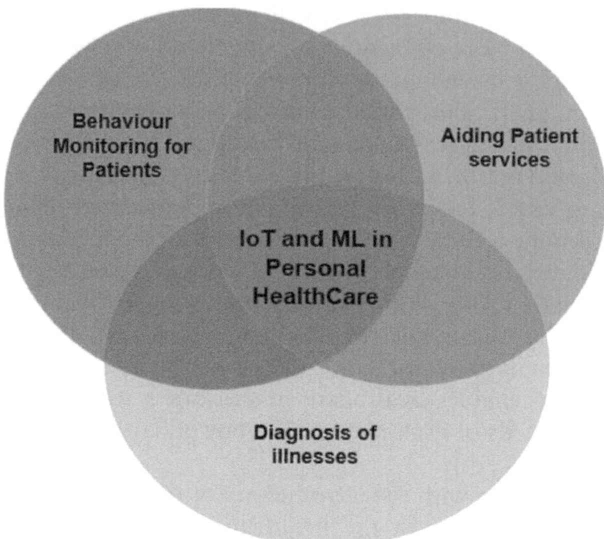

Figure 1.2 The relationship between IoT, ML, and PH.

risk and require extra attention and care. It does this by using IoT devices and sensors, continual (real-time) follow-up, and analysis. These models significantly draw on historical information and subject-matter knowledge. In order to foresee probable future results and begin an action plan to mitigate expected difficulties, the dynamic PH system that would aid in readmission prevention measures must also incorporate dynamic patient data.

The two difficulties as well as a conceptualised picture of the problems and fixes are shown in Figure 1.3. Out-of-date data sources help us make bad judgements, and data security and privacy make IoT devices less reliable. The figure offers us two further related possibilities as an alternative: Federated learning, which allows users to learn from dispersed data, and online education to keep up with knowledge for newly entered data. By describing potential outcomes, we expand on the first problem and the second challenge in this section. We go deeper into the corresponding solutions for providing two solutions in the next section. However, the options have advantages and disadvantages [14].

1.4.1 Problem No. 1: Out-of-date data

Several research initiatives have examined the use of ML in IoT healthcare. Applications for clinical smart systems and healthcare service delivery use analytical models that are provided by ML algorithms. These models are largely evaluated by identifying patient behaviour patterns and different clinical situations utilising data collected from IoT devices. This entails figuring out the patient's improvements, routines, and unusual behaviours when

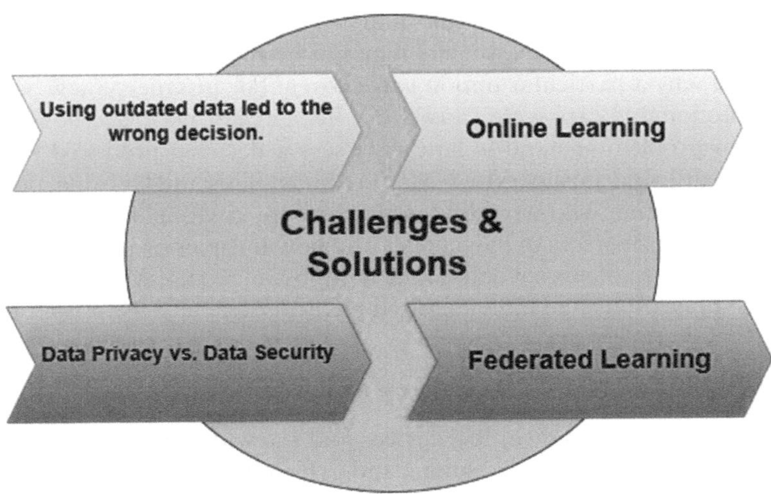

Figure 1.3 Common ML issues in IoT healthcare and related solutions.

engaging in daily activities, as well as different sleeping, digestive, drinking, and eating patterns. Intelligent decision-making algorithms provide particular care plans, lifestyle suggestions, and therapies for the patients based on such patterns. Doctors may also participate further in the process of developing care plans in order to examine and confirm the prescriptions for medication and lifestyle. Due to the sensitivity of medical data, including clinical, lifestyle, and behaviour data, it is extremely likely that biases of various kinds will be present throughout the data collection process, and the data may not be sufficiently diverse to be applicable in all situations. The noisy, imperfect data may also have a negative impact on the likelihood rate for identifying and forecasting a diagnostic and warning notice connected to health. If the training dataset and final model used an out-of-date version of the dataset, even a rich model would be useless.

1.4.1.1 ML in assistive care: Problems

Since ML algorithms produce predictions and conclusions based on prior data (training dataset), we believe they are intimately related to statistical analogies and deduction. The ML-based technique will monitor a patient's condition and evaluate it in light of the training dataset. Consequently, to find the current trend and forecast the future, a training dataset is required. This dataset occasionally exhibits bias and is not as varied as it may be to account for various situations. Consider sleep tracking as an example. Each person may have a distinct sleep pattern depending on their age, health, and other factors. We may estimate PH incorrectly as a result of the absence of a comprehensive dataset of all case studies available during training to monitor sleep patterns.

IoT and ML also provide PH the ability to select a diagnostic or forecast. In some cases, ML-based assessments may not be reliable and may not be able to explain why a particular option was chosen. For instance, a few accidents using autonomous cars were caused by the vehicles' poor decision-making. The main problem at hand is how to assess a decision produced by an AI computer utilising unsupervised ML methods. This might bring up moral concerns regarding who would be responsible for creating a false claim, how to spot or fix such errors in judgement, and how unsupervised ML algorithms operate. These challenges would make it impossible to use ML algorithms for delicate applications like individualised medical care.

1.4.2 Problem No. 2: Accuracy and confidentiality

The development of medical IoT devices and the widespread use of wearable technology, including at work, home, and in hospitals for a variety of reasons, such as childcare and assisted living, have made it possible for us to continuously monitor our own health wherever we are. These gadgets gather electronic health measurements in real time from various items and sensors, send the patient data to an application server for pre-processing and pre-analysis, and then restore the data on a data server.

ML algorithms are employed in this processing and analysis to deliver a variety of services, including motion tracking, which shows the number of steps taken and calories burned, tracking sleep, tracking travel distance, and measuring vital signs like heart rate, electrocardiogram (ECG), skin temperature, and electroencephalogram (EEG). Therefore, when data from an IoT device is analysed and shared with a server through a network connection, difficulties of confidentiality and trust come to light. A server's data and communication networks both are vulnerable to hacking. The need to address privacy and data security is very crucial. There are easy ways to improve data security, like adopting encryption techniques and keeping the data safe. However, if a hacker discovers the decryption algorithm's key and decodes the message, the private information will become publicly accessible. The encryption and decryption processes may also lose some data during the encryption process, and if the decryption techniques are unable to restore all of the original data, the processes become ineffective [15].

1.4.2.1 ML difficulties in tracking patient activities

In a number of research publications, physical activity is defined using data from motion sensors for a variety of case studies in the context of tracking patient behaviour. According to studies, using motion sensors is one of the most reliable ways to keep track of a patient's ongoing physical activity while they are receiving therapy. Due to the characteristics of IoT devices, data gathering from medical IoT sensors and devices for healthcare applications is particularly sensitive. Data gathering and remote real-time monitoring are now improved by recent advancements in wireless communication/transformation and web technology. The lengthy procedure for gathering medical data, however, poses privacy and security issues across the whole data collection life cycle, including data collection, transmission, processing, and storage.

Identification of the data that can safeguard user privacy while being valuable and essential for ML activities is a challenging topic in activity detection using mobile devices rather than wearable devices. In order to approach and resolve this challenging issue, we could address the following two questions: Does the data that has been acquired have robust encryption in place to ensure that no one can access it? How can you tell if the protected data is maintained accurately, just as it was when it was first collected? For secure data transfer, data protection when using mobile devices, and increased end-user trust, it's imperative to strike a balance between data computation and data privacy.

One of the key issues with adopting IoT for healthcare monitoring is ensuring that patient data is secure, and in particular, confidential, during the ML analysis process. Strong user authentication architecture ensures that only users with active accounts may access data and services. Because it exposes them to sensitive hacker access, the accessibility of customer data is a problem. IoT devices will make data interchange challenging given their existing capability [16].

1.5 DIFFERENT IoT HEALTHCARE PROMISES

Statistics on IoT usage have shown that a number of medical and healthcare fields might potentially benefit from access to large volumes of pertinent data gathered by IoT sensors/devices. However, as the healthcare sector increasingly demands high levels of data privacy and security, IoT devices are beginning to be seen as a separate island of data. Due to concerns about obsolete data model issues, data privacy, and security, which are the primary challenges with traditional ML algorithms stated in Sections 1.4.1 and 1.4.2, we also analyse advanced ML promises with IoT healthcare applications in this section. We go into further depth about the promises in the sections that follow. In Section 1.5.1, we discuss the online learning approach, which addresses the problem of incomplete and obsolete data and provides a solution by enabling the classifier to learn from upcoming new data and update the model in real time on each learning iteration. The second technique we provide is called "federated learning," which enables us to learn from scattered data collected from end users without forwarding the data to an application server.

1.5.1 Adaptive or online ML

The basic operation of a ML algorithm has already been explained in Section 1.2. We also discuss the challenges of using traditional ML algorithms in Section 1.1. Thus, the purpose of this section is to offer a strategy that will enable scientists to effectively manage the issue using an online learning algorithm. Even after the training process is over, it is strongly advised to update the best classifier for upcoming data. Online learning or adaptable learning is two terms used to describe this crucial ML technique – unlike the batch learning algorithms, which always start with the best classifier based on what they have learned from the training dataset [17]. In other words, online or adaptive learning treats tasks as flowing in a stream both during and after the training process rather than utilising an offline, constrained dataset. The tasks are more directly tied to the ability to successfully adapt to the current task in the stream with respect to the relevant learning rate rather than on memorising past tasks.

Furthermore, training on training data, such as patient data from therapy sessions, is both logistically and cognitively impracticable, necessitating the development of new data. Online learning is a revolutionary way to ML in this situation. Additionally, it is used when the algorithm must train on all data due to memory restrictions [18].

1.5.1.1 *The process of online ML*

In this section, we try to provide a very brief explanation of an online ML approach shown in Figure 1.4. The three main pieces that make up the online ML schema often work together: The input package also includes IoT devices for wearables or healthcare. Five stages make up the online ML bundle. AI devices are used to generate the findings and projections [19]. With the addition of a step where the learning model is retrained using a learning rate that signals the relevance of new input data, the basic stages of online ML are the same as those of classical ML. The learning rate increases as more significant input data are considered. The model will most probably be susceptible to outliers and might perhaps become stuck in a local minimum or maximum if a greater learning rate is chosen. On the other hand, when the learning rate slows, the outlier exposure also does. The model takes some time to update using new entry data because of the slower learning rate [20].

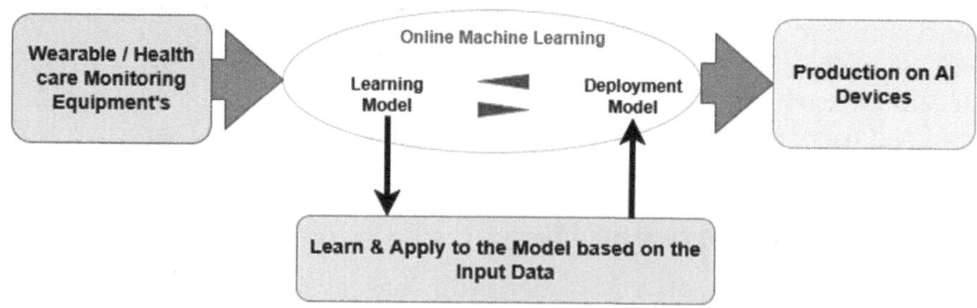

Figure 1.4 An overview of the online machine learning method.

The five steps in the online ML package indicated in Figure 1.4 are essential when implementing online learning in IoT healthcare. Reading input data, training a model, and applying the model are the first three phases of these five steps, which comprise the typical ML learning process. A fresh sequence of data is accepted at the fourth step of an online learning algorithm, which is the initial stage. The algorithm updates the model with a personalised value for the learning rate in the fifth step after learning from the new data [21].

1.5.2 IoT healthcare applications for online learning

The usage of IoT devices and applications has risen across many sectors, thanks to technological advancements like ML and artificial intelligence, but more so and with rising demand in the field of medical and healthcare. Adaptive learning commonly referred to as never-ending learning or online ML is a new fundamental concept in ML. Models develop at a predetermined learning rate while keeping prior knowledge as a function of the input data. The non-static supervised ML technique allows the model to learn from data repeatedly and automatically alter its behaviour in line with the learning rate. How rapidly we pick up new information will limit the range of our behavioural alternatives. In other words, we don't assign the input data we get any greater significance. However, we may need to initialise a very high learning rate that won't be affected by outliers since we want the model to be updated more quickly based on the new data. One example of this online learning is the recommender systems employed by companies like Netflix and Amazon, despite the fact that these systems have their own challenging issues, such as fairness in the ML process [22].

Huge data streaming: A large data streaming computation has been widely used in real-time healthcare analytics. Real-time tracking and monitoring systems, which are essential in the healthcare and medical industries, are only one use of online ML. Mobile apps, sensors, and wearable medical devices/sensors are a few examples of typical rich sources that have been continuously creating a large amount of streaming data. Applying traditional ML algorithms to streaming data to take immediate action in an emergency seems like a difficult task. Huge real-time healthcare analytics frequently take advantage of huge data streaming computations. Online ML is used for a variety of purposes, including real-time tracking and monitoring systems, which are crucial in the healthcare and medical sectors [23]. Examples of typical rich sources that have been continually producing a significant volume of streaming data are mobile applications, sensors, and wearable medical equipment and sensors. It may be challenging to use conventional ML algorithms on streaming data to respond quickly to an emergency.

The second important development in online ML is online meta-learning. An online meta-learning approach is based on the regretful meta-learner. During a task sequence, the approach applies model-agnostic meta-learning for adaptive deep learning, commonly known as MAML. The meta-training and meta-testing phases in this approach come after the training and testing phases, and they allow us to learn from the input data. A training phase is included in the meta-testing stage, even during testing. This capability makes MAML appear strong enough to deliver results that are superior to those attained using other deep learning techniques. The most effective method for FSL and OSL, which allow classifiers to learn from a few examples of each category to precisely predict labels for classes that have not yet been observed, is MAML [24].

Additional challenge in online education even while online ML seems suited for IoT healthcare applications is implementing them with high accuracy. One of the trickiest difficulties is catastrophic forgetting, which happens when new information prevents the model from remembering what it has already learnt. This barrier prevents the classifier from effectively integrating the new input data or utilising the previous data when it regenerates a new model. The bulk of online learning applications that are not medical are less impacted by this limitation. Models for online learning in the healthcare industry address a range of problems when a number of challenging tasks are necessary. The catastrophic interference problem can be easily solved by retraining the model from start each time new data becomes available, but doing so is computationally expensive and prevents the application of real-time conclusions [18].

1.5.3 Federated education

When data is sent to an application server or when the data is recovered on the server, heterogeneous IoT devices with related diverse end-users' (patients') information are more likely to be subject to hacking, which raises concerns about data privacy and security. We provide a very brief overview of the FL process in Figure 1.5. We will discuss these problems in this section and look at a potential remedy to assist us resolve them to a respectable level. This solution must be able to incorporate a model while maintaining user data and training from isolated devices. In a traditional ML-based method, the data gathered by IoT devices is uploaded to an application/data server, where trained models are then applied with ML algorithms. However, as data owners (devices) increase, data privacy becomes more and more important, particularly in the medical and healthcare sectors. In this chapter, we suggest using FL, which was initially proposed by Google, as a fresh approach to handle the privacy need for personally identifiable information. FL is described as a difficult problem of developing a high-quality shared global model using a centralised server and decentralised data spread among several devices or end users [25].

We recommend using FL, a ML technique, that trains a centralised rich model while training data is dispersed among several users and devices with sluggish and unreliable network connections. We employ the FL approach in

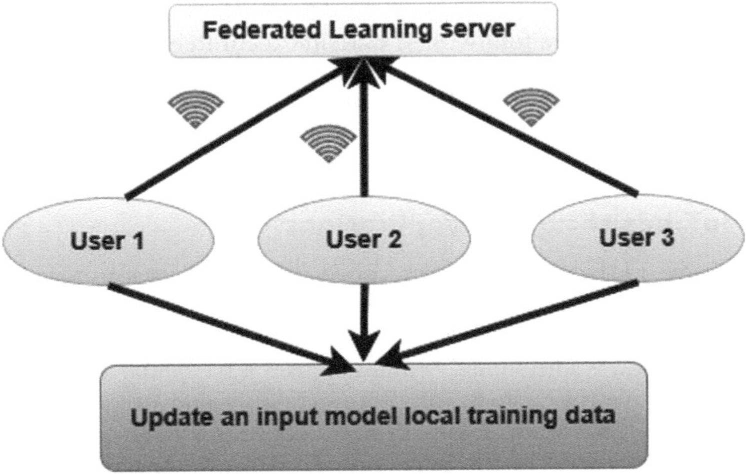

Figure 1.5 Overview of the federated learning process.

this case, where IoT devices autonomously update an input model based on their locally obtained data as needed. After updating this model, we send it to the central server, where the user-side modifications are combined to create/ update a new global or generalised model. The most common technology in this setting, where efficient local collaboration and data transfer are essential, is mobile phones [16].

1.5.4 Federated Learning's wide-ranging process

FL is a technique for building models, as opposed to traditional ML approaches, which demand that all data be given as a single training data-set. In FL, a model is created iteratively by merging collective models that have been collected from several sources (devices – information from users' cell phones). The users' local (training) dataset and privacy are preserved when they participate in a shared FL process. The revised model, which was created using the local training data from the devices, would then be reintegrated once an aggregator had broadcast the aggregated model to all users [26].

The interaction between a FL server and all end users and devices is shown in this figure, which happens before the server begins to broadcast the most current model. The input data (x), parameters, and loss function are transmitted with the model M to the final users or devices [27]. The device then starts learning from the locally acquired training dataset to update the model. The changed model M will be returned, along with revised parameter and loss function values for each device. After compiling the models it has received from devices, the server stores them there, repeats the procedure, and then retrieves the models. With the use of fresh data, this technology lets doctors follow their patients accurately almost immediately. Additionally, sharing of private data is prohibited by this FL. However, FL now only uses smartphones as smart devices, which is one of its logistical disadvantages [21].

1.5.5 IoT healthcare FL applications

A brand-new FL-based framework called FedHealth uses transfer learning for IoT healthcare applications. The transfer learning method has been used by FedHealth to reduce the difference in distribution throughout several different disciplines. Additionally, FedHealth uses a particular encryption technique to increase the security of communicating end user and FedHealth model updates [28]. Additionally, FedAvg has been employed as a federated optimisation approach in the upcoming FedHealth. Although the tailored model in each user does not guarantee that it functions properly locally, the global model changed in the FL centralised server is likely to be available to all end users. To tackle this and enhance the performance of the FL model for end users, the researchers utilised transfer learning to build a personalised model for each user.

Additional problems with FL: FL provides high levels of data security and privacy protection, although some reported assaults discovered that just sharing local data while training and updating the model M was inadequate to give acceptable data privacy. Researchers have suggested a hybrid method called privacy-preserving federated learning in order to create a model with an acceptable level of predictive accuracy as well as the capability to forbid inference over both the messages transmitted during the local training process and the final trained model. Table 1.1 lists the challenges in healthcare system integrated with ML and IoT.

Additionally, FL on IoT devices has the following difficulties:

Device heterogeneity: The technologies and hardware used by IoT devices for medical and healthcare concerns and those used for general reasons both are diverse. This includes the type of CPU, memory storage, and network connections bandwidth, storage capacity, and, last but not least, power. Costs may rise as a result of the difficulty of setting up FL for fault tolerance. Additionally, certain devices could stop participating in different learning processes due to a number of issues, including inadequate network connectivity and battery capacity.

Model heterogeneity and statistical heterogeneity: User behaviour and setting distributions are essential to any ML, but FL in particular, from the standpoint of data collecting. Because FL devices exhibit a wide range of physical properties and behaviours, a complete model may be difficult to develop due to the variety of events and settings that arise. We end up employing several different models in the server application to aggregate them before rebroadcasting [29].

Table 1.1 The challenges in healthcare system integrated with ML and IoT

Application	Description	ML/IoT integration	Challenges
Remote patient monitoring	Distant, continual monitoring of the patient's vital signs and health	IoT devices collect data, and ML algorithms spot trends and warnings	IoT devices gather data, and ML algorithms see trends and warning indicators
Predictive diagnostics	Predicting diseases or conditions based on patient data	ML models trained on patient records, IoT devices for data collection	Data accessibility and quality; ethical concerns (algorithm bias); and the synthesis of many data sources – compliance with laws
Medication adherence	The prompt use of medication by patients	IoT-connected smart pill dispensers that anticipate adherence using ML	User interaction, the confidentiality of medical information, the use of a gadget, and accurate algorithms
Fall detection	Detecting and alerting to falls among older patients	ML algorithms and wearable IoT sensors for fall detection	Positives/negatives that aren't true: The battery life of the wearable sensors; real-time alerts and responses
Hospital asset tracking	Keeping track of medical equipment and hospital assets	Monitoring hospital assets and medical equipment	Upkeep of assets and tagging – compatibility with devices synchronising data in expansive healthcare facilities; scalability
Drug discovery	Expediting the process of medication research and discovery	ML algorithms and IoT for lab automation assess biological data	High computation standards; data integration and curation; safety checks; and regulatory compliance
Disease outbreak prediction	Sickness outbreaks are rapidly located	ML and IoT mixed with epidemiological data for predicting	Correctness and timeliness of the data; privacy concerns; handling enormous volumes of data; and validation of the prediction models

1.6 CONCLUSION

IoT is expanding and gaining strength as ML algorithms are used for network monitoring and user activity management. However, traditional ML techniques might not work well when used to distributed data collected from IoT devices: Due to the nature of the algorithms, which is to collect all of the training data at once and create a rich model capable of anticipating future class labels in a test phase. Distributed data prevents the use of traditional ML techniques from producing promising results. In this study, we discuss IoT, its pipeline, and its use in healthcare, as well as the challenges that ML algorithms may encounter. With better diagnosis, monitoring, and treatment options, thanks to the integration of ML and IoT in biomedical applications, healthcare has substantially improved. It will be important to address problems with data security, interoperability, regulations, ethics, scalability, and user education in order to maintain the sensible growth of this business. A more efficient, patient-focused healthcare system will be made feasible by removing these barriers. This inference summary report highlights the need of holistic solutions and provides a snapshot of the current landscape to allow the suitable and successful integration of ML and IoT in healthcare. In the last section, we examine the methods used to gather data, its constraints, and the implications of big data on IoT health, general IoT concerns, and particularly the difficulties connected with ML in IoT healthcare. We also discuss relevant cutting-edge solutions to these issues.

1.7 SUMMARY

The use of ML and IoT in biomedical applications has ushered a new era in healthcare. This executive summary highlights the necessity for wise expansion and lists impending challenges in this quick-paced sector. Smart growth includes the following: (i) *Enhanced diagnostics:* IoT sensors and ML algorithms have improved diagnostic accuracy, enabling the early detection of disease and the creation of tailored treatment plans. Real-time patient monitoring is provided via IoT devices, which reduces hospital stays and enhances patient care at home. (ii) *Drug discovery:* ML models analyse sizeable biological datasets to expedite the look for novel medications. (iii) *Predictive analytics:* By anticipating disease outbreaks and patient needs, predictive models optimise resource allocation. Upcoming challenges include the following: (i) *Data security:* As data volumes rise, maintaining patient information's security and privacy becomes a major issue. (ii) *Interoperability:* It continues to be challenging to combine different IoT devices and ML systems from different vendors, which limits simple data transmission. (iii) *Regulatory compliance:* Adhering to laws and regulations that are always changing is challenging. (iv) *Considerations of morality:* The ethical use of patient data and AI in the healthcare sector requires rules and oversight. (v) *Scalability:* Scalable infrastructure and trustworthy ML models are needed to handle the massive volume of data produced by IoT devices. (vi) *User education:* Patients and healthcare professionals require more training on effective technology use. With better diagnosis, monitoring, and treatment options, thanks to the integration of ML and IoT in biomedical applications, healthcare has substantially improved. It will be important to address problems with data security, interoperability, regulations, ethics, scalability, and user education in order to maintain the sensible growth of this business. A more efficient, patient-focused healthcare system will be made feasible by removing these barriers. This inference summary report highlights the need of holistic solutions and provides a snapshot of the current landscape to allow the suitable and success-ful integration of ML and IoT in healthcare.

REFERENCES

1. Asali E., Shenavarmasouleh F., Mohammadi F.G., Suresh P.S., Arabnia H.R. DeepMSRF: A novel deep multimodal speaker recognition framework with feature selection. In Advances in computer vision and computational biology (pp. 39–56). Springer, 2021.
2. Blalock D., Ortiz J.J.G., Frankle J., Guttag J. What is the state of neural net-work pruning? arXiv:2003.03033, 2020.
3. Zadtootaghaj P., Mohammadian A., Mahbanooei B., Ghasemi R. Internet of Things: A survey for the individuals' e-health applications. J Inf Technol Manag. 2019;11:102–129. doi: 10.22059/jitm.2019.288695.2398.
4. Kelly J., Campbell K., Gong E., Scuffham P. The Internet of Things: Impact and implications for health care delivery. J Med Internet Res. 2020;22(11):e20135. doi: 10.2196/20135.
5. Verma P., Sood S.K., S. Kalra. Cloud-centric IoT based student healthcare moni-toring framework. Ambient Intell Humaniz Comput. 2018;9:1293–1309. doi: 10.1007/s12652-017-0520-6.
6. Ahamed F., Farid F. Applying Internet of Things and machine-learning for per-sonalized healthcare: Issues and challenges. In 2018 International Conference on Machine Learning and Data Engineering (ICMLDE) (pp. 19–21), Sydney, NSW, Australia, 2018.
7. Qin Z., Sun J., Chen D., Xiong H. Flexible and lightweight access control for online healthcare social networks in the context of the Internet of Things. Mob Inf Syst. 2017:2017. doi: 10.1155/2017/7514867.
8. Kirtana R.N., Lokeswari Y.V. An IoT Based Remote HRV Monitoring System for Hypertensive Patients. In 2017 International Conference on Computer, Communication and Signal Processing (ICCCSP), Chennai, India, 2017. doi: 10.1109/ICCCSP.2017.7944086.
9. Jagadeeswari V., Subramaniyaswamy V., Logesh R., Kumar V. A study on medi-cal Internet of Things and big data in personalised healthcare system. Health Inf Sci Syst. 2018;6(1):14. doi: 10.1007/s13755-018-0049-x.
10. Bloss R. Multi-technology sensors are being developed for medical, manufac-turing, personal health and other applications not previously possible with his-toric single-technology sensors. Sens Rev. 2017;37(4):385–389.
11. Khan R., Plahouras J., Johnston B.C., Scaffidi M.A., Grover S.C., Walsh C.M. Virtual reality simulation training in endoscopy: A Cochrane review and meta-analysis. Endoscopy. 2019. doi: 10.1055/a-0894-4400.
12. Asua E., Etxebarria V., Garcia A., Feuchtwange J. Micropositioning control of smart shape-memory alloy-based actuators. Assemb Autom. 2009;29(3):272–278.
13. Janeh O., Fründt O., Schönwald B. Gait training in virtual reality: Short-term effects of different virtual manipulation techniques in Parkinson's disease. Cells. 2019;8(5): E419. doi: 10.3390/cells8050419.
14. Lai Y.L., Chou Y.H., Chang L.C. An intelligent IoT emergency vehicle warn-ing system using RFID and Wi-Fi technologies for emergency medical services. Technol Health Care. 2018;26(1):43–55.
15. Dai H.N., Imran M., Haider N. Blockchain-enabled internet of medical things to combat COVID-19. IEEE Internet Things Mag. 2020;3(3):52–57.
16. Takabayashi K., Tanaka H., Sakakibara K. Integrated performance evaluation of the smart body area networks physical layer for future medical and healthcare IoT. Sensors. 2018;19(1):E30. doi: 10.3390/s19010030.

17. Vishwakarma L.P., Singh R.K., Mishra R., Kumari A. Application of artificial intelligence for resilient and sustainable healthcare system: Systematic literature review and future research directions. Int J Prod Res. 2023. doi: 10.1080/00207543.2023.2188101.

18. Lomotey R.K., Pry J., Sriramoju S. Wearable IoT data stream traceability in a distributed health information system. Pervasive Mob Comput. 2017;40:692–707.

19. Alzaabi S., Chihabi N. Al H. El, Elsalhy M., Saad M. Istighatha: IoT-enabled emergency response system. Internet of Things. 2023;23:100869. doi: 10.1016/j.iot.2023.100869.

20. Nti I.K., Adekoya A.F., Weyori B.A., Keyeremeh F. A bibliometric analysis of technology in sustainable healthcare: Emerging trends and future directions. Decis Anal J. 2023;8:100292. doi: 10.1016/j.dajour.2023.100292.

21. Mavrogiorgou A., Kiourtis A., Perakis K., Pitsios S., Kyriazis D. IoT in healthcare: Achieving interoperability of high-quality data acquired by IoT medical devices. Sensors. 2019;19(9):E1978. doi: 10.3390/s19091978.

22. Adly A.S., Adly A, Adly S.M.S. Approaches based on artificial intelligence and the internet of intelligent things to prevent the spread of COVID-19: Scoping review. J Med Internet Res. 2020;22(8):e19104.

23. Kumar, M., Kumar, A., Verma, S., Bhattacharya, P., Ghimire, D., Kim, S.-H., Hosen, A.S.M.S. Healthcare Internet of Things (H-IoT): Current trends, future prospects, applications, challenges, and security issues. Electronics. 2023;12:2050. doi: 10.3390/electronics12092050.

24. Rayan R., Tsagkaris C., Romash I. The Internet of Things for healthcare: Applications, selected cases and challenges. In: Marques, G., Bhoi, A.K., de Albuquerque, V.H.C.d., Hareesha K.S. (eds.) IoT in healthcare and ambient assisted living. Studies in Computational Intelligence, vol. 933. Springer, Singapore, 2021. doi: 10.1007/978-981-15-9897-5_1.

25. Vichayanan R., Korejo M.S., Ali J., Thatsaringkharnsakun U. Blockchain-enabled Internet of Things (IoT) applications in healthcare: A systematic review of current trends and future opportunities. Int J Online Biomed Eng. 2023;19(10):99–117. doi: 10.3991/ijoe.v19i10.41399.

26. Shenavarmasouleh, F., Mohammadi, F.G., Amini, M.H., Arabnia, H.R. DRDr II: Detecting the severity level of diabetic retinopathy using mask RCNN and transfer learning. In 2020 International Conference on Computational Science and Computational Intelligence (CSCI) (pp. 788–792), 2020.

27. Shenavarmasouleh, F., Mohammadi, F.G., Amini, M.H., Arabnia, H.R. Embodied AI-driven operation of smart cities: A concise review. arXiv:2108.09823, 2021.

28. Shenavarmasouleh, F., Mohammadi, F.G., Amini, M.H., Taha, T., Rasheed, K., Arabnia, H.R. DRDrV3: Complete lesion detection in fundus images using mask R-CNN, transfer learning, and LSTM. arXiv:2108.08095, 2021.

29. Shaikh R.A., Nikilla S. Real time health monitoring system of remote patient using ARM7. Int J Instrum Contr Autom. 2012;1(3-4):102–105.

Recent advances in ubiquitous sustainable healthcare systems

Shwetha Baliga and Pushkar R. Kulkarni

2.1 INTRODUCTION

2.1.1 Background and context

At the nexus of the Internet of Things (IoT) and machine learning (ML), a groundbreaking synergy in the field of biomedical applications has arisen. This chapter explores the tremendous effects of this merger, which have sparked a revolutionary period in healthcare and medicine. A wide range of opportunities have been opened up by the confluence of IoT with ML, changing illness diagnosis, ongoing patient monitoring, therapy optimization, and more. By examining the core ideas behind IoT and ML, their seamless integration in data collection and preprocessing, and their crucial role in the biological actuation process, this abstract sets the scene.

While ML enables systems to learn, adapt, and make reasoned decisions using data-driven algorithms, IoT is a vast network of networked devices that gather and exchange data on their own. The biomedical industry, where accuracy and real-time data are crucial, is one in which the convergence of IoT and ML has particularly deep ramifications. IoT technologies offer continuous patient monitoring and individualized care, providing an unprecedented amount of real-time health information. These devices range from wearable sensors to cutting-edge medical equipment. In turn, ML algorithms examine this data, revealing patterns, anomalies, and insightful predictions with astounding accuracy.

A crucial component of efficient healthcare, early illness diagnosis has undergone a revolution that now provides options for prompt intervention. With ML models speeding candidate selection and therapeutic results, drug discovery and molecular design have made rapid advancements. As a result of IoT connection, telemedicine platforms have increased access to healthcare by facilitating data sharing and remote consultations. With the use of personalized medicine in the healthcare ecosystem, treatment strategies may now be customized for specific patients based on real-time data. However, this voyage of transformation is not without its difficulties. Data security and patient privacy raise serious ethical issues. IoT-generated data

DOI: 10.1201/9781003487647-2

comes in enormous amounts, thus managing them calls for smart preprocessing and fusion methods. The cost of implementing IoT solutions might be overwhelming, and integrating various IoT devices involves technological challenges.

2.1.2 The convergence of IoT and Machine Learning

IoT and ML coming together denotes a revolutionary synergy between connected devices and intelligent data processing. The IoT is a vast network of connected devices that collect and exchange data. By using this data to learn, ML enables systems to make predictions and decisions without explicit programming. The potential of both technologies is increased by combining IoT and ML. Massive datasets produced by IoT can be analysed by ML algorithms to reveal insights, patterns, and correlations that improve automation, enable predictive maintenance, and support real-time decision-making. By enabling devices to adjust and enhance their performance based on changing data patterns, ML optimizes IoT. By improving efficiency, resource allocation, and user experiences, this convergence affects a number of industries, including healthcare, manufacturing, transportation, and smart cities. However, challenges like data privacy, security, and ethical considerations must be addressed to fully realize the potential of this powerful synergy. The integration of IoT and ML promises a future where smart, autonomous systems intelligently interact with the physical world, revolutionizing industries and shaping the way we live and work.

2.1.3 Effect in transforming biomedical applications

The biomedical field has been significantly impacted by the integration of IoT and ML, revolutionizing patient care and medical research. IoT devices gather real-time health information from medical equipment, implantable devices, and wearable sensors to enable continuous monitoring and individualized care. By analysing this data, ML algorithms can spot anomalies, forecast how a disease will develop, and help with early diagnosis. Through proactive interventions and remote patient management, this synergy improves patient outcomes. ML models speed up candidate selection and improve molecular designs in drug discovery. Telemedicine platforms that are IoT-enabled also make it easier to exchange data and conduct remote consultations, increasing access to healthcare. However, difficulties include data security, privacy, and regulatory compliance. Despite challenges, the fusion of IoT and ML has the potential to fundamentally alter the way healthcare is provided, enhance patient well-being, and spur advances in precision medicine and therapeutic development.

Figure 2.1 explains how satellite technology acts as a vital backbone for connecting the dots in the vast network of IoT devices, enabling data collection,

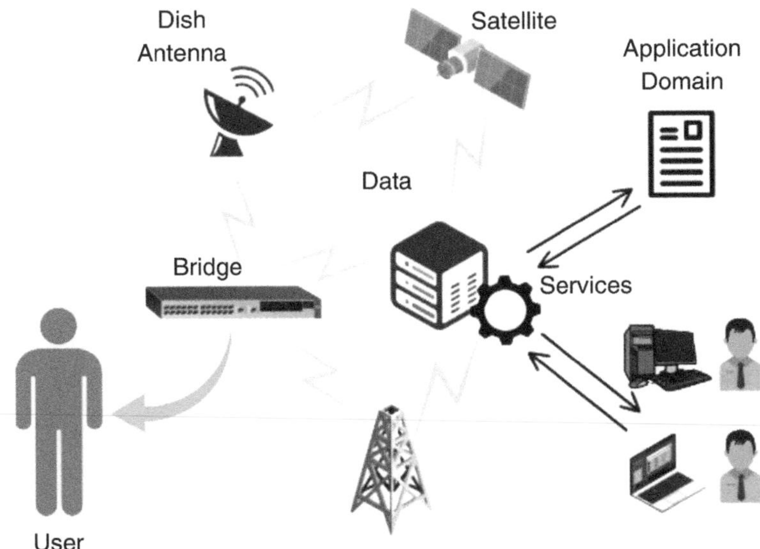

Figure 2.1 Communication in IoT networks.

communication, and powerful applications across the globe, opening doors to a more connected and intelligent future.

2.2 FUNDAMENTALS OF IoT AND ML

2.2.1 IoT architecture and components

IoT represents a network of interconnected devices, often referred to as "things," which have the ability to collect, transmit, and exchange data without human intervention. We discuss the fundamental architecture of IoT systems, encompassing various layers. There are different models in the IoT architecture such as three-, four-, and eight-layered models. The three-layered model has the following:

1. *Perception Layer:* This is where data is collected from sensors and devices, including physiological sensors like heart rate monitors, temperature sensors, and imaging devices.
2. *Network Layer:* Data is transmitted through networks, both local (e.g., Bluetooth, Zigbee) and global (e.g., Wi-Fi, cellular networks), to reach centralized data processing systems.
3. *Application Layer:* Insights are derived from processed data, leading to informed actions or decisions. This layer acts as an interface between the user and the IoT system. A fourth support layer is also seen in the

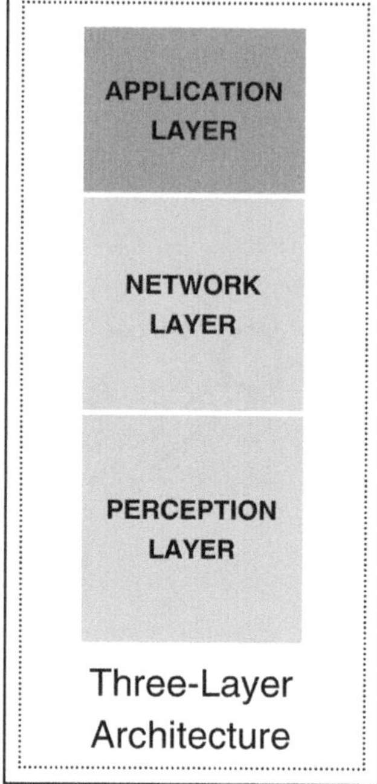

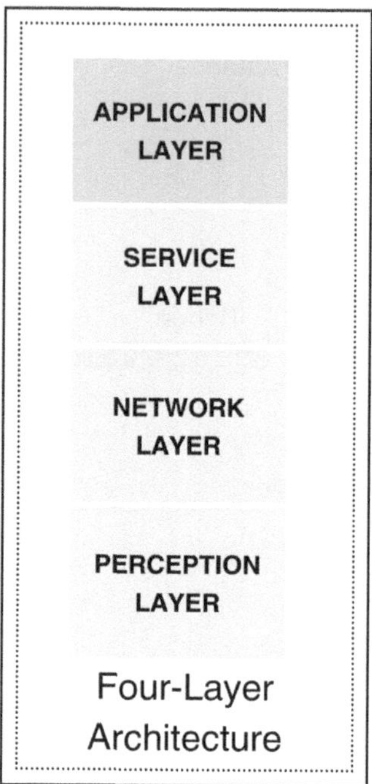

Figure 2.2 Layers of IoT architecture (three- and four-layers).

four-layer model which is responsible for processing and data analysis. An eight-layer model is also proposed by IBM which has few layers related to network-sensing, WAN, etc.

Figures 2.2 and 2.3 show a typical layered architecture for an IoT system. This architecture enables modularity, scalability, and flexibility for developers to build and deploy IoT applications.

2.2.2 ML algorithms and techniques

ML is a branch of artificial intelligence (AI) and computer science which focuses on the use of data and algorithms to imitate the way that humans learn, gradually improving its accuracy (Figure 2.4).

1. *Supervised Learning Algorithms:* Learning methods like decision trees, support vector machines, and neural networks predict based on labelled data. In biomedicine, they detect disease in images or forecast patient outcomes using historical information.
2. *Unsupervised Learning Methods:* Unsupervised techniques, like clustering and dimensionality reduction, are clarified. Clustering groups similar points, aiding patient categorization. Dimensionality reduction, e.g.,

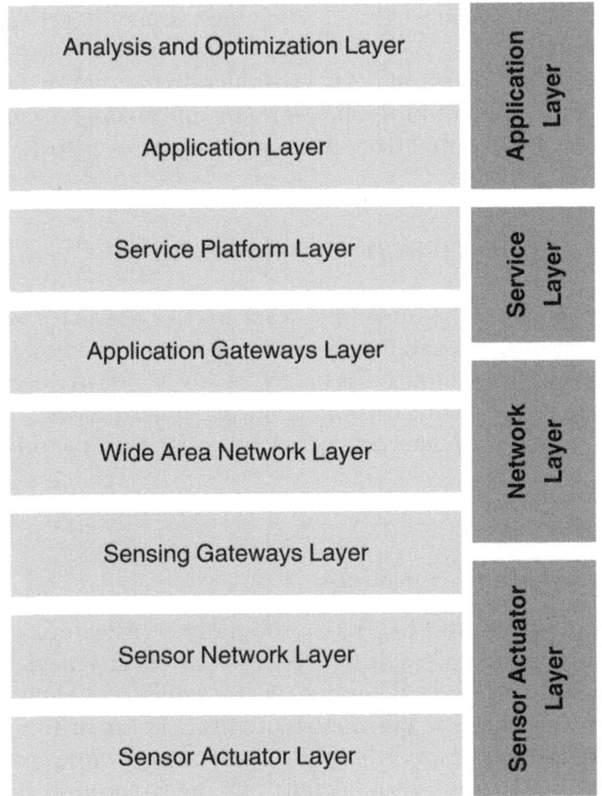

Figure 2.3 Layers of IoT architecture (eight-layer).

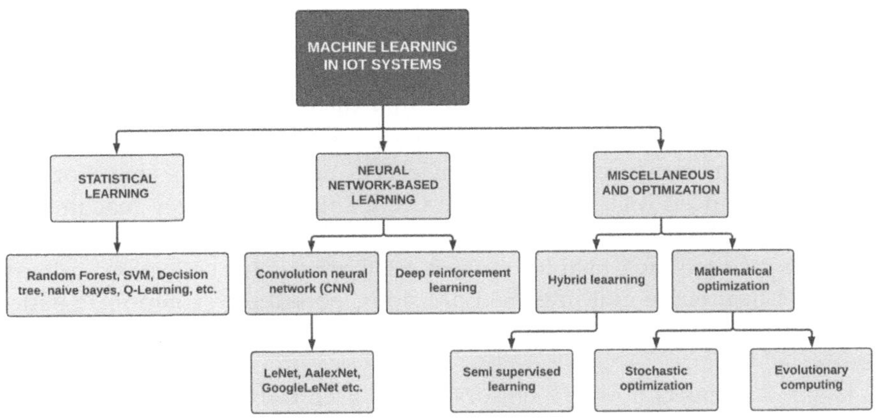

Figure 2.4 ML in various IoT systems.

principal component analysis, trims high-dimensional data, extracting key features.

3. *Reinforcement Learning:* An introduction to reinforcement learning highlights its potential applications in optimizing personalized treatment plans by learning from patient responses over time.

2.3 DATA ACQUISITION IN BIOMEDICAL IoT

Data acquisition forms the most important part of the IoT ecosystem in biomedical applications. The ability to collect real-time, accurate, and comprehensive data from various sources is necessary for healthcare decisions. Sensors can be integrated into medical equipment, personal devices, and even everyday objects, creating an interconnected network that continuously gathers information.

2.3.1 IoT sensors and devices

The integration of IoT and ML has profoundly transformed the biomedical realm, reshaping patient care and medical research. IoT devices gather real-time health data from medical equipment, wearables, and implants, enabling continuous monitoring for personalized care. ML algorithms analyse this data, detecting anomalies, predicting disease progression, and aiding early diagnosis, leading to improved patient outcomes through proactive interventions. ML expedites drug discovery by enhancing candidate selection and molecular design. IoT-enabled telemedicine platforms facilitate remote consultations and data exchange, expanding healthcare access. Challenges include data security, privacy, and compliance. Despite these hurdles, the fusion of IoT and ML holds potential to reshape healthcare, advancing precision medicine and therapeutics.

This synergy can be further enhanced by combining IoT and ML to analyse data patterns, offer predictive insights, and suggest actions. Various sensors are vital in healthcare – blood pressure monitors track cardiovascular health, pulse oximeters measure blood oxygen levels, and ECG sensors monitor heart activity. Advanced imaging tools like CT scanners and X-ray machines aid diagnostics. The humble thermometer remains crucial for precise body temperature readings. IoT-enabled devices harmonize data collection, ushering proactive healthcare and informed decisions, poised to revolutionize patient experiences, diagnostics, and treatments, promising a brighter healthcare future.

Figure 2.5 shows how IoT sensors can be used to measure various human body parameters, providing valuable data for personal health monitoring, remote patient monitoring, sports performance monitoring, and workplace safety monitoring.

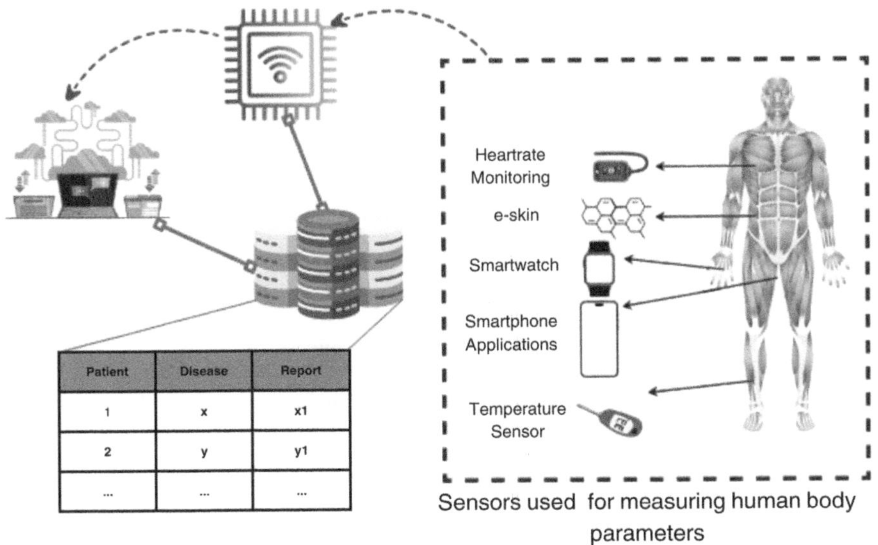

Figure 2.5 Data acquisition of vitals of various patients of different hospitals and passing it to the doctors via the IoT server for necessary actions.

All these sensors are integrated into devices. Some of these devices are simplified so that they can be carried around easily by all the people; these devices are called *wearable devices*.

2.3.2 Wearable devices

The fusion of IoT and ML has revolutionized continuous patient monitoring, led by wearable technology innovation in the biomedical IoT domain. Wearables, spanning from smartwatches to medical devices, reshape data collection, seamlessly merging technology and health. These wearables offer detailed activity monitoring, benefiting patients and healthcare professionals alike. For instance, heart rate monitors track real-time heart rhythm, empowering users to monitor cardiovascular health. Healthcare providers leverage wearable data for informed decisions and tailored interventions.

Sleep trackers exemplify IoT and ML convergence benefits. These trackers analyse sleep patterns, potentially detecting sleep disorders. They facilitate better sleep hygiene by monitoring duration, depth, and disturbances. Wearable technology embodies the synergy of health sciences and technology, harnessing IoT and ML potential for personalized insights, proactive health management, and patient-centric care advancement.

Figure 2.6 showcases how IoT technologies can revolutionize healthcare delivery by seamlessly connecting patients, healthcare providers, and devices, leading to more informed, data-driven, and patient-centric care. Wearable devices and sensors might be used to collect vital signs and other health data.

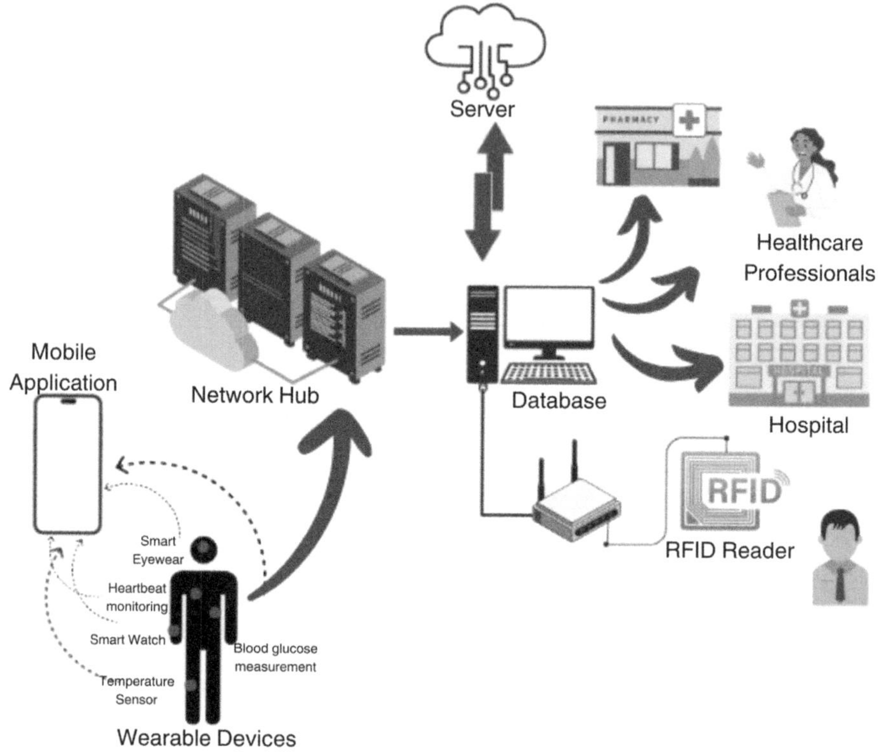

Figure 2.6 Various IoT sensors monitoring a person's vitals via wearable devices and relaying it to the IoT network for analysis by the healthcare professionals.

2.4 DATA PREPROCESSING AND FUSION FOR BIOMEDICAL DATA

Biomedical data collected through IoT devices and ML should be selectively combined to get the most accurate and useful results. The purpose is to integrate multiple data and knowledge of objects with consistent, accurate, and useful application.

2.4.1 Techniques for data fusion

1. *Data-level/Sensor-level Fusion:* Data from different sensors measuring the same or related variables are fused to create a more accurate representation. For example, fusing data from multiple sensors monitoring a particular activity will help us to generate a more accurate result.
2. *Feature-level Fusion:* This involves combining features extracted from individual data sources to create a unified feature set. For instance, combining data from wearable heart rate monitors and glucose sensors to create a specific yet complete profile of a patient's cardiovascular health.

3. *Decision-level Fusion:* Decisions or predictions from multiple sensor systems are combined to arrive at a final decision. In biomedical applications, this could involve aggregating diagnostic predictions from various algorithms to improve overall accuracy.

The fused/final data is then sent to the IoT server, analysed, processed, and stored in the database. This information can be accessed by the doctors for their study and prediction of the future condition of the patient.

2.5 ACTUATION PROCESS BASED ON THE DATA COLLECTED

The integration of IoT and ML technologies in the biomedical field has led to significant advancements in monitoring, diagnosis, treatment, and overall healthcare management. When it comes to the actuation process in the biomedical field, IoT and ML play complementary roles to enhance the capabilities of medical devices and systems. Some of the actuators used in different fields are as follows.

2.5.1 Surgical robots

Surgical robots powered by electromechanical actuators are a cutting-edge breakthrough in medical technology, allowing for delicate and accurate motions during minimally invasive treatments. These robots are piloted by competent surgeons who combine their knowledge with the capabilities of the robot. ML enhances this synergy by improving robotic control algorithms. ML algorithms examine massive information obtained from surgical operations, discovering trends and refining these robots' control systems. As a result, ML integration improves surgical robot accuracy, stability, and overall performance. This symbiotic interaction between electromechanical actuators and ML algorithms has the potential to transform surgical procedures, opening the path for more effective and safer surgeries with less invasiveness and better patient outcomes.

2.5.2 Implantable devices

Modern healthcare is greatly reliant on implantable gadgets that are propelled by electromechanical actuators. These gadgets use electromechanical forces to affect physiological processes, such as pacemakers for controlling heart rhythm and neurostimulators for therapeutic treatments. ML appears as a transformational technology in this setting. By dynamically adjusting stimulation patterns based on real-time monitoring of patient feedback and physiological inputs, ML algorithms can improve implanted device performance. The efficiency of therapy is maximized because of this clever integration, which permits tailored and adaptable treatment techniques. Implantable devices can grow beyond static programming by using ML to comprehend complex patterns and interactions within the body. This results in a dynamic and patient-centred approach. This synergy has the potential to improve implantable medical therapies' accuracy, effectiveness, and customizability, improving patient care and well-being.

2.5.3 Ultrasound transducers

Medical technology is not complete without ultrasound transducers, which use piezoelectric materials to generate high-frequency sound waves. When these waves are focused within the body, they interact with the tissues and organs, producing echoes that are then recorded to produce finely detailed pictures for medical imaging. This non-invasive method is now crucial for making diagnoses, seeing within the body, and keeping track of fetal growth. Beyond imaging, therapeutic uses for ultrasonic waves include dissolving kidney stones and accelerating wound-healing. The operation of the transducer is supported by the piezoelectric effect, in which certain materials transform mechanical energy into electrical impulses. Modern medicine now has access to safer and more accurate diagnoses and treatments, thanks to this cutting-edge technology.

2.5.4 Hearing aids

The combination of IoT and ML in hearing aids is a classic example of cutting-edge medical developments. These gadgets can record external audio input, thanks to tiny microphones. Advanced ML algorithms then analyse this data, identifying subtle sound patterns and tailoring amplification levels to each listener's specific aural requirements. These customized modifications are then sent to actuators inside the hearing aid through seamless IoT connectivity, delivering the best possible sound transmission to the ear. Hearing aids become individualized aural improvement tools, thanks to the seamless integration of IoT's real-time data transfer and ML's pattern detection, improving users' auditory experiences and quality of life.

2.5.5 Artificial limbs

Artificial limbs, usually referred to as prosthetic appliances, are made to mimic the motions of real limbs. ML and IoT technology integration has significantly improved the usability and functionality of these devices. By converting the data from wearable sensors and brain interfaces into commands that operate the actuators in prosthetic limbs, ML plays a crucial role. Movements are made more naturally and intuitively, more like those of biological limbs, thanks to this synergy. For those who have lost limbs, ML-driven prosthetic limbs improve mobility, comfort, and quality of life by continually learning from user interactions and adjusting to changing surroundings.

2.6 REAL-TIME MONITORING AND PREDICTIVE MODELLING

In the world of healthcare and medicine, the ability to monitor patients in real time and predict potential health issues is a boon to the doctors. Advancements in IoT-enabled ML are propelling the field of personalized medicine to unprecedented heights. The most important thing for real-time monitoring is early disease detection with IoT and ML.

2.6.1 Early disease detection with IoT and ML

It is a critical factor in improving patient outcomes and reducing healthcare costs. By combining the capabilities of IoT devices with ML algorithms, healthcare professionals can identify changes in the human body due to developing disease before noticeable symptoms appear.

IoT devices, such as wearable sensors and implantable monitors, continuously collect and transmit data about a patient's vital signs. ML algorithms can analyse this data to establish a database and creates a pattern of health for individuals. When deviations from this pattern is seen, the system can generate alerts or notification. Early detection facilitated by IoT and ML not only enhances patient outcomes but also reduces the burden on healthcare systems by addressing medical issues before they escalate into more complex and costly conditions.

2.6.2 Research and population health management

The integration of real-time monitoring through the convergence of IoT and ML has introduced a paradigm shift in the realms of research and population health management. The copious volumes of data generated by continuous patient monitoring offer a vast canvas for researchers to paint a comprehensive understanding of health dynamics. This abundance of information provides an extensive sample size for intricate studies, enabling researchers to explore a multitude of variables and conditions to derive insightful conclusions. Furthermore, the synergistic potential of IoT and ML empowers researchers to engage in intricate simulations.

This predictive capacity proves invaluable in anticipating future trajectories and planning effective interventions. For example, ML algorithms can analyse data patterns to forecast viral mutations, facilitating proactive strategies such as the development of targeted treatments. In the realm of population health management, real-time monitoring equips healthcare authorities with the tools to track and respond to health trends swiftly. Timely data analysis enables the identification of disease hotspots, resource allocation optimization, and the implementation of preventive measures. This synergy fosters a data-driven approach to healthcare, enhancing decision-making and enabling the customization of interventions based on population health needs.

2.7 FUTURE TRENDS AND EMERGING APPLICATIONS

The future of healthcare is bright, thanks to the convergence of IoT and ML. These two technologies are already being used to improve patient care in a variety of ways, and their potential is only just beginning to be realized.

One of the most promising applications of IoT and ML in healthcare is remote patient monitoring. IoT devices, such as wearable sensors and implants, can be used to collect real-time data on a patient's vital signs, activity levels, and other health metrics. This data can then be analysed by ML algorithms to identify any potential problems early on. For example, an ML algorithm could be used to detect a patient's heart rate increasing before they experience an arrhythmia. This would allow the patient to receive treatment sooner, potentially preventing a more serious health event.

Another area where IoT and ML are having a major impact is in diagnostic imaging. ML algorithms can be used to analyse medical images, such as X-rays and CT scans, to identify diseases and abnormalities that would be difficult or impossible to spot with the naked eye. This is already being used in clinical practice to improve the accuracy of cancer diagnoses and other life-threatening conditions.

In the future, IoT and ML are also likely to play a role in drug discovery and development. ML algorithms can be used to analyse large datasets of medical data to identify new drug targets and design new drugs that are more effective and less toxic. This could revolutionize the way we treat diseases and improve patient outcomes.

Of course, there are also some challenges that need to be addressed before IoT and ML can be fully realized in healthcare. One challenge is data privacy. As more and more health data is collected and stored electronically, it is important to ensure that this data is secure and protected from unauthorized access. Another challenge is the cost of implementing IoT and ML solutions. These solutions can be expensive, and it may be difficult for some healthcare organizations to afford them.

Despite these challenges, the future of healthcare is bright. IoT and ML have the potential to revolutionize the way we deliver care, making it more personalized, predictive, and effective. With careful planning and execution, we can ensure that these technologies are used to improve patient care and advance the field of medicine.

Here are some additional thoughts on the future of IoT and ML in healthcare:

- Wearable health devices will become more common and affordable, making it easier for people to track their own health data.
- ML algorithms will be used to develop personalized treatment plans for patients.
- IoT-connected devices will be used to monitor patients in real time, even when they are not in a hospital or clinic.

- AR and VR will be used to provide surgeons with more precise guidance during procedures.
- Telemedicine will become more widespread, allowing patients to receive care from doctors who are located far away.
- AI-powered chatbots will be used to answer patients' questions and provide support.

2.8 CHALLENGES AND LIMITATIONS

The healthcare IoT contains various applications, and it allows us to determine the deep connections. However, we face some critical issues (Figure 2.7):

i. *Data Security and Privacy*
   Safeguarding sensitive patient data stands as the most important concern. The network of healthcare IoT raises fear about data breaches and unauthorized access. Implementing robust security measures and encryption protocols is necessary to uphold patient confidentiality and privacy.

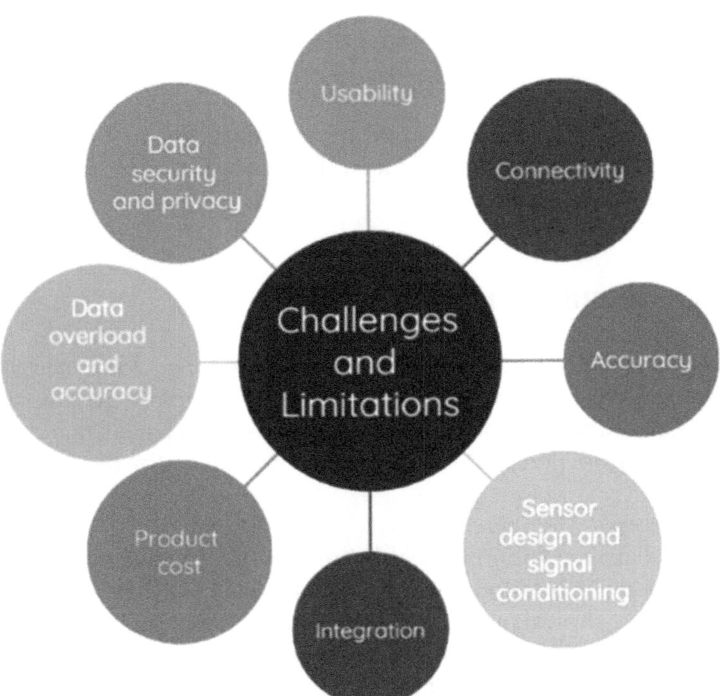

Figure 2.7 Challenges faced in implementation of ML and IoT in medical field.

ii. *Data Overload and Accuracy*
   The influx of data from IoT devices can overwhelm healthcare systems, potentially leading to data misinterpretation or oversight. Striking a balance between the quantity and quality of data is crucial to ensure accurate analysis and meaningful insights.

iii. *Product Cost*
   Implementing and maintaining healthcare IoT solutions can entail substantial costs, including device procurement, infrastructure setup, and ongoing maintenance. Balancing the potential benefits with financial feasibility is a challenge that requires careful resource allocation.

iv. *Sensor Design and Signal Conditioning*
   The effectiveness of healthcare IoT hinges on sensor design and accurate signal conditioning. Ensuring sensors are reliable, accurate, and capable of capturing relevant health metrics is vital for generating trustworthy data for analysis.

v. *Integration*
   There are many different types of IoT devices and medical applications in use today, and they often use different communication protocols and data formats. This can make it difficult to integrate these devices and applications together to create a cohesive system.

vi. *Accuracy*
   IoT devices and medical applications are only as good as the data they collect. If the data is inaccurate, the results of the analysis will be inaccurate as well.

vii. *Usability*
   IoT devices and medical applications must be easy to use for both patients and healthcare providers. If they are not user-friendly, they will not be adopted widely.

2.9 LITERATURE REVIEW

In recent years, ML has emerged as a transformative force across various domains, including healthcare. This chapter aims to explore the diverse applications of ML in healthcare, focusing on the cited research papers that cover a wide range of topics, from personalized medicine to virtual reality therapy (Table 2.1).

1. *Personalized Medicine*
   A paradigm revolution in healthcare is being ushered in by personalized medicine, which tailors therapies to each patient based on their particular genetic, clinical, and lifestyle traits. By evaluating massive datasets to forecast patient reactions to certain therapies or interventions, ML plays a crucial role in this sector. The study by Khan [1] emphasizes how crucial ML is becoming in obtaining genuinely customized healthcare and how it has the ability to completely transform disease prevention and treatment.

Table 2.1 A few papers and studies on IoT- and ML- involved research in biomedical industry

Application	Use case	Benefits	Research paper
Personalized medicine	Predicting patient risk of heart disease	Early intervention and prevention	[1]
Remote patient monitoring	Tracking patient vital signs	Early detection of health problems	[2]
Wearable devices	Monitoring exercise and sleep patterns	Personalization of healthcare	[3]
Medical imaging	Diagnosing diabetic retinopathy	Early detection and treatment	[4]
Drug discovery	Screening potential drugs for safety and efficacy	Speeding up the drug discovery process	[5]
Intelligent medical systems	Automating tasks	Reducing human error	[6]
Real-time mental health monitoring	Tracking patient mental health data	Early detection of mental health problems	[7]
Medical image analysis	Classifying different types of medical images	Improved accuracy of diagnosis	[8]
Personalized nutrition	Recommending personalized diets	Improved health outcomes	[9]
Virtual reality therapy	Treating mental health disorders	Reduced symptoms and improved quality of life	[10]

2. *Predicting Patient Risk of Heart Disease*

   Worldwide, heart disease continues to be one of the top causes of death. To forecast a person's risk of developing heart disease, ML models can examine patient data, including medical history, lifestyle variables, and genetic information. Through early intervention and preventative actions made possible by these prediction models, lives may be saved and the cost of healthcare may be decreased. The relevance of ML in cardiovascular healthcare is emphasized by Khan's review [1].

3. *Early Intervention and Prevention* [1]

   In order to stop the course of the disease and enhance patient outcomes, early intervention is essential. Medical professionals may take proactive action by identifying health issues early on, thanks to ML-driven risk prediction models. By avoiding costly therapies linked to severe illness stages, this strategy improves patient care while also lowering healthcare expenditures.

4. *Remote Patient Monitoring*

   Remote patient monitoring made possible by IoT is becoming more popular, particularly in light of the COVID-19 epidemic. The importance of IoT in remotely gathering patient's vital signs is highlighted by Hossain's comprehensive study [2]. This technology is a vital tool in contemporary healthcare since it permits continuous monitoring, early diagnosis of health concerns, and prompt medical actions.

5. *Wearable Devices*
   Smartwatches and fitness trackers are only two examples of the wearable technology that has proliferated in recent years. In Ref. [3], Khan highlights their potential for healthcare and highlights how important it is for them to track their sleep and exercise routines. In order to deliver individualized healthcare suggestions, promote better lives, and avoid chronic illnesses, ML algorithms can assess the data produced by these devices.

6. *Medical Imaging*
   Another industry that benefits from ML improvements is medical imaging. Asif's review [4] focuses on the diagnosis of diabetic retinopathy, a condition for which retinal pictures may be examined by ML algorithms for early identification and treatment planning. ML-powered image analysis improves screening efficiency while simultaneously improving diagnosis accuracy, perhaps avoiding diabetes patients from losing their vision.

7. *Drug Discovery*
   The process of discovering new drugs is labour- and time-intensive. By speeding the evaluation of possible medications for efficacy and safety, ML provides a solution. In Ref. [5], Khan describes how ML algorithms can forecast drug–target interactions and find good candidates, possibly cutting down on the time and expense needed to get novel medications to the market.

8. *Intelligent Medical Systems*
   Intelligent medical systems use ML to automate a variety of healthcare processes, lowering human error and increasing efficiency. These systems, which include anything from administrative assistance to diagnostic tools, improve the standard of patient care overall. The review by Imran [6] emphasizes the various ways that intelligent medical systems are used in various healthcare settings.

9. *Real-time Mental Health Monitoring*
   A vital part of total well-being is mental health. Patient mental health data can be continuously tracked using real-time mental health monitoring utilizing ML. According to Santos' study [7], this technology has the ability to identify mental health issues early, allowing for prompt treatment and better patient outcomes.

10. *Medical Image Analysis*
    The area of radiology has undergone a revolution, thanks to ML-based medical image analysis. Singh's paper [8] describes how ML algorithms can categorize several medical picture types, including X-rays and MRIs, improving diagnostic precision. These developments enable speedier and more accurate diagnosis, which directly affects patient care.

11. *Personalized Nutrition*
    Diet is essential to overall health. To suggest individualized diets, ML may assess people's dietary choices, nutritional demands, and health objectives. Khan's analysis [9] highlights how ML-enabled tailored diet might help with illness prevention and better health outcomes.
12. *Virtual Reality Therapy*
    A novel method of treating mental health illnesses is VR treatment. The systematic review by Santos [10] examines the use of VR in mental health therapies, highlighting its potential to lessen symptoms and improve quality of life for those who are dealing with mental health problems.

2.10 CONCLUSION

There is no denying the fact that IoT and ML have combined to change the healthcare and medical industries. These technologies have come together to create new opportunities for personalized patient care, complex analysis, and real-time data collecting. The enormous potential of IoT-driven ML applications covering a broad range of biological settings has been made clear by this synergy. These applications include, but are not limited to, early-stage disease detection, ongoing patient monitoring, and individualized therapy improvement.

However, ethical issues, particularly those relating to the protection of data privacy and security, loom large as we traverse this historic advancement. Comprehensive frameworks that guarantee the security and integrity of sensitive patient information are required for the seamless integration of these technologies. Looking into the distance, a promising trajectory emerges with ongoing enquiry and investigation in this area. AI-enhanced healthcare ecosystems have the potential to greatly improve diagnosis accuracy, give patients more control over their treatment, and fundamentally alter the healthcare landscape. It makes sense that the collaborative relationship between IoT and ML provides a strong and effective route for magnifying accomplishments within the biomedical field, thereby improving the human experience in a palpable and long-lasting way.

REFERENCES

1. A. M. Khan, *"Machine learning for personalized medicine: A review,"* IEEE Access, vol. 7, 136254–136275, 2019.
2. S. M. S. Hossain, *"Internet of Things (IoT) enabled remote patient monitoring: A systematic review,"* Sensors, vol. 20, 7310, 2020.
3. R. A. Khan, *"Wearable devices for healthcare: A review,"* Sensors, vol. 19, 4248, 2019.
4. S. M. Asif, *"Machine learning for medical imaging in diabetic retinopathy: A review"* IEEE Access, vol. 7, 102135–102150, 2019.

5. M. A. Khan, "*Machine learning for drug discovery: A review,*" IEEE Access, vol. 7, 54772–54792, 2019.
6. S. M. Imran, "*Intelligent medical systems: A review,*" IEEE Access, vol. 7, 107860–107876, 2019.
7. R. M. N. Santos, "*A real-time mental health monitoring system using machine learning,*" IEEE Access, vol. 8, 140411–140424, 2020.
8. A. V. Singh, "*Medical image analysis using machine learning: A review,*" IEEE Access, vol. 8, 88242–88260, 2020.
9. M. A. Khan, "*Personalized nutrition using machine learning: A review,*" IEEE Access, vol. 9, 62602–62621, 2021.
10. R. M. N. Santos, "*Virtual reality therapy for mental health disorders: A systematic review,*" IEEE Access, vol. 9, 100122–100135, 2021.

IoT-enabled healthcare system using machine learning

P. Jothi Thilaga, K. Vignesh Saravanan, S. Kavi Priya, and K. Vijayalakshmi

3.1 INTRODUCTION

Before the advent of the Internet of Things (IoT), patients could solely engage with their doctors through in-person meetings, telephone calls, or text messages. There was no practical means for healthcare professionals or institutions to continuously oversee patients' well-being and provide guidance. Thanks to the introduction of IoT-connected devices in the healthcare industry, remote monitoring has become a reality. This has unleashed the potential to maintain the safety and well-being of patients while enabling healthcare providers to deliver exceptional treatment. The ease and efficiency of doctor–patient interactions have improved, leading to increased patient participation and satisfaction [1]. Furthermore, by constantly monitoring patients' health, remote patient monitoring has curtailed hospital stays and minimized the likelihood of readmissions. The utilization of IoT has substantially enhanced patient outcomes and simultaneously reduced healthcare system expenses.

The healthcare industry is undergoing a transformative change through IoT, reshaping the way devices and individuals interact in the delivery of healthcare solutions, all while maintaining trust. IoT healthcare applications bring advantages to a diverse range of stakeholders, including patients, physicians, hospitals, and insurance providers. [2, 3].

IoT for Medical Use: Wearable technologies, such as fitness bands, and wirelessly connected medical devices, including blood pressure and heart rate monitoring cuffs and glucometers, are empowering patients to access personalized healthcare. These gadgets can be customized to send users reminders for tracking changes in their blood pressure, upcoming appointments, and various other healthcare-related tasks. IoT has significantly transformed people's lives by enabling the continuous monitoring of medical conditions, particularly among elderly patients [3]. This has a profound impact on both individuals living alone and families. Any disruptions or alterations in a person's daily activities are promptly detected by their alarm system, which in turn notifies concerned family members and healthcare professionals.

DOI: 10.1201/9781003487647-3

IoT for Medical Professionals: Medical professionals can enhance patient health monitoring by integrating wearables and other IoT-enabled home monitoring devices. This allows them to closely monitor a patient's adherence to their treatment plan and respond promptly to any urgent medical needs. With the help of IoT, healthcare staff can now engage more actively with patients and maintain a heightened level of vigilance. The data collected from IoT devices can assist clinicians in choosing the most appropriate treatment strategies for patients, ultimately leading to the achievement of desired outcomes [4].

Hospital IoT Applications: In hospital management system, IoT applications extend beyond patient health monitoring to serve various additional functions. IoT devices equipped with sensors are employed to provide real-time tracking of medical equipment such as wheelchairs, defibrillators, nebulizers, oxygen pumps, and other monitoring devices. Furthermore, real-time evaluation of the locations of medical staff is made possible [3, 4]. To alleviate patient concerns regarding infections in healthcare facilities, IoT-enabled hygiene monitoring technology can be employed, effectively contributing to infection prevention. Additionally, IoT devices find utility in managing various assets, such as pharmacy inventories, monitoring refrigerator temperatures, and regulating environmental conditions like humidity and temperature.

The swift evolution of smart object technology has paved the way for significant strides in application development for wireless sensor-based distributed communication systems. This advancement has fostered the creation and integration of diverse, innovative, on-demand, and real-time IoT services in daily life. These services leverage the contactless nature and data retrieval efficiency of contemporary smart devices [5, 6]. When designing IoT-based applications, it is essential to carefully consider key data processing parameters, including volume, velocity, diversity, and, most importantly, data accuracy. While IoT-focused approaches open the door to the development of novel applications, they also introduce new risks that need to be managed.

At the core of the security challenge within the realm of IoT lies the integration of camera and voice interaction, which facilitates the operation of IoT products and their interactive applications [7]. Presently, IoT has emerged as an exceptionally promising communication paradigms. Within this framework, all intelligent objects that we encounter daily, capable of communication and computation, connect to the internet. While this offers new possibilities for IoT applications, it also introduces fresh security challenges. Regarding system vulnerability, any smart object or sensor in the IoT ecosystem can potentially pose a security risk. In other words, every intelligent device could become a potential point of vulnerability for malicious attacks [8].

Consequently, two primary security concerns have surfaced: (1) ensuring the physical security of smart devices and (2) preserving data confidentiality, integrity, and privacy during data exchange among these smart objects. There is a widespread expectation for an innovative and groundbreaking security solution tailored specifically to the unique characteristics of IoT technology, given its novelty [9]. Conventional security measures may not be suitable for smart objects, as they often possess limited resources and narrowly defined objectives. For instance, firewalls with network management control protocols can oversee high-level internet traffic, but such application-level solutions may not be adequate for IoT applications.

Wireless body sensor networks (WBSNs) is a particular class of wireless sensor networks (WSNs)used in healthcare applications. A WBSN is made up of tiny biological sensor nodes that can be implanted inside human tissues or strategically positioned on the body. They are designed to diagnose a variety of life-threatening disorders at an early stage, offering cost-effective and immediate options for health monitoring. WBSNs are used for both medical and non-medical purposes, including many others in the fields of sports, entertainment, the military, and healthcare [10–12]. The goal is to offer them better, more affordable options for their quality of life. In addition to sharing traits with WSNs and MANETs, WBSNs also face several particular limitations, including node heterogeneity, local energy awareness, transmission range, postural body movement, the influence of radiation on tissue heating, and global network longevity.

3.2 ROLE OF ARTIFICIAL INTELLIGENCE (AI) AND IoT IN HEALTHCARE AND FUTURE

IoT comprises a network of smart objects and devices that seamlessly integrate into a practical information network. These devices possess distinct identities, physical characteristics, and the ability to self-configure based on established communication protocols. The primary goal of IoT is to connect billions of everyday items to the internet, enabling them to interact and communicate with one another [13]. Examples of such objects include smart watches, vehicles, washing machines, and various household applications. The integration of RFID and sensors serves as the cornerstone for IoT, allowing diverse devices and objects to link to the internet and collaborate to achieve common objectives.

IoT connects a multitude of devices, a task that is either infeasible or impractical with traditional network architecture. To effectively manage and oversee these data-rich IoT networks, new protocols and structures are required [14, 15]. Taking a broader perspective, the centralized functionality of software-defined networking (SDN) can be harnessed to govern these networks. This approach enhances IoT network performance by optimizing bandwidth utilization, load balancing, and reducing latency, thereby improving overall network functionality [16].

Medical research studies reveal that approximately 80% of adults aged 65 and older suffer from at least one chronic illness, which can make self-care challenging for many elderly individuals. Consequently, ensuring a good quality of life for the elderly has become a significant societal challenge. The rapid proliferation of information and communication technologies has paved the way for cutting-edge healthcare tools and solutions capable of addressing these issues. In the 21st century, IoT stands as one of the most powerful communication paradigms. With their communication and computational capabilities, all the everyday items integrated into the IoT ecosystem become part of the internet. IoT expands and extends the concept of the internet itself [17, 18].

3.3 DATA COLLECTION, MINING, AND ANALYTICS IN THE HEALTHCARE SECTOR

Security stands out as one of the most vital components in any system, and its definition can vary since people have different perspectives on it. Generally, security and system safety are closely related concepts [19]. The practice of collecting, examining, and making conclusions based on data has a long history in the field of healthcare. This appears to be a result of regulatory agencies' requirements. In the coming years, it's expected that the overall volume of healthcare data will surpass the Yottabyte mark. In the past, a variety of AI-based methods have been employed to assess injury risk and forecast performance. Medical diagnostics have also made use of vision-based motion analysis. The vast potential of big data continues to be an invaluable resource for enhancing various aspects of clinical processes, public health, preventive care, precision medicine, evidence-based medicine, remote monitoring, patient profiling, and preventive healthcare. These enhancements bring about cost reductions, faster analysis, and a decrease in error rates [20]. To foster innovation in the field of smart medicine, critical components include refining data collection techniques and harnessing data mining from existing sources.

Architectural frameworks empowered by AI and machine learning (ML) have been proposed for assessing the wealth of vital data available in different healthcare sectors. However, the gradual and fragmented integration of comprehensive data across diverse healthcare applications remains a notable challenge. The variability in data structures and features from various healthcare environments can present hurdles for trained algorithms [21]. Thanks to the availability of affordable, near-standard sensor technology, integrating multiple sensors to gather well-organized, time-synchronized data now serves as the initial step in creating a pipeline for diverse medical and diagnostic applications. Wearable sensors have emerged as particularly effective tools for collecting high-quality data. Smartphones have evolved into versatile instruments for capturing a wide array of data, including health-related information in daily life, thanks to their practicality, mobility, and robust computing capabilities [22]. These devices provide an ideal platform for streamlining data transmission from various sensors using technologies like Wi-Fi and Bluetooth. Data can be collected using the smartphone's built-in sensors, external sensors, and the device that can also serve as a hub for data transfer, processing, information gathering, and interaction. Due to its features that facilitate input, output, and interactive activities, the smartphone is a vital component of data management systems.

Today, most sensor network applications in healthcare, like body sensor networks (BSNs), rely on wireless communication. However, this wireless communication can introduce security risks to these systems, including significant vulnerabilities associated with cloud-based data storage [23]. This section addresses the primary security requirements for an IoT-based healthcare system using BSN.

Data Confidentiality: Much like in WSNs, data privacy is considered the most significant concern in BSNs. Safeguarding data against unauthorized disclosure is of utmost importance. It is crucial to ensure that essential patient information remains shielded from any inadvertent exposure to nearby or external networks through BSNs. In the context of an IoT-based healthcare system, sensor nodes are responsible for gathering sensitive data and relaying it to a central coordinator. Nonetheless, there is a concern that malicious actors might intercept this communication, potentially obtaining access to critical data. Eavesdropping poses a significant risk, as it could lead to severe harm to the patient, with the adversary potentially exploiting the acquired information for illicit purposes.

Data Integrity: Privacy measures do not inherently safeguard information from external tampering or alterations. Content can still be modified by an adversary, either by adding extra elements or by operating the data within a packet. The coordinator may unknowingly receive these altered data. This can be particularly perilous in situations where data integrity is of paramount importance.

Data Tint: To confuse the controller, the adversary may occasionally intercept data in transfer and replay it in future by means of an outdated key. Data tint indicates that data is current and that previous messages cannot be played back.

Data Authentication: Authentication is indeed a critical requirement for any IoT healthcare system based on BSNs to effectively thwart impersonation attacks. In a healthcare system relying on BSN, all sensor nodes communicate their data to a coordinator, which subsequently updates a server about the patient's status at regular intervals. In this context, verifying the identities of both the coordinator and the server is crucial. Authentication mechanisms can be employed to allow each party to confirm the other's identity, thereby enhancing security.

Intractability: It ensures that the adversary cannot determine who the patient is nor determine whether two chats originate from the same patient, this is a more satisfying aspect of anonymity. Thus, anonymity during wireless communication conceals a packet's source. It is a service that can promote privacy.

Nonvulnerable Localization: Many BSN applications require accurate patient location estimation, but they can be vulnerable to attacks where an adversary provides false signal intensities, potentially leading to the transmission of precise but deceptive patient location data, even without the need for a sophisticated tracking system. To establish a secure IoT-based healthcare system using BSN, it is essential for the system to adhere to the security standards mentioned earlier and be resilient against various security threats and attacks, such as data manipulation, impersonation, eavesdropping, replay attacks, and more.

3.4 WEARABLE BIOSENSORS

In the pursuit of creating efficient health monitoring and support tools, this system combines the deeply trained real-time BSN environment with a computer diagnosis environment. The following phases of implementation make up the proposed system.

- Implementing the recommended data processing techniques
- Implementing the body sensor computing environment
- Constructing a testbed for comparative experiments

Wearable sensors have emerged as highly effective tools for collecting physiological and critical data. They've garnered significant popularity in various sectors, including medical, entertainment, security, and business [24]. A recent review in *Nature Biotechnology* delves into the growing interest in wearable biosensor technology, spanning academia, sports, and the healthcare industry. These wearables have the potential to offer continuous, real-time physiological data by noninvasively monitoring biochemical and physiological indicators. Pioneering applications in the military, precision medicine, and the fitness sector are harnessing these sensors to gather precise, high-fidelity data tailored to their specific needs.

Wearable biosensors present an opportunity to advance the diagnosis, treatment, and research of various medical conditions, including substance use disorder. They provide discreet, increasingly capable, and cost-effective continuous health data from the wearer's natural environment [25]. However, real-time anomaly detection using ML necessitates novel techniques to extract clinically relevant insights from fast, noisy, multidimensional data streams. The review discusses current algorithms for monitoring drug usage in wearable biosensor data streams and explores the anticipated impact of the evolution of 5G and 6G wireless communications on this field's progress [26]. The work also highlights ongoing challenges inadequately addressed by current ML algorithms and emerging trends.

To create a revolutionary health monitoring and assistance system, an appropriate computing environment is crucial for real-time responses. This environment comprises a compact CPU, integrated volatile memory, read-only memory, a general-purpose input and output system (GPIO), various interfaces, a Wi-Fi module, a Bluetooth module, a rechargeable battery unit, and body sensors. This computing environment enables more efficient sensing of biological indicators related to both motor and non-motor activities. Medical data is processed to detect symptoms of illness, and the OHPAS processor unit utilizes various AI techniques, including VAER, K-means clustering, and LSTM, for symptom categorization. This approach facilitates the development of an active, automated decision-making system for disease management [27].

3.5 BODY SENSOR NETWORK

A BSN is a specialized network designed for connecting various medical implants and sensors placed both inside and outside the human body. Integrating BSN into medical monitoring offers operational flexibility and cost-saving options, benefiting both patients and healthcare providers [28]. BSNs enhance mobility and reduce user discomfort, with applications including patient monitoring within hospitals, medication administration, and the tracking of human physiological data. Vital signs are utilized to assess an individual's fundamental bodily functions, which is crucial for evaluating their overall health.

In recent years, numerous WBSNs have been developed, aimed at monitoring specific medical conditions or physiological signals from patients in a home environment. Some WBSNs have been designed to recognize daily physical activity and monitor heart rate as well [29]. These systems must meet specific requirements while operating within strict hardware resource constraints. The system faces a dual challenge in its design – the imperative need to safeguard the security and privacy of the collected personal medical data, while concurrently striving to minimize power consumption for prolonged operational life. Crafting solutions that address these constraints represents a formidable undertaking.

This research significantly influences the development of preventive healthcare applications built upon WBSNs. Within healthcare facilities, patients routinely undergo health monitoring using a prescribed health monitoring system, which relies on a WBSN architecture with a mobile data collector. To conserve sensor resources, the system optimally deploys the mobile collector, activating sensor nodes solely when they anticipate the collector's presence. Most prevailing guidelines for WBSN system development primarily address implementation challenges and often lack an automated method for ascertaining the behavior of system components. Typically, the development process involves selecting the appropriate target platform, followed by the specific operating system and programming language [30].

The primary objective of the healthcare sector is to provide high-quality medical care to people worldwide, around the clock [31]. This should be accomplished more affordably and with a focus on patients' well-being. Therefore, there is a need to upgrade patient monitoring devices to enhance the effectiveness of patient care. Patient monitoring faces two key issues – the requirement for caregivers and healthcare professionals to be present at the patient's bedside and the fact that patients are often confined to their beds and connected to cumbersome devices.

For individuals with chronic conditions, in particular, the provision of healthcare services is crucial. These patients require ongoing care that is typically provided within hospital settings. Numerous factors influence urge for the work:

- *Freeing Up Medical Staff:* By streamlining administrative tasks and automating processes, healthcare providers can allocate more time to patients who require intensive care and attention.
- *Swift Information Delivery:* Rapid transmission of patients' medical information to healthcare providers is crucial, especially in emergency or accident situations, where every moment counts.
- *Reducing Manual Data Entry:* Automation reduces the need for manual data entry, minimizing errors and saving time.
- *Expanding Access:* Improved healthcare accessibility benefits not only those who lack access to healthcare providers but also individuals who face challenges in accessing public transportation to reach hospitals.

These measures contribute to a more efficient and equitable healthcare system, ultimately improving patient outcomes and overall healthcare delivery.

The wireless body area network (WBAN) is another cutting-edge innovation that offers a remote system for monitoring and collecting patient health information through wearable sensors [32, 33]. Maintaining robust system security and protection is considered crucial in safeguarding this data during its use by healthcare professionals and ensuring that patient information remains secure against potential threats from intruders.

Discussing security and privacy concerns related to WBANs is an exciting and important topic. In this context, this chapter examined WBAN communication technology, security, privacy requirements, and security risks, taking into account the most recent standards and developments. It also delved into the fundamental challenges facing WBANs in these aspects, aiming to enhance the protection of patient data and the integrity of healthcare systems.

3.6 AI AND ML ALGORITHMS FOR BIOSENSOR DATA ANALYSIS

Artificial neural networks (ANNs), a category of ML models, simulate the learning process of the human brain. They are comprised of three main layers – an input layer that receives data for processing, multiple hidden layers that carry out data processing, and an output layer that delivers the results. In these ANNs, the hidden layers receive intermediate inputs, apply random weights and biases to each input, and compute weighted sums. These sums then propagate through successive layers, each having its own set of weights and sums, until they reach the final layer. In the final layer, an activation function is employed to generate the output. If the output results are not sufficiently accurate, adjustments are made by modifying the weights, guided by a cost function. This iterative process refines the model until it achieves the desired level of accuracy.

In the realm of multidimensional signal processing, various time series analysis tools and methods are available. Recent advancements in AI and ML have expanded the range of time series analysis algorithms that can be employed as data mining and analytical tools [34]. These algorithms offer a versatile tool for handling multivariate data and have numerous applications.

In the field of AI/ML-based time series analysis, new algorithms are continually being developed, with many libraries in R and Python, as well as open-source projects on platforms like GitHub. These techniques enable the analysis and interpretation of multivariate data gathered from various sensors, even though some sensors in different domains may be univariate or purely theoretical. Continuous, time-synchronized physiological vital data, real-time location system (RTLS) data, and AI/ML algorithms have a broad spectrum of applications in sports and medicine [35].

This analysis aims to underscore the existing tools within the realms of wearable biosensors, RTLS, and AI/ML. Furthermore, the authors introduce the AIBSNF, a framework designed for BSNs, which seamlessly integrates RTLS with wearable sensor technologies to continuously collect multifaceted physiological and real-time location data, potentially in a synchronized manner [36]. AI/ML algorithms are ideally suited to harness this data for knowledge discovery, with the AIBSNF serving as the fundamental framework for data acquisition. Within the scope of this chapter, the authors accentuate the framework's application in two distinct contexts – team sports and medical diagnostics, with a specific focus on monitoring and researching patients with rheumatoid arthritis. This highlights the adaptability and profound impact of such integrated systems across diverse fields.

3.7 AI- AND IoT-BASED BSN FRAMEWORK

The internet is commonly used to connect healthcare applications for IoT. The number of IoT applications is continuously increasing, with devices connecting to the global information network. For example, a heart monitor or body temperature sensor connected to the internet can relay a user's medical information to their healthcare provider. IoT applications generate a significant amount of data [37]. Users are linked to the internet when they are at home and using their home network, but they switch to the office network when at work. This scenario requires a robust security approach that can adapt to various network configurations, particularly for healthcare applications.

In the realm of IoT healthcare, devices commonly establish connections through a wide array of wireless standard protocols, such as Wi-Fi, GSM, WiMax, Bluetooth, Bluetooth Low Energy (BLE), Zigbee, and 3G/4G. Leveraging IoT technology, medical devices are equipped to transmit data across an IP network utilizing specific network protocols, facilitating interactions with other devices [38]. These health devices possess the capability to link up with an IoT health network from virtually anywhere and at any given time. Moreover, IoT healthcare devices have the capacity to transmit data within a network, either in a secure and legitimate manner or potentially with malicious intent, all contingent on the network's particular topology. As a result, devising a security model that accommodates the dynamic nature of network topology presents a formidable challenge.

The choice of sensors and their location on the body is essential, considering the restrictions on the number of sensors that can be attached to an individual. Furthermore, different sensors may have varying sampling rates, which need to be considered based on the specific healthcare applications in use [39].

The proposed method allows for the derivation of the behavior of WBSN components from the requirements model. The behavior of the components, as depicted in Figure 3.1, is then systematically modified based on the requirements model. It is crucial that the derived behaviors of these components are synchronized because WBSNs typically operate in a distributed environment. These synchronized behaviors should collectively meet the initial requirements outlined in the model. This process ensures that the behavior of the WBSN components aligns with the desired functionality and objectives defined in the requirements model.

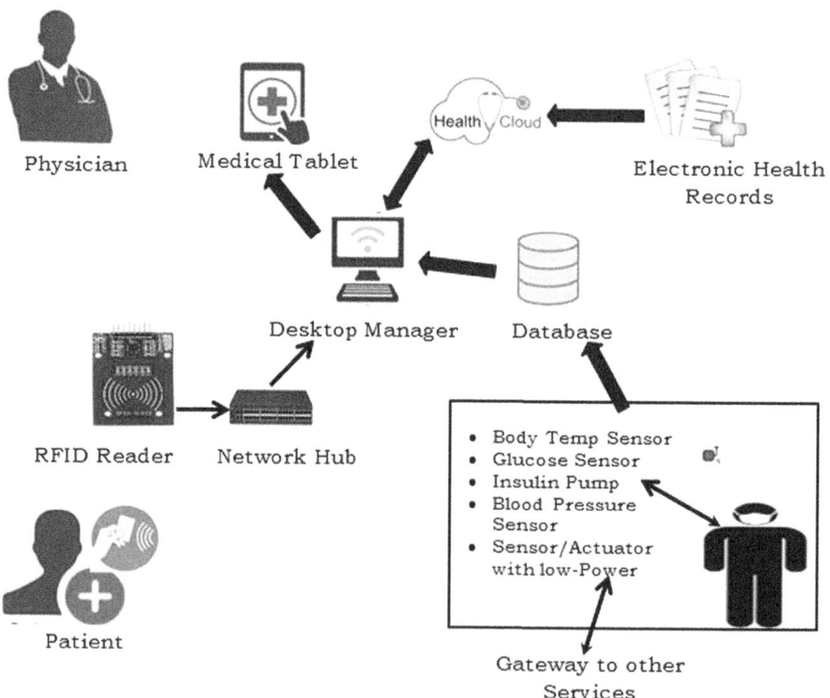

Figure 3.1 Components of proposed system.

The core objective of this strategy is to delineate the process of derivation, which encompasses the following integral elements:

a. *Formulation of the Requirements Meta-model:* This meta-model offers a high-level abstraction of the WBSN system, enabling the encapsulation of the system's comprehensive behavior. Models constructed using this meta-model should provide a conceptual-level representation of the system's behavior.

b. *Description of the Design Meta-model:* This meta-model captures the localized or regional behavior of each individual system component. Once the requirements are established, the resultant behavior models are automatically generated from this design meta-model.

c. *Model-to-model (M2M) Transformation:* This transformation process maps conceptual elements from the requirements meta-model to the design meta-model. The derivation process is meticulously guided by this transformation, ensuring that the requirements are precisely translated into specific design behaviors.

d. *Platform-specific Meta-model Description:* This is a specific meta-model for the chosen platform, detailing the platform's capabilities and constraints.

e. *Transition from M2M:* This phase facilitates the connection between concepts within the design meta-model and platform-specific meta-model concepts, ensuring harmonization of the design behavior with the capabilities of the selected platform.

f. *Transformation from Model to Text (M2T):* This transformation utilizes platform-specific models to automatically generate code. It translates the design and behavior models into executable code for the selected platform.

In summary, the strategy outlined involves a systematic approach for deriving the behavior of a WBSN system. It encompasses various stages, from establishing high-level requirements to generating platform-specific code, emphasizing the importance of abstraction, transformation, and alignment with the chosen platform.

This strategy draws upon previous successful applications and is in accordance with the conceptual framework illustrated in Figure 3.2.

This approach involves the utilization of sample sensors, ensuring their optimal arrangement, and focusing on data collection and preprocessing to

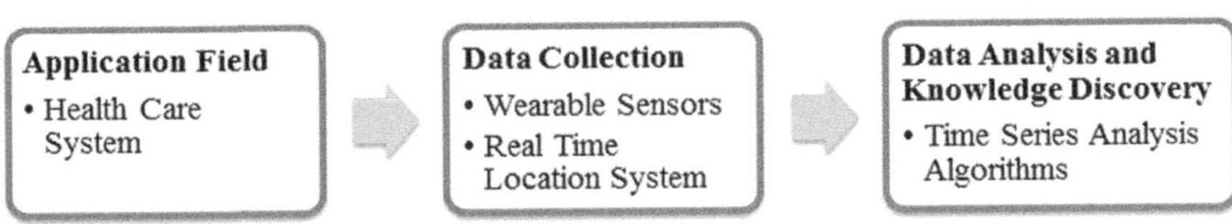

Figure 3.2 Conceptual framework.

synchronize the data. Time series analysis algorithms are then employed for specific sport-specific event detection.

While numerous architectures and techniques have been proposed for managing WSNs, it appears that there is a lack of effective and reliable designs specifically tailored to healthcare systems [40–42]. Currently available configurations often adapt WBSNs to existing IoT architectures, which may not be suitable for the unique requirements of healthcare systems. Therefore, it is crucial to consider factors such as real-time responsiveness, alignment with the application's needs, and energy efficiency when designing WBSN architectures.

In response to these challenges, a novel architecture called SENET has been proposed. SENET leverages AI techniques and IoT-based programmable devices to address the issues associated with healthcare-oriented WBSNs [43]. This architecture aims to provide a more effective and dependable solution by tailoring WBSNs to the specific demands of healthcare systems.

The methodologies used in existing work related to the healthcare systems and the limitations were discussed in Table 3.1.

3.8 LIMITATIONS AND ISSUES

It appears that various methods, including ANNs, support vector machines (SVMs), decision trees (DTs), and more are employed to create a prediction model. These prediction models are designed and tested to ensure their accuracy before being embedded in programmable IoT-based devices [45]. The use of live data analysis methods, while valuable for real-time reporting of essential data, may not be suitable for predicting undesirable outcomes. However, these real-time models can provide critical information within predefined time frames.

The programmable IoT-based devices play a crucial role in the suggested architecture. First, they utilize the real-time models integrated into them to predict suspicious events. Second, these devices can serve as head cluster nodes for covering WBSNs, which are integral for health monitoring and other applications. This architecture leverages IoT devices to enhance predictive capabilities and real-time monitoring in a variety of domains.

The head clusters in this architecture are characterized by their reliance on stable energy sources. They primarily operate using a stable energy source but can switch to battery power in case of an energy source problem. This dual-source setup enhances the overall lifetime of the architecture, making it more durable than previous designs.

In SENET's initial layer, mobile wireless body sensors are deployed to collect predefined data, which is then transmitted to the head clusters for analysis. The head clusters process this data and promptly alert the relevant specialists in case of any undesirable events. Additionally, SENET employs the concept of k-coverage to enhance sensor reliability, addressing a critical concern in healthcare systems.

Table 3.1 Existing systems and its limitations

Research work	Methodology	Limitations
Real-time cloud-based patient-centric monitoring using computational health systems [6]	ML classification algorithms are employed for heart disease prediction	The cloud-fog layer in IoMT is utilized in heart disease applications
Congestion-free routing mechanism for IoT-enabled WSNs for smart healthcare applications [9]	Distributed congestion control algorithm is used to resolve the congestion for IoT-enabled WSNs healthcare applications	Disease warning system without any analysis
SENET: A novel architecture for IoT-based BSNs [3]	SENET, comprising three layers, leverages AI, WBSNs, and IoT-based programmable devices to create a decision support system	Reliability of the SENET depends on the head clusters which covers the WBSNs
A secure IoT-based healthcare system with BSNs [24]	IoT-centric BSN infrastructures incorporate a two-step authentication process for implementation	Computation cost is more and system efficiency is less
Healthcare IoT-based affective state mining using a deep convolutional neural network [44]	Recognition of affective state from wearable biosensors done through CNN	Better framework can be used for affective state mining
A multi-sensor data fusion enabled ensemble approach for medical data from BSNs [11]	Kernel random forest is used in a fog computing environment for heart disease prediction	Customized fusion mechanism based on the individual sensor capabilities can be improved
Open knowledge accessing method in IoT-based hospital information system for medical record enrichment [45]	Link open data–based knowledge accessing method for IoT-based HIS system is used	Compatible knowledge accessing method can be implemented for different diseases
Improving IoT-based architecture of healthcare system [14]	IoT-based human healthcare services framework is discussed	Many advances in the IoT-based medicinal services network is not discussed
IoT as a service system for eHealth [39]	Communication platform for QoS-aware delivery of complex services is discussed	Efficiency of proposed signalization schemes is less

Heuristic and metaheuristic algorithms have been developed to address problems fairly, but they have limitations. First, the solutions proposed by heuristic algorithms are typically not more accurate than those of meta-heuristic algorithms. Furthermore, these methods do not leverage advanced metaheuristic techniques. To overcome these limitations, the WCC algorithm has been developed and applied to solve the problem. The results demonstrate the superiority of cutting-edge algorithms for optimizing head cluster node placement, which helps minimize energy consumption in WSNs and maximize the coverage of the environment. While all algorithms perform well in determining head cluster node locations in small environments, their performance diverges as the issue size increases.

3.9 CONCLUSION AND FUTURE WORK

The market for wearable Internet of Medical Things (IoMT) is indeed expanding rapidly, especially for health status monitoring and sports training. Wearable biosensors play a significant role in this expansion. These sensors not only help monitor physical health but also have the potential to benefit mental health. One interesting application of wearable biosensors is their ability to recognize affective states, which refers to the emotional and mood states of individuals. When combined with context-aware recommendations, these sensors can contribute to mood stabilization and even assist in the treatment of stress and depression. By observing data from these biomedical sensors, which are often small and easily integrated into everyday consumer products, it becomes possible to infer and understand human emotions.

This intersection of technology, health, and emotion has promising implications for both healthcare and personal well-being, as it enables individuals to gain greater insight into their emotional states and potentially receive recommendations and interventions tailored to their mental health needs. The suggested affective state mining method has demonstrated a notable accuracy of 87.5%, which is a significant improvement compared to the most advanced physiologically based emotion recognition systems. This enhanced accuracy can be attributed to several factors, with depth-level characteristics generated by a convolutional neural network playing a pivotal role in distinguishing affective states.

However, it is worth noting that there is always room for further improvement in performance. One strategy that holds promise is the utilization of time-sequence AI architecture, such as a deep recurrent neural network. Given the continuous and sequential nature of biological sensor data, employing a deep recurrent neural network can enhance classification accuracy even further. This approach allows the system to consider the temporal aspect of the data, which can be crucial in understanding and accurately classifying affective states, particularly in real-time scenarios.

Continued research and development in this area have the potential to yield even more accurate and robust affective state recognition systems, which could have a wide range of applications in mental health, well-being, and human–computer interaction.

REFERENCES

1. Sudip Misra, Pradyumna Kumar Bishoyi and Subhadeep Sarkar, "i-MAC: In-body sensor MAC in wireless body area networks for healthcare IoT," IEEE Systems Journal, vol. 15, no. 3, pp. 4413–4420, 2020. doi: 10.1109/JSYST.2020.3020306.
2. Ashwin A. Phatak, Franz Georg Wieland, Kartik Vempala, Frederik Volkmar and Daniel Memmert, "Artificial intelligence based body sensor network framework – Narrative review: Proposing an end-to-end framework using wearable sensors, real-time location systems and artificial intelligence/machine learning algorithms for data collection, data mining and knowledge discovery in sports and healthcare," Sports Medicine, vol. 7, pp. 79, 2021.
3. Zohre Arabi Bulaghi, Ahmad Habibi Zad Navin, Mehdi Hosseinzadeh and Ali Rezaee, "SENET: A novel architecture for IoT-based body sensor networks," Informatics in Medicine, vol. 20, 100365, 2020.
4. M. N. Bhuiyan, M. M. Rahman, M. M. Billah and D. Saha, "Internet of Things (IoT): A review of its enabling technologies in healthcare applications, standards protocols, security, and market opportunities," IEEE Internet of Things Journal, vol. 8, no. 13, pp. 10474–10498, 2021. doi: 10.1109/JIOT.2021.3062630.
5. Ali Raza Bhangwar, Adnan Ahmed, Umair Ali Khan, Tanzila Saba, Khaled Almustafa, Khalid Haseeb and Naveed Islam, "WETRP: Weight based energy & temperature aware routing protocol for wireless body sensor networks," IEEE Access, vol. 7, pp. 87987–87995, 2019. doi: 10.1109/ACCESS.2019.2925741.
6. C. Chakraborty and A. Kishor, "Real-time cloud-based patient-centric monitoring using computational health systems," IEEE Transactions on Computational Social Systems, vol. 9, no. 6, pp. 1613–1623, 2022. doi: 10.1109/TCSS.2022.3170375.
7. Rajasoundaran Soundararajan, A. V. Prabu, Sidheswar Routray, Prince Priya Malla, Arun Kumar Ray, Gopinath Palai, Osama S. Faragallah, Mohammed Baz, Matokah M. Abualnaja, Mohamoud M. A. Eid and Ahmed Nabih Zaki Rashed, "Deeply trained real-time body sensor networks for analyzing the symptoms of Parkinson's disease," IEEE Access, vol. 10, pp. 63403–63421, 2022.
8. Y. Ma, R. Li, J. Lei, M. Zhang and L. Yin, "Design of a wireless compact implantable electrochemical biosensor system for health monitoring application," In: IEEE International Conference on Integrated Circuits, Technologies and Applications (ICTA), 2020. doi: 10.1109/icta50426.2020.9332135.
9. P. Chanak and I. Banerjee, "Congestion free routing mechanism for IoT-enabled wireless sensor networks for smart healthcare applications," IEEE Transactions on Consumer Electronics, vol. 66, no. 3, pp. 223–232, 2020. doi: 10.1109/TCE.2020.2987433.
10. J. Rumbut, D. Singh, H. Fang, H. Wang, S. Carreiro and E. Boyer, "Poster abstract: Detecting kratom intoxication in wearable biosensor data," In: 2019 IEEE/ACM International Conference on Connected Health: Applications, Systems and Engineering Technologies (CHASE), 2019. doi: 10.1109/chase48038.2019.00028.
11. M. Muzammal, et al. "A multi-sensor data fusion enabled ensemble approach for medical data from body sensor networks," Information Fusion, vol. 53, pp. 155–164, 2020.
12. M. M. Miran and F. Arifin, "Design and performance analysis of a miniaturized implantable PIFA for wireless body area network applications," In: 2019 International Conference on Robotics, Electrical and Signal Processing Techniques (ICREST). IEEE, 2019.
13. K. Vignesh Saravanan, P. Jothi Thilaga, S. Kavipriya and K. Vijayalakshmi, Data protection and security enhancement in cyber-physical systems using AI and blockchain. In: Bhushan, B., Sangaiah, A.K., Nguyen, T.N. (eds), AI models

for blockchain-based intelligent networks in IoT systems: Engineering cyber-physical systems and critical infrastructures, vol. 6. Springer, Cham, 2023. doi: 10.1007/978-3-031-31952-5_13.

14. I. Singh and D. Kumar, "Improving IoT based architecture of healthcare system," In: 2019 4th International Conference on Information Systems and Computer Networks (ISCON), 2019. doi: 10.1109/iscon47742.2019.9036287.

15. I. A. Sawaneh, I. Sankoh and D. K. Koroma, "A survey on security issues and wearable sensors in wireless body area network for healthcare system," In: 2017 14th International Computer Conference on Wavelet Active Media Technology and Information Processing (ICCWAMTIP), 2017. doi: 10.1109/iccwamtip.2017.8301502.

16. E. B. Hamida, R. D'Errico and B. Denis, "Topology dynamics and network architecture performance in wireless body sensor networks," In: 2011 4th IFIP International Conference on New Technologies, Mobility and Security. IEEE, 2011.

17. C. Bayilmis and M. Younis, "Energy-aware gateway selection for increasing the lifetime of wireless body area sensor networks," Journal of Medical Systems, vol. 36, no. 3, pp. 1593–601, 2012.

18. S. Pushpan and B. Velusamy, "Fuzzy-based dynamic time slot allocation for wireless body area networks," Sensors, vol. 19, no. 9, p. 2112, 2019.

19. R. M. Aileni, et al. Body area network (BAN) for healthcare by wireless mesh network (WMN). In: Body area network challenges and solutions. Springer, 2019. pp. 1–17.

20. M. Mukherjee, et al., "Sleep scheduling for unbalanced energy harvesting in industrial wireless sensor networks," IEEE Communication Magazine, vol. 57, No. 2, pp. 108–115, 2019.

21. W. Balzano, et al., "A smart compact traffic network vision based on wave representation," In: Workshops of the International Conference on Advanced Information Networking and Applications. Springer, 2019.

22. M. Abdel-Basset, et al., "Internet of things in smart education environment: Supportive framework in the decision-making process," Concurrency Computer Practices Experience, vol. 31, no. 10, p. e4515, 2019.

23. D. Pozo, et al., Remote monitoring air quality in dangerous environments for human activities. International Conference on Applied Human Factors and Ergonomics. Springer, 2019.

24. Ye Kuo-Hui, "A secure IoT-based healthcare system with body sensor networks," IEEE Access, vol. 4, pp. 10288–10299, 2017. doi: 10.1109/ACCESS.2016.2638038.

25. A. Farooq and T. Iqbal, "An exposition of wireless sensor network area coverage and lifetime based on meta heuristic and particle swarm optimization algorithms," VAWKUM Transactions on Computer Sciences, vol. 15, no. 2, pp. 92–8, 2018.

26. Niharika Kumar, "IoT Architecture and System Design for Healthcare Systems," In: International Conference on Smart Technology for Smart Nation, 2017.

27. J. Tian, M. Gao and G. Ge, "Wireless sensor network node optimal coverage based on improved genetic algorithm and binary ant colony algorithm," EURASIP Journal on Wireless Communication Network, vol. 1, p. 104, 2016.

28. F. Sallabi and K. Shuaib. "Internet of Things network management system architecture for smart healthcare." In: Digital Information and Communication Technology and its Applications (DICTAP), 2016 Sixth International Conference on, pp. 165–170. IEEE, 2016.

29. S. Raza, P. Misra, Z. He and T. Voigt, "Building the Internet of Things with bluetooth smart," Ad Hoc Networks, 2016.

30. Farag Sallabi, Faisal Naeem, Mamoun Awad and Khaled Shuaib, "Managing IoT-based smart healthcare systems traffic with software defined networks." In: 2018 International Symposium on Networks, Computers and Communications (ISNCC), IEEE, 2018.

31. M. A. R. Abdeen, M. H. Ahmed, H. Seliem, T. Rahil Sheltami and T. M. Alghamdi, "Smart health systems components, challenges, and opportunities," IEEE Canadian Journal of Electrical and Computer Engineering, vol. 45, no. 4, pp. 436–441, 2022. doi: 10.1109/ICJECE.2022.3220700.

32. N. Malathy, S. K. Priya and K. V. Saravanan, "Pedestrian safety system with crash prediction," International Journal of Health Sciences, vol. 6, no. S2, pp. 8707–8717, 2022. doi: 10.53730/ijhs.v6nS2.7247.

33. S. M. Riazul Islam, Daehan Kwak, Md. Humaun Kabir, Mahmud Hossain and Kyung-sup Kwak, "The Internet of Things for health care: A comprehensive survey," IEEE Access, vol. 3, 678–708, 2015.

34. Prosanta Gope and Tzonelih Hwang, "BSN-care: A secure IoT-based modern healthcare system using body sensor network," IEEE Sensors Journal, 2015. doi: 10.1109/JSEN.2015.2502401.

35. Vikas Vippalapalli and Snigdha Ananthula, "Internet of Things (IoT) based smart health care system," International Conference on Signal Processing, Communication, Power and Embedded System (SCOPES), 2016.

36. K. Habib, A. Torjusen and W. Leister, "Security analysis of a patient monitoring system for the Internet of Things in eHealth," In: Proceedings of the International Conference on eHealth, Telemedicine, and Social Medicine, 2015.

37. G. Fortino, S. Galzarano, R. Gravina and W. Li, "A framework for collaborative computing and multi-sensor data fusion in body sensor networks," Information Fusion, vol. 22, pp. 50–70, 2015.

38. S. C. Mukhopadhyay and N. Suryadevara, "Internet of Things: Challenges and opportunities," in Internet of Things, Springer, 2014, pp. 1–17.

39. P. Swiatek and A. Rucinski, "IoT as a service system for eHealth," In: 2013 IEEE 15th International Conference on e-Health Networking, Applications and Services (Healthcom 2013), 2013, pp. 81–84.

40. A. Harbouche, M. Erradi and A. Kobbane, "A flexible wireless body sensor network system for health monitoring," 2013 Workshops on Enabling Technologies: Infrastructure for Collaborative Enterprises, 2013. doi: 10.1109/wetice.2013.17.

41. R. Gravina, P. Alinia, H. Ghasemzadeh and G. Fortino, "Multi-sensor fusion in body sensor networks: State-of-the-art and research challenges," Information Fusion, vol. 35, pp. 68–80, 2017.

42. P. Khan, A. Hussain and K. S. Kwak, "Medical applications of wireless body area networks," International Journal of Digital Content Technology and Its Applications, vol. 3, no. 3, pp. 185–193, 2009.

43. G. Fortino, R. Giannantonio, R. Gravina, P. Kuryloski and R. Jafari, "Enabling effective programming and flexible management of efficient body sensor network applications," IEEE Transactions on Human-Machine Systems, vol. 43, no. 1, pp. 115–133, 2013.

44. M. G. R. Alam, S. F. Abedin, S. I. Moon, A. Talukder and C. S. Hong, "Healthcare IoT-based affective state mining using a deep convolutional neural network," IEEE Access, vol. 7, pp. 75189–75202, 2019. doi: 10.1109/ACCESS.2019.2919995.

45. C. Xie, P. Yang and Y. Yang, "Open knowledge accessing method in IoT-based hospital information system for medical record enrichment," IEEE Access, vol. 6, pp. 15202–15211, 2018.

An efficient architecture for classification of super-resolution enhanced human chromosome images

D. Menaka and K. S. Subhashini

4.1 INTRODUCTION

The genetic information of an individual is stored on chromosomes. Chromosomal aberrations are more common among newborn babies, hence automated analysis is very much essential. Chromosome analysis through manual labor is labor-intensive and heavily reliant on special expertise when utilized for diagnosis. Karyotyping refers to the arrangement of chromosomes in a particular order based on its characteristics like size, shape, and banding patterns. In recent years, deep learning techniques, particularly those based on convolutional neural networks (CNNs), have become increasingly popular for chromosome segmentation and classification tasks. Several CNN-based methods have been proposed and adopted, leveraging the power of deep learning for more accurate and efficient chromosome analysis.

Karyotyping involves preprocessing, segmentation, and classification of chromosomes into 24 classes [1–3]. The impact of deep learning in the medical society is truly remarkable. Many cutting-edge deep learning models have demonstrated outstanding performance in chromosomal recognition, which helps to speed up the karyotyping procedure and detect any aberrations.

EfficientNets have emerged as a highly effective model for image classification tasks across various domains, including iris recognition, scene classification, and other image classification applications. The strength of EfficientNets lies in their compound scaling approach, which involves scaling the width, depth, and image resolution dimensions of the model. In a variety of classification problems, this approach usually results in increased accuracy.

The significant contributions in this research work are given as follows:

1. A simple CNN model was built and tested using a variety of hyperparameters and optimizer parameters. It had a small number of convolutional and max pooling layers. It was discovered through experimentation that using the ADAM optimizer with step decay generated the best quality.
2. Experimental results have shown that applying the Laplacian pyramidal superresolution network (LaPSRN) to enhance all input images leads to a noticeable improvement in accuracy. Specifically, the utilization

DOI: 10.1201/9781003487647-4

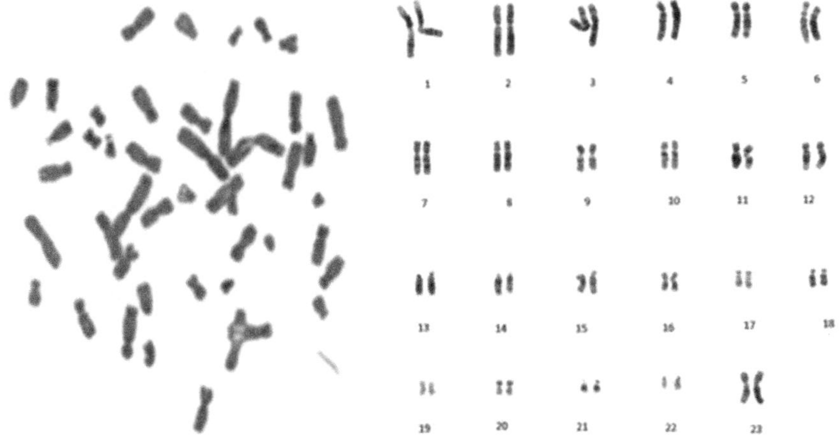

Figure 4.1 (a) Metaphase chromosome. (b) Karyotyped image.

of superresolution (SR) techniques has been demonstrated to increase the accuracy by 3%, validating its positive impact on the classification process.

3. In this proposed work, the Swish activation function was employed instead of the commonly used ReLU activation. To our knowledge, the application of the EfficientNet model in chromosome classification tasks had not been explored prior to this study.

The novelty of this research lies in the utilization of the LaPSRN, ADAM with step decay as optimization function, and the Swish activation function. As a result of these key components, an impressive accuracy of 96% is achieved using the EfficientNet architecture. This accuracy surpasses other CNN-based architectures previously explored for chromosome classification.

Figure 4.1 (a) and (b) shows a metaphase image and its corresponding karyotype. It became evident through the karyotyping analysis that any aberrations or abnormalities can be readily diagnosed. This is due to the fact that chromosomes are organized and arranged according to their size, allowing for easy identification and detection of any deviations.

4.2 RELATED WORKS

The impact of deep learning in medical society is truly remarkable. Several advanced deep learning models [8–10] have demonstrated exceptional performance in detecting chromosomes, leading to significant improvements in the efficiency of the karyotyping process and contributed to speeding up the categorization of chromosome images and enhancing the detection of any abnormalities or irregularities.

Swati et al. [7] presented a research paper "Automatic Classification of Low-resolution Chromosomal Images." In their paper, they introduced a Super-Xception network designed to categorize low-resolution images into 24 different chromosome class labels. The network combines SR models with the traditional classification systems, such as the Xception network. The training process is conducted in an end-to-end manner, where the SR layers assist in converting the low-resolution images into high-resolution counterparts. These high-resolution images are then passed through deep classification layers for label assignment. They evaluated its performance on a publicly available bioimage chromosome classification dataset consisting of healthy chromosomes. They compared the results against baseline models created using traditional deep CNNs, specifically ResNet-50 and Xception network architectures.

Chengchuang Lin et al. [12] developed the automatic classification system CIR Net, which uses an improved version of the CNN Inception-ResNet. The metaphase chromosomes can be bent or distorted, so the authors created a module called the image adaptive interface to accept any shaped metaphase chromosome images as input adaptively, obviating the need for preprocessing activities such as straightening. Affine transformation was used to increase the amount of the training dataset by chromosome data augmentation (CDA), which improved the classifier's robustness and categorization accuracy. Additionally, it eliminates deformations like input chromosomes' unpredictable positions and directions. The pretrained inception-ResNet model acquired the split augmented data in an 8:2 ratio. On a dataset of 2,990 images, the model was trained and validated using an RMSprop optimizer, and by utilizing the CDA instead of the same CIR Net model with straightening augmentation, it improved accuracy by 8.57%.

Al-Kharraz et al. [4] suggested an ensemble CNN for chromosome image categorization in which the authors fine-tune the standard models that had been trained like MobileNetV2, ResNet 50, and VGG 19. Better categorization results are obtained by merging the results from the pretrained models using average voting and majority voting. The model was trained using the above three CNN models individually, and every model will output its prediction output on the validation data. After taking the voting outcomes from the ensemble of various models, the authors have proved that the results are comparatively better than those produced by the individual pretrained models. This method was trained and validated on two standard datasets: BioImLab and Genomic medical unit, and attained a better categorization accuracy of 97.01% and 94.97%, respectively.

In a research work proffered by Wei et al. [13], the G-stained metaphase images are categorized using content-aware probabilistic prediction CNN. The authors used three essential stages in their research work: The input-aware module zooms the raw images into multiscale images (global, portion, and object scale) using an attention approach. The attributes are extracted from all these images using three feature extractors. The feature maps extracted are given to different layers like average pooling and fully connected layers. The network uses a probabilistic module to interpret the result of each CNN separately, and the final output decision is based on the combined votes of all the three deep CNNs. This method was evaluated on a dataset containing 13,800 images using a SGD optimizer and the following hyperparameters are utilized: initial learning rate – 0.02; batch size – 26 – 50 epochs. They presented a higher categorization accuracy, precision, F1 score, and recall in contrast with the other methods stated in the recent literature. The limitation of the suggested model is its higher complexity as all the input chromosome images have to be processed in three different scales to obtain the final outcome.

Swati et al. [6] have presented a research paper "Automatic Chromosome Classification Using Deep Attention-based Sequence Learning of Chromosome Bands." They presented a residual convolutional recurrent attention neural network (Res-CRANN), which was created specifically to take advantage of the chromosomal band sequences' inherent sequential structure for classification. Res-CRANN is an end-to-end trainable architecture that takes a sequence of feature vectors extracted from the feature maps generated by the convolutional layers of residual neural networks (ResNet) as input. These are then fed into recurrent neural networks (RNN), and an attention mechanism is added on top of the RNN output sequences to allow the network to selectively focus on the band sequence and create connections with various classes of chromosomes. The output sequences from the attention mechanism are further classified into one of the 24 labels. The researchers demonstrated the effectiveness of the proposed Res-CRANN architecture on a standard bioimage chromosome classification dataset and it was found that the model achieves an improvement in Top-1 accuracy in classification of about 3% when compared to baseline models made using conventional deep CNNs and ResNet-50.

Mona Salem Al-Kharraz et al. [14] have presented a research paper "Automated System for Chromosome Karyotyping to Recognize the Most Common Numerical Abnormalities Using Deep Learning." They have applied deep learning algorithms to automate the process of karyotyping and recognize frequent numerical anomalies. The King Abdulaziz University Center of Excellence in Genomic Medicine Research provided the researchers with a dataset of 147 nonoverlapping pictures of metaphase cells for their study. The metaphase images underwent three stages of analysis. In the first stage, individual chromosome detection was performed using the YOLOv2 CNN, followed by chromosome post-processing. This step achieved a mean Intersection over Union (IoU) of 0.84, an average precision (AP) of 0.9923, and 100% accuracy in individual chromosome detection. The second stage involved feature extraction and classification. Two alternative methods were used to fine-tune the VGG19 network: one involved adding more fully connected layers, and the other involved swapping out fully connected levels for a global average pooling layer. The best accuracy achieved was 95.04%.

In the final stage, abnormality detection was performed, achieving an accuracy of 96.67%. To further validate their classification method, they examined the publicly available Biomedical Imaging Laboratory dataset and obtained an accuracy of 94.11%.

The research paper "A New Multiple-Distribution GAN Model to Solve Complexity in End-to-End Chromosome Karyotyping" was presented by Yirui Wu et al. To create chromosomal candidates based on visual traits, they initially used the extremal regions (ER) technique. In order to group pixels with similar characteristics and approximate chromosomal shapes in the presence of extreme occlusion and cross-overlapping, they used the ring radius transform. The usage of a multi-distributed generated advertising network (MD-GAN) was suggested as a solution to the issue of an unbalanced and short dataset, as well as to cover various data patterns. Through the creation of extra training samples, this network enhanced the data. They then incorporated the created and enhanced training images for fine-tuning a CNN for the chromosomal categorization task. The suggested method showed great accuracy in chromosomal detection, segmentation, and classification tasks through experiments carried out on self-collected datasets. Additionally, according to the experimental results, a small amount of data augmentation made by the MD-GAN helps the CNN's classification outcomes.

Mingxing Tan et al. [15] have presented a paper "EfficientNet: Rethinking Model Scaling for Convolutional Neural Networks." They have put forth a novel model scaling technique that scales up CNNs in a more organized way by employing a straightforward yet incredibly potent compound coefficient. Contrary to traditional methods, which scale network dimensions like width, depth, and resolution arbitrarily, this technique scales each dimension evenly using a predetermined set of scaling factors.

For chromosomal categorization, Zhang et al. developed a CNN-based deep learning approach in which 4 convolution layers, 2 pooling layers, a dropout of 0.5, a flattening layer, a dense layer that is fully connected with 120 neurons, and a single output layer were all used. This network would generate the labels for 24 classes with a learning rate of 0.0001. The model used the Adam optimization method and the softmax activation function and cross-entropy as objective functions. On a dataset of 10,304 chromosomal images, this method's training and testing were carried out. To validate the results, testing was also conducted on a separate dataset containing 4,830 chromosomes, achieving an accuracy above 90%. However, it should be noted that this method is specifically applicable to vertical chromosomes and may not be suitable for bent or curved chromosomes.

Based on the survey conducted, it is apparent that several different chromosomal segmentation and classification approaches have been constructed. With the advancement of computational capabilities and the growing need for improved accuracy, it has been demonstrated that efficient nets offer superior outcomes for various applications, primarily due to their compound scaling capability.

4.3 MATERIALS AND METHODS

CNNs have emerged as a significant advancement in image recognition, finding applications in various fields such as automation, natural language processing, medical domains, and autonomous navigation systems [17–18]. These networks are inspired by biological systems, with information flowing unidirectionally from inputs to outputs. A CNN is used in the proposed approach to categorize chromosomes into 24 distinct categories. Input, hidden, and output layers make up the CNN architecture, which uses convolution, pooling, subsampling, and nonlinear activation functions in the hidden layer to extract high-level features from the data.

The convolution layer captures features from the input data by applying the convolution operation, which involves convolving the input with a predefined kernel. The weights of the kernel are adjusted during the backpropagation algorithm. The filter parameters are shared across local positions, and the hyperparameters define the filter size and strides. The key benefit of the convolution operation is the reduction of parameters, as the output is influenced by a sparse set of input connections. Mathematically, the output of the convolution layer can be expressed as follows:

$$Y_k = f(w_k * x)$$

where x denotes the input and w_k denotes the weights corresponding to the Kth convolution filter. Let I denote the input size, F the filter length, P the amount of zero padding, S the stride, then the size of the feature map along that dimension is given by

$$o = \frac{I - F + P_{start} + P_{end}}{S} + 1$$

Pooling refers to the subsampling operation in CNNs, where computations can be performed using either the maximum or average operation. Typically, max pooling is employed, where the maximum pixel value within a specific patch is selected. This pooling technique is commonly used as it helps preserve the extracted features. The stride in both the convolution and pooling layers indicates the number of pixels by which the window is shifted after each operation.

After the pooling operation, the next step in the CNN is the flattening operation. This process converts the multidimensional data into a single-dimensional vector, which is then passed as input to the final layer, known as the fully connected layer. In the fully connected layer, all of the inputs from the preceding layer's neurons are used to do computations with the neurons in the current layer, much like a conventional neural network. This allows the generation of the desired output. Figure 4.2 provides a visual representation of a typical CNN architecture, illustrating multiple layers of convolution and pooling as an example.

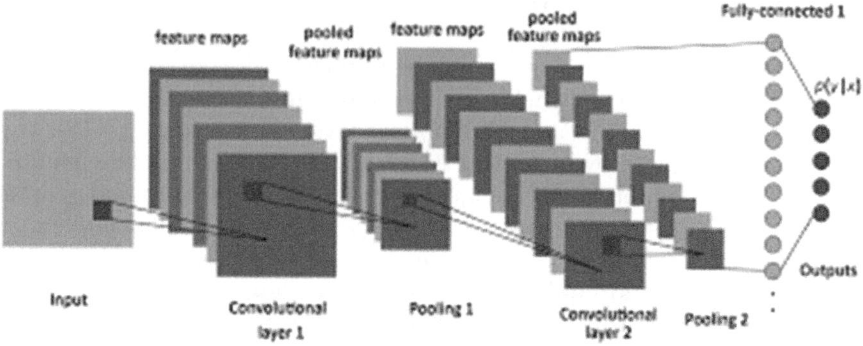

feature maps

pooled feature maps

feature maps

pooled feature maps

Fully-connected 1

Input

Convolutional layer 1

Pooling 1

Convolutional layer 2

Pooling 2

Outputs

Figure 4.2 A general CNN architecture model.

4.4 PROPOSED METHOD

4.4.1 Dataset used

In order to validate the proposed architecture, a dataset from the BioImLab was utilized. This dataset consisted of 5,256 chromosome images from healthy individuals, which were manually segmented by trained cytogeneticists. All the chromosomes were polarized according to ICSN (International System for Human Cytogenetic Nomenclature) standards and stored in bitmap format. The dataset was divided into a 70:30 proportion, with 70% of the images used for training and the remaining 30% for testing.

Before using the images in the dataset, a simple preprocessing pipeline was applied, including adaptive median filtering and data normalization. Due to the limited number of available images in the dataset, basic data augmentation techniques were employed to increase the dataset size and improve the classification accuracy.

A sample chromosome image used for classification is visualized in Figure 4.3.

4.4.2 Workflow

The entire work module can be split into four parts (Figure 4.4):

- Localization
- Superresolution
- Classification
- Abnormality detection

4.4.2.1 Localization

4.4.2.1.1 COCO annotator

COCO Annotator is a web-based annotation tool specifically designed for image segmentation tasks. It offers an intuitive and customizable interface,

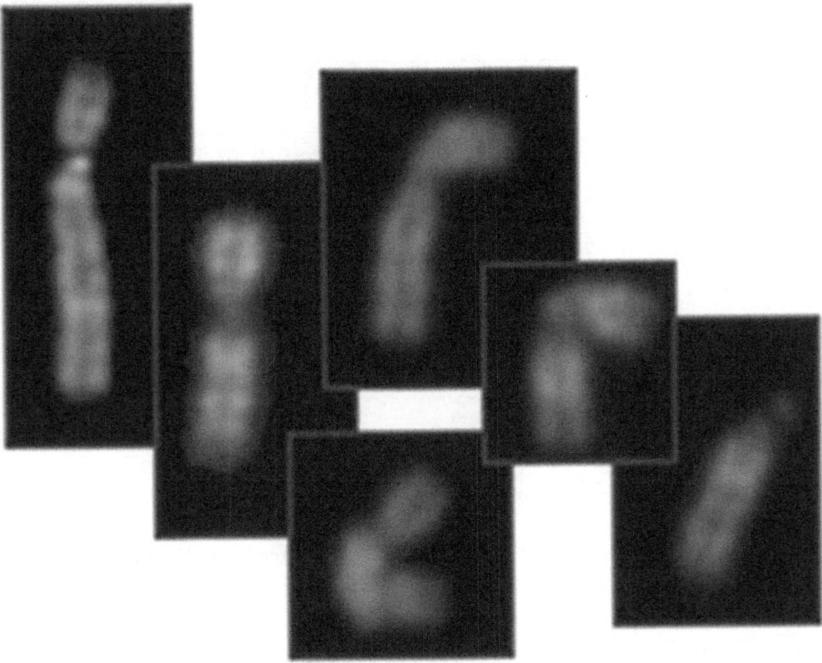

Figure 4.3 BiolmLab dataset (sample chromosome data for classification).

making the annotation process more efficient and accurate. This tool provides various features such as the ability to label image segments or specific parts within a segment, supports tracking object instances, labeling objects with disconnected visible parts which is particularly useful when annotating videos or sequences of images where objects move or change over time, stores,

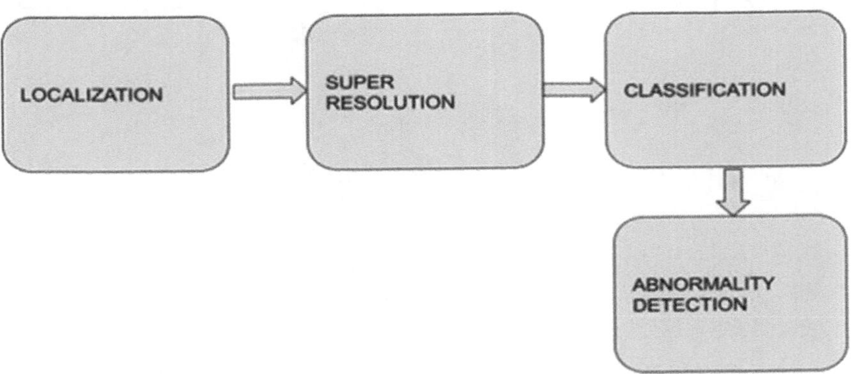

Figure 4.4 Workflow.

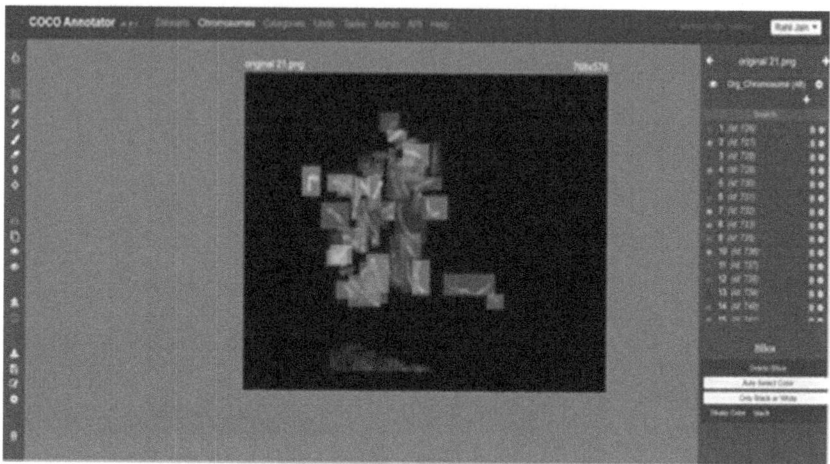

Figure 4.5 Manual segmentation of all the chromosomes using COCO annotator.

and exports annotations in the popular COCO format. Docker applications are used to run COCO annotator. The User Interface of the application can be seen in Figure 4.5. Using COCO annotation, 62 chromosome images are annotated and 2,480 individual chromosome strands are segmented. These individual strands will be used as training and testing data for the Detectron2 model. Figure 4.6 shows the annotated images of chromosomes.

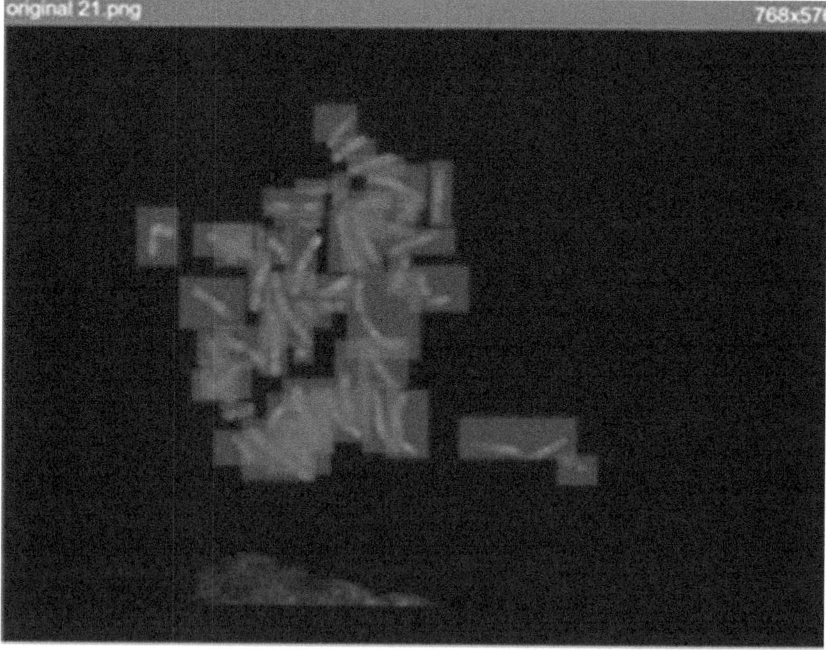

Figure 4.6 Annotated images of chromosomes.

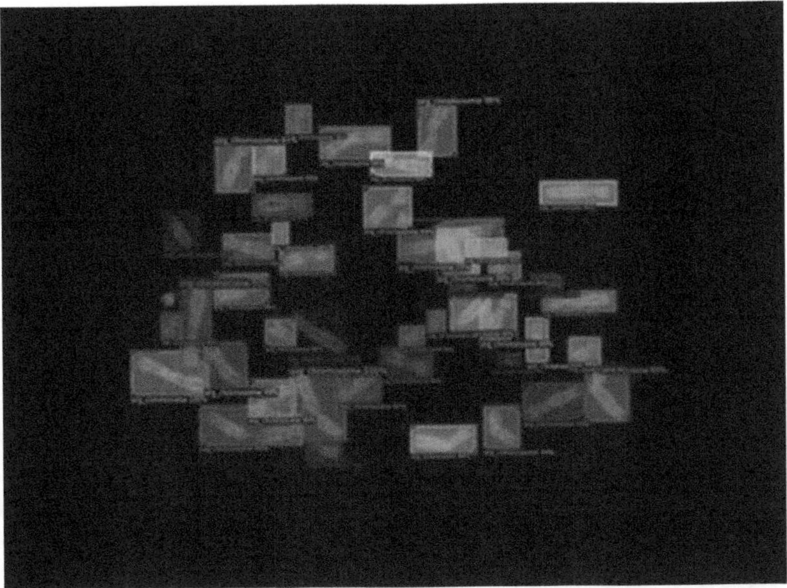

Figure 4.7 Chromosomes identified using Detectron.

4.4.2.1.2 Detectron2

Detectron2 is an advanced computer vision framework developed by Facebook Artificial Intelligence Research (FAIR). It offers a comprehensive set of tools and state-of-the-art models, including Fast R-CNN, Faster R-CNN, and Mask R-CNN, that can be utilized for various object detection tasks. Indeed, Detectron2 provides a valuable model zoo that includes a wide range of pretrained models. These models have been trained on the popular COCO (Common Objects in Context) dataset, which consists of a diverse set of object categories [19–21].

In the proposed workflow, the Detectron model is responsible for both detecting and segmenting each chromosome in the input images. Figure 4.7 shows the chromosomes identified using the Detectron model. These segmented images will be given to the classification model (EfficientNet) to classify all 24 chromosomes.

4.4.2.1.3 Yolo V4

The You Only Look Once (YOLO) series is a collection of one-stage object detectors known for their speed and accuracy. YOLOv4, an enhancement of YOLOv3, introduces significant improvements by incorporating a new architecture in the backbone and making modifications to the neck. These changes have resulted in a 10% increase in mean average precision (mAP) and a 12% improvement in the number of frames per second (FPS). YOLOv4 has made

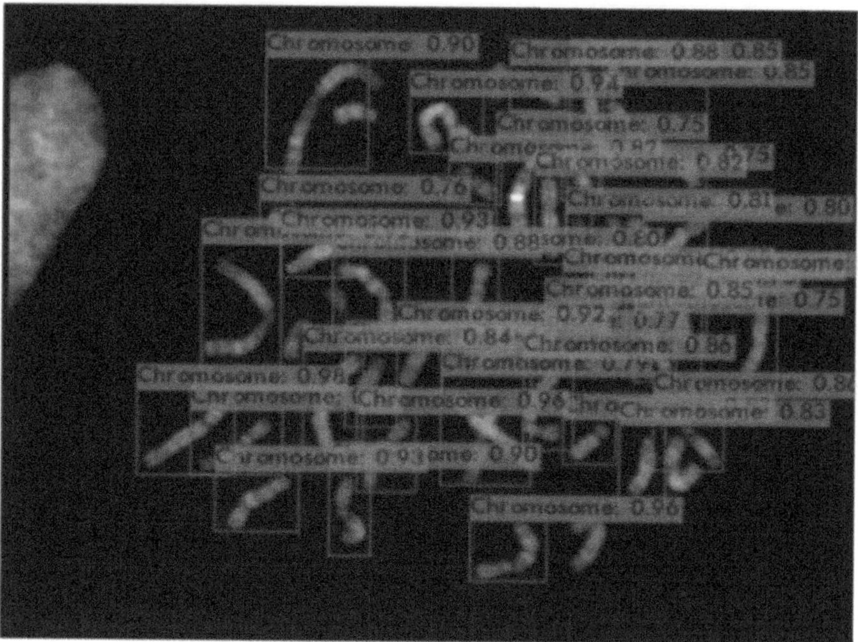

Figure 4.8 Chromosomes identified using Yolo V4 model.

the training process more accessible, as it can now be efficiently trained on a single GPU. YOLOv4, in comparison to the Detectron2 model, exhibits relatively lower accuracy and faces challenges in detecting every chromosome present in an image, as shown in Figure 4.8.

4.4.2.1.4 SR models

OpenCV, an open-source computer vision library, offers a vast array of powerful algorithms. With a recent merger, OpenCV now includes a user-friendly interface for implementing deep learning-based SR methods [22–23]. This interface incorporates pretrained models that can be readily and efficiently utilized for inference.

Within the SR module of OpenCV, there are four distinct models available:

Enhanced deep residual network
Efficient subpixel convolutional network
Laplacian pyramid SR network

4.4.2.1.5 Laplacian pyramid SR structure

Through the use of Charbonnier loss functions and a progressive recon-struction approach for subband residuals, the LapSRN model, as shown in Figure 4.9, surpasses other models such as SRCNN (SR convolutional neural

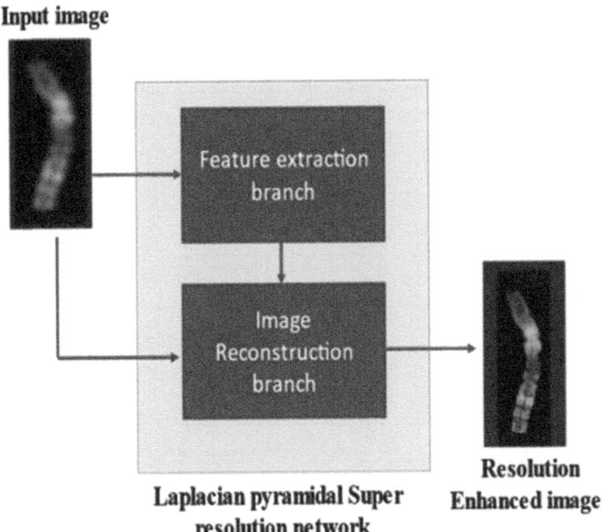

Figure 4.9 Architecture of Laplacian pyramid SR structure.

network), FSRCNN (fast SR convolutional neural network), VDSR (very deep SR), and DRCN (deeply recursive convolutional network) in terms of performance. The LaPSRN model leverages parameter sharing, local residual learning (LRL), and multiscale training to further enhance its capabilities and the MS-LaPSRN model even outperforms the DRRN (deep recursive residual network) model in terms of SR quality and accuracy. Two branches make up the network's architecture: feature extraction and image reconstruction.

The network used in this method gradually reconstructs the subband residuals of high-resolution images, in contrast to a single-step upsampling approach. This reconstruction is performed at multiple pyramid levels, typically corresponding to log2(S) levels, where S represents the scale factor (e.g., 2, 4, 8). An advantage of this method is that without using bicubic interpolation, it directly extracts features from the low-resolution input image.

4.4.2.1.6 *Feature extraction*

One transposed convolutional layer (or deconvolutional layer) and "d" convolutional layers are present at level "s" of the network, and they are both in the position of scaling up the extracted features by a factor of 2. Two separate layers receive the output from each transposed convolutional layer: (1) Reconstructing a level "s" residual image using a convolutional layer. (2) A second convolutional layer is used to extract features at the level "s + 1," which is more accurate. The feature representations acquired at lower levels are shared by higher levels. Due to the network's increased nonlinearity from

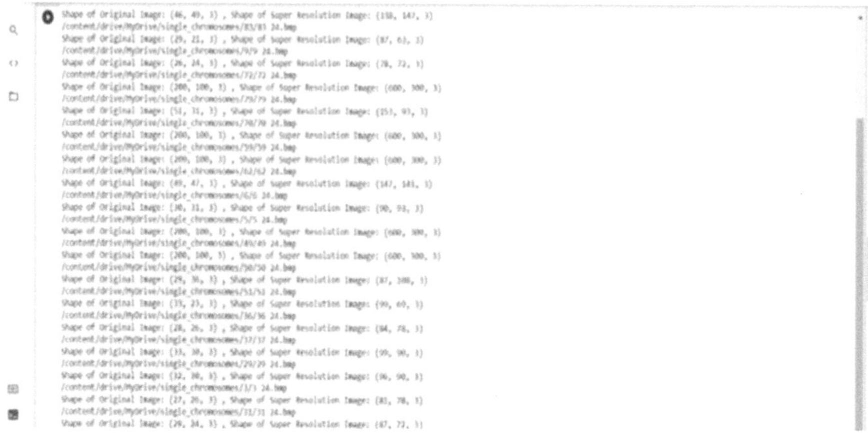

Figure 4.10 Output of LaPSRN.

the sharing of feature representations, it is now able to learn complicated mappings at finer scales.

4.4.2.1.7 Image reconstruction

At level "s," an upsampling (transposed convolutional) layer is used to scale the image being processed up by two times. The projected residual image from the feature extraction branch is combined with the initialized bilinear kernel of this particular layer to produce a high-resolution output image.

The images in Figure 4.10 represent individual strands of chromosomes that have been successfully segmented after identification and segmentation using Detectron2 object detection model. The output of LaPSRN is also shown in Figure 4.10.

The output of the LaPSRN for the example images from the 24th class selected from the dataset is displayed in Table 4.1. The resolution of the input chromosomal images is found to have increased three times after taking SR for all sample images. Similar to this, all of the input chromosomal images are improved using LaPSRN, and the improved images are saved in a separate folder that will be used as input for the DL model.

Table 4.1 Output of LaPSRN block for sample images in the dataset

Reference number of images with class label 24 in the dataset	Shape of the original image	Shape of SR-enhanced image
83	46,49,3	138,147,3
9	29,21,3	87,63,3
72	26,24,3	78,72,3
79	200,100,3	600,300,3
70	51,31,3	153,93,3
31	29,24,3	87,72,3

4.5 EFFICIENTNETS

A structured way for scaling all dimensions, including depth, width, and resolution, is provided by the CNN design and scaling method known as EfficientNet. In contrast to conventional techniques, which scale these variables separately, EfficientNet uses a compound coefficient to consistently scale the network's width, depth, and resolution using a preset set of scaling coefficients.

4.5.1 Basic structure

EfficientNet-B0 consists of a total of 237 layers, while EfficientNet-B7 has a total of 813 layers. To simplify the understanding of these layers, they can be organized into five distinct modules, as illustrated in Figure 4.11.

The first module is utilized as the foundation for the subsequent blocks. All seven of the main blocks, with the exception of the first, use Module 2 as their starting point for the first sub-block. All of the sub-blocks are connected to Module 3 as a skip connection. The skip connection in the initial sub-blocks is combined in Module 4, which is used for that purpose. Module 5 combines all of the sub-blocks after they have been connected in a skip connection to their preceding sub-blocks.

These modules are then put together to create sub-blocks, which are then used in the blocks in a certain fashion.

We have worked with three models of EfficientNet:

- B0
- B5
- B6

4.5.1.1 B0 model

There are 237 layers in EfficientModel-B0 (Figure 4.12). This acts as a baseline model for the remaining EfficientNet models.

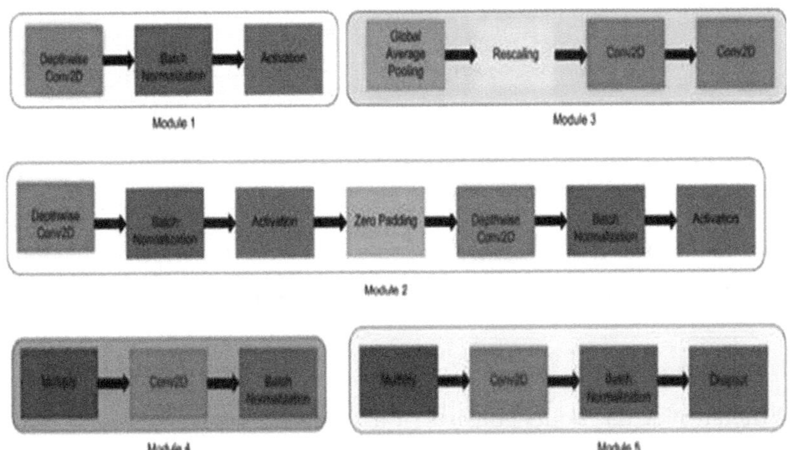

Figure 4.11 Base structure of EfficientNet.

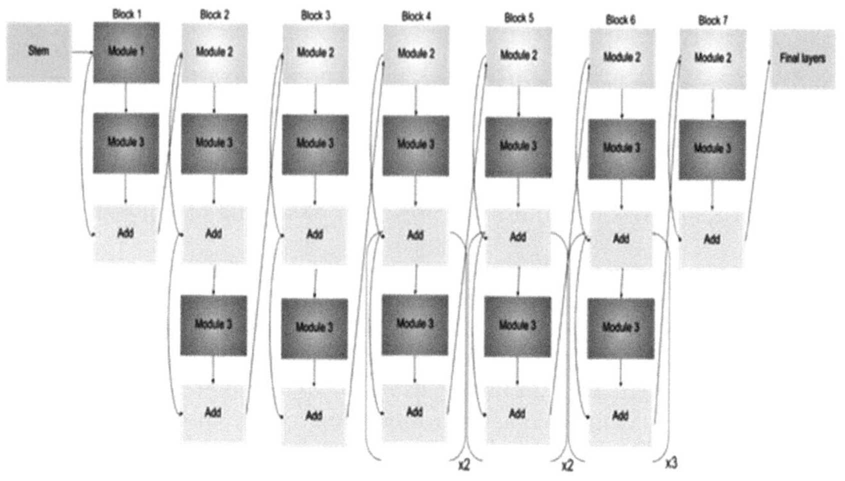

Figure 4.12 Architecture of EfficientNet-B0 model.

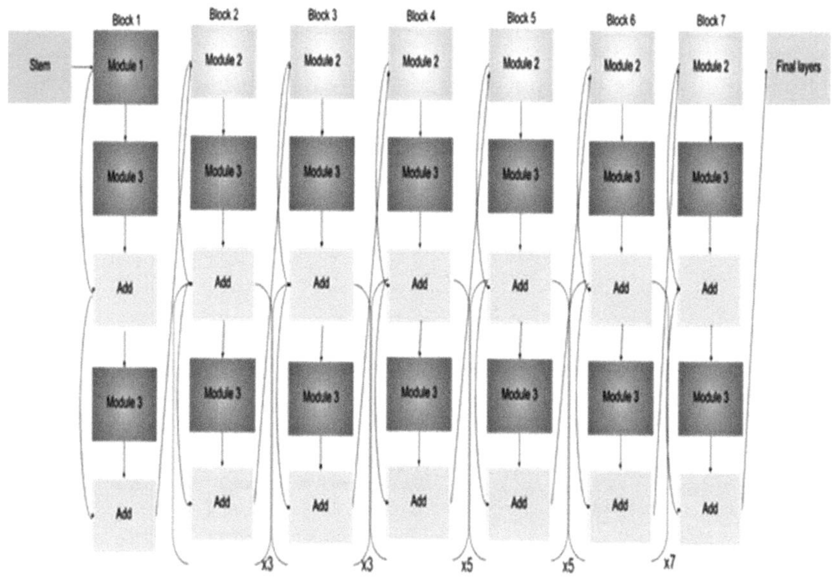

Figure 4.13 Architecture of EfficientNet-B5 model.

4.5.1.2 B5 model

The EfficientNet-B5 model consists of 521 layers (Figure 4.13).

4.5.1.3 B6 model

The EfficientNet-B5 model consists of 671 layers (Figure 4.14).

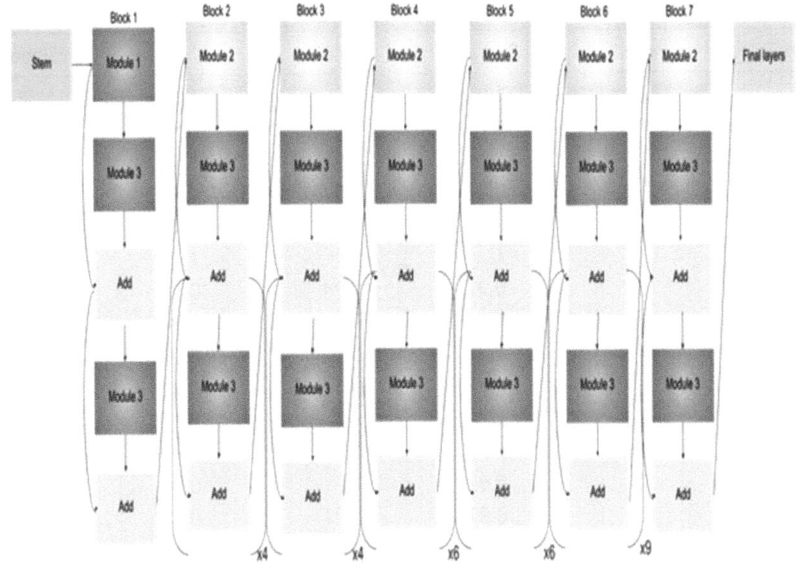

Figure 4.14 Architecture of EfficientNet-B6 model.

4.6 RESULTS AND DISCUSSION

In the suggested work, the initial learning rate was found to be 0.0001 after numerous iterations. The training process was carried out for a total of 30 epochs with a dropout rate of 0.95. The learning rate schedule consisted of specific epochs at 10, 15, 20, and 30.

The classification report for the B6 + Custom last layers model can be found in Table 4.2.

From Table 4.3, it can be inferred that the highest accuracy is achieved using EfficientNet-B6. The difference between the classification accuracy results of the EfficientNet-B6 model and Custom model is notable.

4.6.1 Accuracy calculation formula and calculation

- No. of correct predictions/Total No. of predictions = 804
- No. of correct predictions = 77

Therefore, accuracy = 1,930/2,000 = 0.966. The proposed EfficientNet-B6 model achieved an impressive accuracy of 96.6%. This accuracy outperforms the performance of cutting-edge methods for chromosomal image karyotyping that have recently been published in literature.

4.7 CONCLUSION

The main goal of this research was to create a modern classification model for correctly classifying chromosomes using a variety of deep learning models,

Table 4.2 Classification report on B6 + custom last layers model

Chromosome number	Precision	Recall	F1 score	Support
1	1	1	1	35
2	0.9	1	0.95	35
3	1	0.91	0.96	35
4	0.92	0.97	0.94	35
5	0.97	0.94	0.96	35
6	1	1	1	35
7	0.97	0.94	0.96	35
8	0.94	0.94	0.94	35
9	1	0.94	0.97	35
10	0.97	0.94	0.96	35
11	1	1	1	35
12	1	0.97	0.99	35
13	0.97	1	0.99	35
14	0.97	0.91	0.94	35
15	0.94	0.97	0.96	35
16	0.91	0.91	0.91	35
17	0.97	0.91	0.94	35
18	1	1	1	35
19	1	0.91	0.96	35
20	0.9	1	0.95	35
21	0.95	1	0.97	35
22	0.94	0.94	0.94	35
23	0.9	0.96	0.93	28
24	1	1	1	6
Accuracy			0.96	804
Macro-average	0.96	0.96	0.96	804
Weighted average	0.96	0.96	0.96	804

including ResNets, VGG-16, a customized model, and EfficientNets (B0, B5, B6). Following model training, it was observed that the EfficientNet-B6 model achieved the highest accuracy, reaching an impressive 96.66%. Comparing the results with existing chromosome classification models on the market, the proposed model also outperformed them.

Table 4.3 Model summary

Model	Accuracy
EfficientNet-B0 (without SR)	88.75
EfficientNet-B0	92.06
EfficientNet-B5	95.2
EfficientNet-B6	96.6
VGG16	94
Custom model	88

In addition to classification, the research also focused on chromosome detection using two object detection models: YOLOv4 and Detectron2. While YOLOv4 struggled to detect each individual strand of the chromosome, Detectron2 successfully accomplished this task. The detected chromosome strands were subsequently used as training and testing sets for the classification model.

The significant improvement in accuracy was attributed to the utilization of SR techniques. When non-super resolution images were given as input data for the classification model, the accuracy dropped by 1–2% compared to the images enhanced with SR. With sufficient data collected, the proposed approach allows for the detection of abnormalities in chromosomes. This can greatly expedite the karyotyping process and aid doctors in identifying any irregularities or anomalies present.

Overall, this study successfully developed a high-accuracy classification model for chromosomes, leveraging SR techniques and benefiting from effective chromosome detection through the Detectron2 model. The findings have the potential to significantly enhance chromosome analysis and expedite the diagnosis of abnormalities by medical professionals.

For the purpose of validating the effective net architecture, chromosomal images from the BioImLab dataset are used. Before being used in clinical practice, the designs must be carefully validated using numerous datasets because chromosomal analysis is crucial for diagnosing tumors and locating genetic anomalies. As human chromosomal data from patients is particularly difficult to collect, there are fewer images accessible in many datasets. In order to further improve the categorization accuracy, the data may be enhanced by utilizing modern methods like generative adversarial networks (GAN).

REFERENCES

1. Roshtkhari, M. J., and Setarehdan, S. K., 2008, 'A novel algorithm for straightening highly curved images of human chromosomes', Pattern Recognition Letters, vol 29, no. 9, pp. 1208–1217.
2. Menaka, D., and Ganesh Vaidyanathan, S., 2022, 'ChromeNet: A CNN architecture with comparison of optimizers for classification of human chromosome images', Multidimensional Systems and Signal Processing, vol 33, no. 3, pp. 747–768.
3. Zgang, W., et al., 2018, 'Chromosome classification with convolutional neural network based deep learning', 2018 11th International Congress on Image and Signal Processing, BioMedical Engineering and Informatics (CISP-BMEI). IEEE.
4. Al-Kharraz, M. S., Elrefaei, L. A., and Fadel, M. A., 2020, 'Automated system for chromosome karyotyping to recognize the most common numerical abnormalities using deep learning', IEEE Access, vol 8, pp. 157727–157747.
5. Al-Kharraz, M., Elrefaei, L.A., and Fadel, M., 2021, 'Classifying chromosome images using ensemble convolutional neural networks', In Applications of Artificial Intelligence in Engineering, pp. 751–764, Springer, Singapore.
6. Wang, X., Zheng, B., Li, S., Mulvihill, J. J., Wood, M. C., and Liu, H., 2009, 'Automated classification of metaphase chromosomes: Optimization of an adaptive computerized scheme', Journal of Biomedical Informatics, vol 42, no. 1, pp. 22–31.
7. Swati, S., Sharma, M., and Vig, L., 2018, 'Automatic classification of low-resolution chromosomal images', Proceedings of the International Joint Conference on Neural Networks, pp. 1–8, IEEE.

8. Swati, S., Gupta, G., Yadav, M., Sharma, M., and Vig, L., 2017, 'Siamese networks for chromosome classification', in Proceedings of the IEEE International Conference on Computer Vision Workshops, pp. 72–81, IEEE, Venice, Italy.

9. Swati, Sharma, M., and Vig, L., 2018, 'Automatic chromosome classification using deep attention based sequence learning of chromosome bands', Proceedings of the International Joint Conference on Neural Networks, pp. 1–8, IEEE.

10. Abid, F., and Hamami, L., 2018, 'A survey of neural network based automated systems for human chromosome classification', Artificial Intelligence Review, vol 49, no. 1, pp. 41–56.

11. Sharma, M., Saha, O., Sriraman, A., Hebbalaguppe, R., Vig, L., and Karande, S., July 2017, 'Crowdsourcing for chromosome segmentation and deep classification', in Proceedings of the IEEE Conference on Computer Vision and Pattern Recognition Workshops, pp. 786–793, IEEE, Honolulu, HI.

12. Ji, L., 1994, 'Fully automatic chromosome segmentation', Cytometry, vol. 17, no. 3, pp. 196–208.

13. Minaee, S., Fotouhi, M., and Khalaj, B., 2014, 'A geometric approach to fully automatic chromosome segmentation', in Proceedings of the Signal Processing in Medicine and Biology Symposium, pp. 1–6, IEEE, Philadelphia, PA.

14. Balaji, V. S., and Vidhya, S., 2015, 'Separation of touching and overlapped human chromosome images', In Advancements of Medical Electronics, pp. 59–65, Springer, Berlin, Germany.

15. Menaka, D., and Ganesh Vaidyanathan, S., 2023. 'A hybrid convolutional neural network–support vector machine architecture for classification of super-resolution enhanced chromosome images', Expert Systems, vol. 40, no. 3, p. e13186.

16. Ooi, Y. K., and Ibrahim, H., 2021, 'Deep learning algorithms for single image super-resolution: A systematic review', Electronics, vol 10, no. 7, p. 867.

17. Luo, C., Yu, T., Luo, Y., Wang, M., Yu, F., Li, Y., Tian, C., Qiao, J., and Xiao, L., 2020, 'DEEPACC: Automate chromosome classification based on metaphase images using deep learning framework fused with prior knowledge', arXiv:2006.15528.

18. Lin, C., Zhao, G., Yang, Z., Yin, A., Wang, X., Guo, L., Chen, H., Ma, Z., Zhao, L., Luo, H., and Wang, T., 2020, 'CIR-Net: Automatic classification of human chromosome based on inception-ResNet architecture', IEEE/ACM Transactions on Computational Biology and Bioinformatics, vol 19, no. 3, pp. 1285–1293.

19. Wang, Z., Chen, J., and Hoi, S., 2020, 'Deep learning for image super-resolution: A survey', IEEE Transactions on Pattern Analysis and Machine Intelligence, vol 43, no. 10, pp. 3365–3387.

20. Wei, H., Gao, W., Nie, H., Sun, J., and Zhu, M., 2022, 'Classification of Giemsa staining chromosome using input-aware deep convolutional neural network with integrated uncertainty estimates', Biomedical Signal Processing and Control, vol 71, p. 103120.

21. Hernández-Mier, Y., Nuño-Maganda, M. A., Polanco-Martagón, S., and García-Chávez, M. d. R., 2020, 'Machine learning classifiers evaluation for automatic karyogram generation from G-banded metaphase images', Applied Sciences, vol 10, no. 8, p. 2758.

22. Arora, T., and Dhir, R., 2019, 'A novel approach for segmentation of human metaphase chromosome images using region based active contours', International Arab Journal of Information Technology, vol 16, no. 1, pp. 132–137.

23. Balagalla, U. B., Samarabandu, J., and Subasinghe, A., 2022, 'Automated human chromosome segmentation and feature extraction: Current trends and prospects', F1000Research, vol 11, https://doi.org/10.12688/f1000research.84360.1.

Chapter 5

Applications of machine learning to the impact of IoT in biomedical applications

Shwetha Baliga, Rakshita Basarakod, Kalathmika G., Nandana P. Pillai, Jayashree Shivakumar, and Preeti Yadav

5.1 CHAPTER OBJECTIVES

1. The chapter aims at highlighting the interlaying importance of Internet of Things (IoT) and machine learning (ML) in present-day biomedical applications.
2. Studying deeply case studies in the field to understand and deduce the effectiveness and limitations of IoT and ML applications in the field.
3. Providing clear idea on the various applications such as Diagnosis using IoT and ML, image-guided surgery (IGS), robot-assisted surgery, electrocardiogram (ECG) analysis, and ML in drug discovery.

5.2 BACKGROUND AND DRIVING FORCES

IoT and ML have revolutionized the world with their magical power to ease the life of humans. They have juddered the biomedical fields and its application, changing the lives of millions in a celestial way. In simple terms, IoT could be attributed to a device whose major function is to amass data about patients' health. What shoots this star to fame is its supreme ability of early detection and frequent monitoring. ML encompasses within itself the unshakeable and indomitable power of artificial intelligence (AI). What started out as a picayune has now changed human lives forever. ML is a towering domain under AI engirdling algorithms to find relations and design received data, and to determine the best prediction based on analysis of the result. With their ever-growing importance, they have replaced the conventional surgical processes. A lot of problems in traditional healthcare has been overcome by IoT and ML inclusions in the medical field. The fact that the biomedical field and IoT are an encouraging sign of advancement and evolution in this field. The perks of this groundbreaking change are much debated and their effectiveness is still surrounded by clouds of uncertainty. Hence, it is pivotal to explore the various existing applications of IoT and ML in the biomedical field and thus deduce their success. The chapter deals with some of the major areas in the medical field tended and strengthened by IoT and ML. Such an excursion of

DOI: 10.1201/9781003487647-5

their advantages and limitations will help us understand deeper and decide the probable areas of development provided by IoT and ML in the biomedical applications. The chapter also deals with the various impacts, pros and cons of IoT and ML through various extensive case studies, their analysis, and conclusions.

5.3 DIAGNOSIS USING ML MODELS

5.3.1 Breast cancer diagnosis

Cancer is the root cause of the demise of people all around the globe. It is caused by unusual cells in the body that spread from its initial region to all other sectors of the body. This is diagnosed when a malignant tumor is detected in the breast tissue. Magnetic resonance imaging and thermal imaging can be used for its diagnosis, but it is way too costly and requires wholesome knowledge to interpret the result. ML offers an alternative to the diagnosis of human diseases, particularly for cancer detection. Integrating this with the IoT enables wireless and remote device communication through the internet. This involves three stages. It starts with the collection and testing of histopathological breast samples from the patients followed by analysis of the sample features acquired from the first step using hyperparameter-optimized CNN classifier and finally the results are verified and finalized by the therapists to provide the patients with the proper medications.

Apart from this, various machine algorithms like decision tree, random forest, support vector machines (SVMs), k-nearest neighbor, and deep learning through Adam gradient descent can be used for breast cancer diagnosis [1]. Dataset that had information of 30 different measurements was taken into consideration to create a model. This model's work was to measure and classify the cells as malignant (cancerous) or benign. Deep learning and Adam gradient descent learning were used to build the model, which was quite successful in giving accurate predictions of 98.24% [1]. Other methods like SVMs and random forests were also used to build this model, which had an accuracy of 97.2%. In short, it can be concluded that Adam gradient descent leaning with deep learning can be integrated to get more the best results. Exploring this method would provide new doors to improve breast cancer diagnosis.

5.3.2 Lung cancer prediction and treatment

The preliminary stage of cancer prediction is necessary to treat diseases like cancer. Machine-based technology provides techniques to improve lung cancer and provide important perceptions on decision-making in the medical field. The further information provides one with the methodology to subdue the self-preservation of the lung cancer disease prediction with diabetes and smoking using ML which has been in concern over the past few decades.

The process includes three stages, i.e., data collection diagnosis followed by analysis, and finally comparison of algorithms with visualization. Initially, the data of the patient is collected from which necessary data is extracted. This extracted data is fed to the MLT which involves further analysis in which the feature data extracted is reduced to provide precision; these features are stored in databases through which prediction is performed. Finally, the third stage involves the comparison of three different algorithms: SVM, decision tree algorithm (C4.5), and naive Bayes (NBs) algorithm – within which the best-predicted result is taken into consideration [2]. Predictions are made based on the classifier algorithms. To mention, two labels are considered more and less, where more indicates a person will live for more than a year and less indicates a person will live less than a year. Assessment is made on the prognosis with the different algorithm's test input.

The three algorithms mentioned are compared based on the parameters such as accuracy, precision, and area under the curve. With the consideration of all these parameters, it is found that the C4.5 algorithm provides the best result in predicting cancer. The main intention of this was to provide doctors with diagnosing cancer and to invent treatments for patients' better results. There is still more research scope in this as SVM kernel methods or other such algorithms can be used for the evaluation. The prediction is presently done for lung cancer patients with diabetes and smoking features, but this is not limited only to these two parameters. This proposed model can be further improvised by opting for other parameters or even considering different types of cancers. To make this application more endurable, this can be developed as a mobile application.

To consider another approach in the domain of ML in cancer diagnosis, many standards are considered for evaluating the cancer diagnosis that includes RECIST-Response Evaluation Criteria in Solid Tumors [3]. This process involves imaging data, particularly computerized tomography (CT) and magnetic resonance imaging (MRI), which detects the growth or shrink of the tumors in patients. A CNN model is designed to track changes in the volume of the tumor from CT imaging. To enhance the prediction performance, the model is unified with patient data obtained from EGFR mutant drug complex. In recent years, a study proposed that tumor proportional scoring (TPS) is calculated as the percentage of tumor cells in digital pathology images, to evaluate the lung cancer treatment response. More recently is developed phenotype representation learning (PRL) via self-controlled learning and group spotting for the dimensional assembly of cell type annotation on biopsy report of logical images. Their assembly results can be used for tracing tumor growth trends and its reoccurrence. Ultimately, this work can certainly bring a positive impact on the patient's life as early prediction and diagnosis through this can save many lives (Figure 5.1).

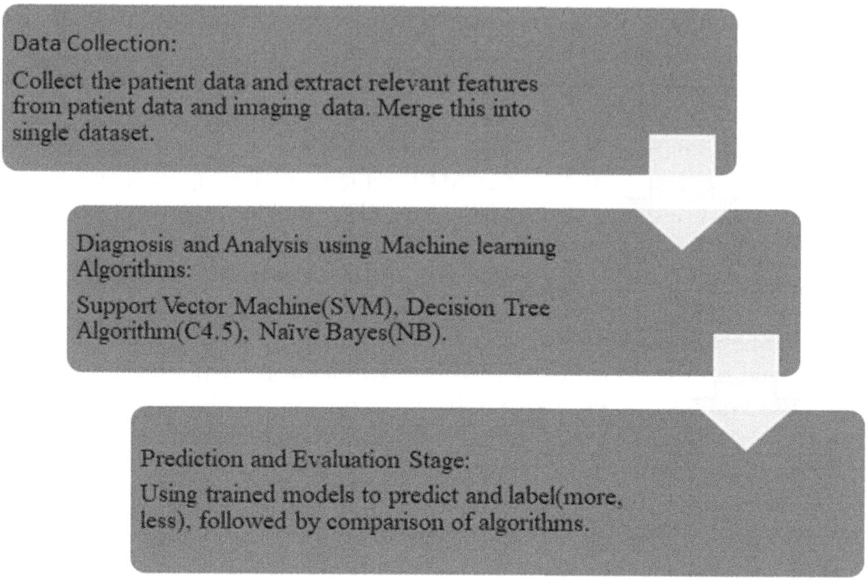

Data Collection:

Collect the patient data and extract relevant features from patient data and imaging data. Merge this into single dataset.

Diagnosis and Analysis using Machine learning Algorithms:

Support Vector Machine(SVM), Decision Tree Algorithm(C4.5), Naïve Bayes(NB).

Prediction and Evaluation Stage:

Using trained models to predict and label(more, less), followed by comparison of algorithms.

Figure 5.1 Methodology of lung cancer detection.

5.4 IMAGE-GUIDED SURGERY

IGS has grown to be one of the most integral technologies in the field of medicine and surgery. It has transformed the conventional surgical methods to pave the way to efficient surgeries that are not only faster but also promises higher rates of survival [4].

IGS can be defined as any surgical procedure in which the efficiency and success rate of the surgeries are boosted by tracking of surgical instruments which function in concurrence with pre-procedural images to assist surgery.

5.4.1 Advantages of IGS

The application of this technology varies from open surgery to minimally invasive spinal surgeries and tumor surgeries. Advanced equipment establishes that least number of tissues are affected during the surgery effectively just as much as necessary for the surgical instruments to pass through.

What is minimally invasive spinal surgery and why is it important?

In contrast to conventional open spine surgery, minimally invasive spinal surgery ensures not only faster and secure surgeries but also reduces the recovery time, thus making a favorable impact [5].

Minimally invasive spinal surgery in elementary words mean that there is no appalling or critical invasion involved in the surgery. This involves minimal and small incisions on the surface of the skin.

5.4.2 Working of IGS

As discussed earlier, it is imperative that the surgical instrument must be tracked at all times. Optical tracking system are usually adorned with this responsibility. This is usually established by fiducial markers often referred to as fiducials. The instruments might either be manufactured with them as a key part of their composition or be provided with a universal tracker, which is nothing but a set of such fiducials which can be attached to any comprehensive instrument.

These markers later establish a coordinate reference frame (CRF) which ensures the repositioning of the patient as well as the optical position sensor [6].

The optical position sensor is one of the most important parts of the technology. Its primary function is to track the markers and map them to the CRFs established by the calibrations in the instrument. Thus, it ensures the effective tracking of the instrument edge in the physical space that is occupied by the patient.

The CRF or the markers are often fastened to the patients.
They are used in cranial, ENT (ear nose throat), as well as spinal surgeries.

Cranial Surgery

- Here the CRF is attached to a head clamp.
- The patient's head is attached to this head clamp.
- The head is invasively attached.

ENT Surgery

- Involves a not invasively attached head frame.

Spine Surgery

- It is attached to a spinous process.

The CRF establishes a common coordinate system which encompasses the position of all interior surgical systems and instruments.
This system gives rise to three major errors:

Fiducial Localization Error (FLE): It highlights difference between the positions of a marker, namely, its true and measured position.
Fiducial Registration Error (FRE): It is the difference in positions of corresponding fiducial points after registration.
Target Registration Error (TRE): It is the difference in positions between other corresponding points excluding the fiducial points after registration [6,7].

5.5 ROBOTIC-ASSISTED SURGERY

The collaboration of IoT with robotic-assisted surgery had enabled surgery process more unambiguous and accurate. Computer-aided surgery requires the expertise of surgeons in handling the robots. The combination of IoT technology with computer-aided surgery had facilitated the existing system to communicate and connect the IoT devices such as smart devices and mobile phones. Surgeons can link for remote operation through the internet in IoT-aided robotic surgery.

Many studies have witnessed that IoT-aided robotic systems have facilitated many applications such as microsurgery and remote surgery. Ishak and Kit have developed the robotic arm which helps the doctor during the surgery and it can be controlled through motion and posture information [9]. To increase the efficiency and safety of surgery, it is necessary to build a more precise model of both the human body and the robot characteristics [10]. There are many challenges for the IoT-aided robotic technology which affects the accuracy and safety of surgery. Some of these challenges are slow internet speed and service quality.

The computer-aided surgery integrated with IoT operates by creating the link between physical, network, and application layers. The physical layer deals with the sensors which collect information about the patients such as temperature and heartbeat through smart devices. The sensors or actuators connect with the robots to form the multi-robot network. The network layer establishes the link between the controllers and network protocols. The application layer takes the information from the physical layer and recuperates via the network layer and performs the specified task according to the information.

Robotic-assisted surgery technology consists of the following:

1. Surgical arms with tiny instruments.
2. Special camera which gives magnified 3D images of the surgical areas.
3. Surgical console through which surgeon controls and operates each move.

This technology is used by urologists, gynecologist surgeons, general surgeons, cardiothoracic surgeons, and colorectal surgeons. The major difference between traditional surgery and robotic-assisted surgery is that surgeon makes small incision instead of large incision and the surgical instruments require less space to do their job.

In conclusion, the future developments of robotic-assisted surgery are expected to improve surgical precision and reshape the way the surgeries are performed. Advancements in robotics, AI, and data analytics are expected to expand surgery applications and improve patient outcomes.

5.6 BIG DATA INTEGRATED WITH IoT HEALTH CARE

The big data concept deals with the analytic approaches required to gather, analyze, store, and speculate data. In the time of COVID-19, the researchers used the data analytic method to study the virus and its spread. In the context of big data implementation, the researchers studied patients' health conditions, diabetes diagnosis, sleep monitoring, and infectious diseases such as tuberculosis. Big data analytics with IoT technology had enabled various IoT devices to auto-monitor the patient's condition.

At present, many sensors monitor and gather a large amount of information regarding patients. This large amount of data is called big data which is continuously generated by smart devices and sensors. It is difficult to analyze and process this huge amount of data into valuable information. Therefore, an organization needs to have methodical and secure architecture to operate this big data. Currently, medical sensors are emerging with more memory and diagnosis efficiency that can make use of improved particle swarm optimization algorithms which help in sensing whether the required amount of drug had reached a particular part of our body or not. These medical sensors gather huge amounts of data per second which are interconnected and this data is called big data. This data is analyzed and sent to the concerned authority or organization.

The patient suffering from diabetes needs regular checkup of their blood glucose level and insulin dosage. Generally, this involves regular visit to the hospital. However, with the integration of IoT and big data, remote patient monitoring becomes more effective. The patient with diabetes wears continuously glucose monitoring device, which is an IoT-enabled wearable. This device produces a stream of real-time data. This data consists of blood glucose reading, timestamps, and other contextual information like physical activity levels and meals. This data is collected from several patients' using similar devices and this data is gathered in a centralized cloud database. This database is able to handle large volume of data and can accommodate different types of data such as numerical readings, timestamps, and textual notes. Big data analytics algorithms process the aggregated data. They can detect patterns, anomalies, and trends overtime. If the analytics system detects a significant deviation from the patient's normal range or a potentially dangerous situation (e.g., severe hypoglycemia), it triggers the automated alerts. The doctor or patient's healthcare provider receives an alert through dedicated application or a web portal. The system might also suggest dietary modifications or meditation adjustments by considering the patient's historical data and responses. The patient also can go through their own data through their mobile data.

This integration of IoT devices with big data enhances the patient care by continuously monitoring, early detection if any changes in their health, and timely interventions. It reduces the periodic visit to hospitals, making healthcare more convenient for the patient. There are some challenges such as ensuring data security and privacy is critical. Additionally, interoperability between different IoT devices and data sources can be a challenge.

In conclusion, the integration of IoT and big data in biomedical applications holds immense promise for transforming healthcare delivery, research, and patient outcomes. As these technologies continue to advance, they will contribute to more proactive personalized and effective approaches to managing health and treating diseases [14].

5.7 ECG ANALYSIS

As per a report from the World Heart Federation (WHF), deaths globally due to cardiovascular diseases have seen an increase from 12.1 million in 1990 to 20.5 million in 2021.

Analyzing ECG using IoT and ML has the ability to transform the healthcare sector. This concept will give rise to remote monitoring of the individuals. This requires the usage of ECG sensors which can be incorporated into wearables like smartwatches or chest straps. The information gathered from the sensor is then transmitted to the cloud for further analysis. ML algorithms can be used to examine and detect abnormalities such as heart blockages and other conditions.

The graphical representation of the electrical activity of the heart during a cardiac cycle is known as electrocardiogram. Three electrical leads, one to each wrist and other to the left ankle, are connected to the electrocardiograph which monitors the heart activity. For more accurate results, multiple leads are attached in the chest region.

In a standard ECG, multiple peaks are identified starting from P to T waves. The P wave corresponds to depolarization of the atria, which refers to the contraction of both the atria. Following this, we have the QRS complex which refers to the depolarization of the ventricles which causes contraction of the ventricles and hence the beginning of systole. Then, we have the T wave that corresponds to the repolarization of the ventricles. This also marks the end of systole. The shape of the ECG is mostly the same for all individuals, hence any deviation from the standard indicates an abnormality.

The combination of IoT and ML will allow for customization of healthcare by collecting data on the individual's heart rate and their activity levels, and hence will provide a complete image of one's health.

Rahman et al. [12] have employed the following steps for the analysis of ECG:

1. The heart data is read from the human chest by the ECG sensor Ad8232.
2. The data is now sent to Arduino Mega 2560 and then to ESP8266 which is a Wi-Fi module.
3. The data is then uploaded to IoT cloud with the help of HTTP (hypertext transfer protocol) and MQTT (message queuing telemetry transport) servers.
4. These results are then uploaded to the prediction stage for pre-processing.
5. The data is analyzed using correlation and covariance to pin point the attributes behind heart conditions.
6. To this, linear regression algorithm is applied to predict the diseases.
7. The result is then sent to the application interface for further analysis.

To identify the attributes which are behind the heart condition using correlation and covariance, the following formulas are used:

$$r = \frac{\Sigma(x_i - \bar{x})(y_i - \bar{y})}{\sqrt{\Sigma(x_i - \bar{x})^2\,\Sigma(y_i - \bar{y})^2}}$$

$$\mathrm{cov}_{x,y} = \frac{\Sigma(x_i - \bar{x})(y_i - \bar{y})}{N-1}$$

Here, r is the correlation coefficient, $\mathrm{cov}_{x,y}$ is the covariance of x and y, x_i is the value of x variable, y_i is the y variable, $\bar{x}$ is the mean of x_i, $\bar{y}$ is the mean of y_i, and N is the number of data in the dataset.

The ECG identifiers P,Q,R,S, and T waves are used to identify heart diseases using linear regression method. To calculate slope and intercept, the following formulas are used:

$$\mathrm{Slope} = m = \frac{n(\Sigma\,xy) - (\Sigma\,xy)(\Sigma\,y)}{n(\Sigma\,x^2) - (\Sigma\,x)^2}$$

$$\mathrm{Intercept} = b = \frac{\Sigma\,y - m(\Sigma\,x)}{n}$$

The variable to be predicted is abbreviated as y. The predictor variable, on which the predictions are based, is abbreviated as x.

Just like a coin has two sides, even though there are many benefits of the usage of IoT and ML in analyzing ECG, there are also some drawbacks. The most important one is privacy of the data gathered and the problems faced while ensuring its security. The data of patients has to be confidential.

Additionally, the accuracy and dependability of the data which is collected and final results obtained should be confirmed before it can influence clinical decision-making.

Thus, the integration of IoT and ML in ECG analysis has the ability to enhance accuracy and diagnosis of cardiovascular diseases which can ultimately lead to lesser loss of lives to these diseases (Figure 5.2).

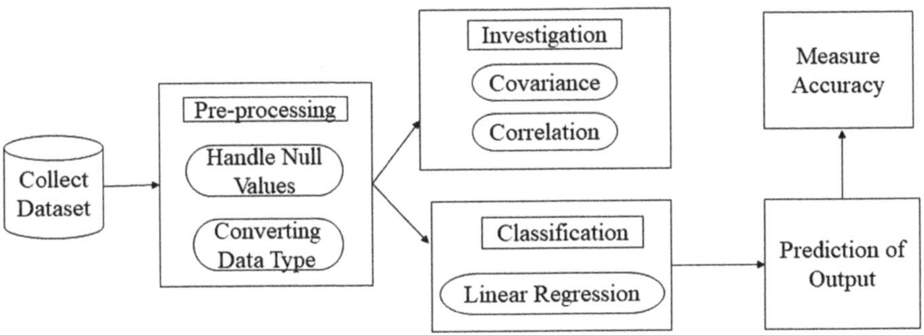

Figure 5.2 Heart disease prediction system.

5.8 PREDICTION OF RISK LEVEL OF CARDIOVASCULAR DISEASES

The researchers adopted IoT and ML techniques to classify the users into three risk levels that include high, moderate, and low risks of having cardiovascular diseases, which had a F1 score of 80.4%. The two risk levels which involved high and low had a F1 score of 91%.

The system developed by them allows users to monitor the possibility of having cardiovascular diseases in the future. This system is assessed from the human–computer interaction (HCI) point of view and also provides a new face to the present biomedical sector.

5.9 ML APPLICATIONS IN DRUG DISCOVERY

The pharmaceutical industry faces numerous challenges in drug discovery and development, including long pipelines, complex processes, and high failure rates in clinical trials. In recent years, ML techniques have emerged as powerful tools to address these challenges. This chapter explores the feasible literature on drug discovery through ML tools and techniques, emphasizing their applications across various phases of drug development. From target validation and hit discoveries to *de novo* drug architectures, ML offers the potential to retrieve accurate outcomes, improve decision-making, and deduce risk failures in clinical trials. However, interpretability issues remain a significant obstacle to the widespread adoption of ML in drug discovery. To tackle these challenges, systematic and comprehensive high-dimensional data needs to be generated. Nevertheless, with ongoing efforts to overcome these limitations and an increasing awareness of the factors required to validate ML approaches, the application of ML holds the promise of promoting data-driven decision-making and accelerating the drug discovery process.

Drug discovery and development in the pharmaceutical industry are complex processes that rely on a multitude of factors. However, the advent of high-throughput approaches, such as "omics" technologies, has created both challenges and opportunities for identifying plausible therapeutic hypotheses to develop new drugs. ML approaches have gained traction within the pharmaceutical industry, offering tools that improve discovery and decision-making processes with abundant and high-quality data. This chapter explores the applications of ML in various stages of drug discovery, from target validation to digital pathology analysis in clinical trials. The potential of ML in addressing attrition and cost issues in drug development is highlighted, along with the challenges that hinder its widespread adoption. *ML Toolbox:* Fundamentally, ML involves using algorithms to parse data, learn from it, and make predictions about future data. Unlike traditional hand-coding of software routines, ML algorithms are trained on large datasets to learn how to perform specific tasks. Two main types of ML techniques are supervised and unsupervised learning. Supervised learning involves training models to predict future values of data categories or continuous variables, while unsupervised learning is used for exploratory purposes to cluster data in meaningful ways. Model selection is critical in ensuring ML models generalize well to new data, considering prediction accuracy, training speed, and the number of variables handled. *Applications in Drug Discovery:* ML has found applications in various stages of drug discovery and development, presenting new opportunities for the pharmaceutical industry. Some notable applications include target validation, where ML can provide stronger evidence for target–disease associations and hit discoveries, where ML helps improve small-molecule compound design and optimization. Furthermore, ML aids in understanding disease mechanisms, developing new prognostic biomarkers, and analyzing biometric and wearable device data from patient monitoring. Additionally, ML has shown promise in enhancing digital pathology imaging, extracting high-content information from images, and resolving disease and non-disease phenotypes.

Despite the potential benefits of ML in drug discovery, several challenges need to be addressed to maximize its impact. The primary challenge lies in the lack of interpretability and repeatability of ML-generated results, limiting their application in critical decision-making processes. Another concern is the need to generate comprehensive and high-dimensional data systematically to support ML research. However, ongoing efforts to address these issues and increasing awareness of the factors necessary to validate ML approaches are paving the way for broader implementation.

ML techniques offer a promising avenue for accelerating drug discovery and reducing failure rates on clinical trials. By leveraging abundant and high-quality data, ML enables data-driven decision-making at various stages of drug development. Challenges related to interpretability and data generation are being addressed through systematic efforts and increasing industry awareness. As the pharmaceutical industry continues to invest in ML resources and technologies, collaboration with technology giants, biotechnology start-ups, and academic centers can further advance the application of ML in drug discovery and development. With the continuous progress in ML algorithms and data management, the future holds immense potential for transforming the drug discovery landscape.

5.10 IoT- AND ML-BASED DEVICES USED IN MEDICAL APPLICATIONS

5.10.1 Wearable devices

These consist of sensors embedded within them which may be temperature sensors, optical sensors, accelerometers, or biometric sensors. IoMT devices incorporated with sensors are the root for data extracted through ML algorithms. There is a research effort required in this field. There is a tremendous growth in smartwatches in recent years. The sensors continuously collect data from the environment, and the collected data is transmitted via wireless technologies. Collected data is stored in databases, and ML algorithms are used to extract patterns, trends, and correlations, ultimately providing personalized recommendations. These devices also act on the analyzed data and user preferences (display notifications, vibrate to alert users). But it has to overcome many challenges like system efficiency, cost, user insight, and security issues. There is a need for further research in these domains. Thus, we need to find a solution to all this to use these devices at their fullest potential possible.

As per research conducted by the Icahn School of Medicine at Mount Sinai in New York, it has been found that using data from smartwatches like the Apple watch could aid in training ML models. This data can include heart rate which will help in regulating patient well-being. In March 2023, JMIR Formative Research published a paper which emphasized how the data from Apple Watch could be used to predict pain scores in hospitalized sickle cell disease patients. This data can be helpful to build ML algorithms [13].

5.10.2 Implantable devices

These devices are placed below the patient's skin and help monitor, diagnose, and nurse various diseases. These are broadly used in many medical applications such as radiology, heart attack stent, neuron, and microchips. These devices are often embedded with sensors to collect data. ML algorithms analyze this data to provide insights for personalized treatment. They even include a microprocessor or microcontroller accountable for collecting and processing data from sensors incorporated into implantable devices and finally controlling actions based on it. Some of the challenges faced by implantable devices are as follows: The materials selected should be compatible with the human body and should not cause any damage to tissues. These devices collect delicate information. This data should be secured; ML algorithms and accuracy should be simultaneously maintained, and should possess a long lifetime.

5.11 CASE STUDY

5.11.1 Wearable device in arrhythmia detection

Smartwatches and wristbands track heart rates. Using such wearable devices, Apple, Huawei, and Fitbit have tried to detect irregular heartbeats, like atrial fibrillation. The approach of the author involves a ML model called SVM that helps to identify the raw heartbeats. This is further followed by DTW (dynamic time warping) method with K-medoid clustering that aims to clean and find any distorted heartbeats. The other approach involves SVM and bagging trees to detect the same disease using ECG signals. PPG signal, recorded by a Cardiotracker ring or Oximeter can also be adapted to serve the same purpose. CNN ML algorithm can be used to compare the PPG and ECG signal, providing higher accuracy and effective diagnosis for atrial fibrillation. Research is still going on to detect the disease using other ML algorithms to analyze the heart rate received via wearable devices.

The device used to detect irregular heartbeats termed arrhythmias is called a Holter monitor. This is used when ECG does not provide sufficient information on the heart's condition. The damage to this device can be caused by water. As sensors attached to the device may provide discomfort to the patients, it is not affected by other electrical devices. The user needs to avoid magnets, electric blankets, cell phones, and other such devices as these signals may interrupt signals given from the Holter monitor.

It has gained a lot of attention in recent years as it is noninvasive. This device is to be worn for one to two days even while sleeping. During this period of time, the heartbeats of the patient will be recorded. The Holter monitor's data is compared with the record of symptoms given by the patient, which helps in accurate diagnosis.

5.11.2 Use of IGS in minimally invasive esophagectomy

The major challenge in developing an efficient navigation system with respect to the minimally invasive esophagectomy is the prevailing uncertainty in the tumor or lymph nodes or any other sensitive tissues positions [5].

Hence the need of the hour is a more systematic navigational system for tumor surgeries and analysis in the chest.

Materials and Methods Involved

1. *Immobilization*
   - The elementary step in this was to ensure that the patient is immobilized. As movement of any kind might cause organ deformation or any other inconsistency in the surgery.
   - For this purpose, an immobilization device was created. It is comprised of a dual computerized-numeric control stretcher.
   - The top part of the stretcher consisted of a short vacuum mattress which was predominantly composed of polyvinylchloride and was highly desired as it avoids the formation of any CT artefacts, i.e., inconsistencies in the CT numbers between the true and reconstructed images.
   - The device also saw the embedding of CT markers over the stretcher specifically in the thoracic region. These CT markers were composed of a chemical- and temperature-resistant material which also showed the desired properties of radiation resistivity – polyetheretherketone, which was desired due to its characteristic to not form CT artefacts.
2. *CT Acquisition and Segmentation*
   - The next important step was to analyze the acquired CT and segment in accordance to the needs.

- The CT is acquired and the target and risk areas are segmented using segmentation software, like the one provided by MITK.

3. *Marker Configuration and Optical Tracking*
   - The next step included the measuring of the spatial positions of the optical markers, which was done using the Polaris tracking system.

4. *Operating Room Setup*
   - The da Vinci Surgical System consisted of three parts:
     i. The robot arms and the other surgical instruments were carried by a telemanipulator.
     ii. The augmentative interface between the camera movements and the instruments was provided on the surgeon's console aiding an efficient and safe surgery.
     iii. It was also provided with other essentials for a surgery such as lights and control monitors or panel for others assisting the surgery.

5. *Image Registration*
   One of the most fundamental steps of the surgery is that it basically refers to the procedure of finding or establishing the relations between the CT image taken initially and the real-time conditions in operating room. This is done by mapping the corresponding images of the two.

6. *Calibration*
   The surgical instruments are calibrated prior to the surgeries using software (NDI 6D Architect software) in order to establish a relation between the instrument tip and its marker plate.

7. *Navigation and Visualization*
   It is necessary to ensure that active tracking of the instruments happen throughout the course of the surgery. It requires the constant tracking of the instruments as well as the patient stretcher. The information derived was then transferred to the #D coordinate system acquired by the pre-operative CT. In case of a deviation from its usual path or obstruction, the system highlights the error by changing the instruments' color and displaying its last known position.

8. Operative Workflow Test
   For this, one previously segmented esophageal carcinoma dataset was loaded to the system. The 53-year-old male patient had distal adenocarcinoma. All the risks and targets were segmented.

The setup and operation of the system was successful. Though the stretcher was made immobilizable. Its position could be changed during the course of the surgery without affecting the organs much internally. The system achieved a precision of 0.94 ± 0.76 mm.

5.11.3 Healthcare robots enabled with IoT and AI for elderly patients

Nowadays there is drastic increase in the number of people who are above the age 60. The population of elderly persons is expected to shoot up from

605 million (in 2000) to 2 billion (in 2050) [11]. Therefore, there is need of caretaker in the future. Even though there are plenty of nursing homes and care centers which help them to take care of their health and also provides the social support, but they lack the feeling of independence. Usually, old-age people feel more comfortable in their houses rather than care centers, but to have good health without any support is difficult as aging is cognates with health issues. To obliterate these problems, there are some service robots which act as companion for old-age people. Some of the popular service robots are Care-o-Bot, Aibo, CAESAR, JoHOBBIT, and PT2. When these service robots are integrated with IoT devices, they help to connect old-age people with doctors as well as family members. This also helps in maintaining level of well-being by setting reminders and fall detection.

The health of elderly people can be taken care of if healthcare sensors are incorporated in service robots. These sensors help in analyzing the old-age people health condition by detecting the heart rate, blood pressure, and brain activities. The robotic system also records patient-reported outcome measure (PROMs) at the time of their interaction with the robots. The information from PROMs and sensors is gathered to form a health report of elderly people which is available for doctors, caretakers, and family members. At present, there are many old-age people who get affected by the mild cognitive impairment, which is one of the social challenges for elderly people. This affects the physical and intellectual activities of older people. "Robotic assistant for MCI patient at home (RAMCIP)" is the project designed by Kostavelis et al. It is a service robot that helps the older people with MCI. The designed system has the ability to perform high-level intellectual activities through advanced human and environment perception mechanism that succor the robot when to help the patient. Elderly people are facing another major problem of depression who are living alone. Randall et al. have checked the viability of social-assistive robots (SARs) as in-home alleviative support for older people who are facing with depression. After comparing the mental health state of the older people after and before the installation of SARs in-home, the results indicate that it gives some possible solutions for in-home depression of the elderly people. Marques et al. have invented "AirBot" for elder persons to monitor the quality of air inside the home using IoT devices and also cautions the caretakers or family members. It is helpful in maintaining the healthy environment for the aged people [8].

Additionally, animal-robots can be developed which act as pets and provide amity to depressed people to overcome their psychological issues. A major problem in installation of these robots is that elder are not adapted with the technology in comparison with present generation. The aspiration is to review the capabilities of robots in maintaining the healthy environment and lay the basic work for future advancement, perform multiple functions, and promptly alert the ambulance in case of emergencies (Figure 5.3).

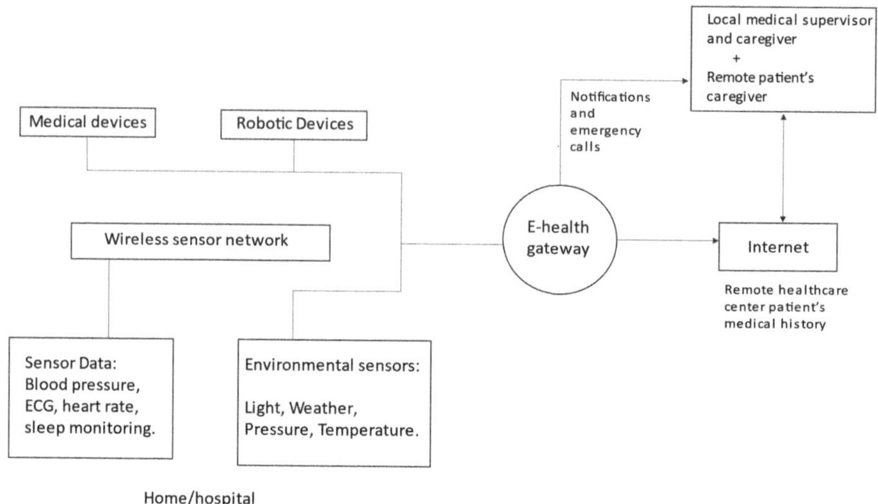

Figure 5.3 IoT-aided robotic healthcare system for elderly patients.

5.11.4 Neural circuit reconstruction for memory formation

Scientists are interested in understanding how memories are formed and stored in the brain. They choose to focus on a specific region of the brain called the hippocampus, which is known to play a crucial role in memory formation.

The objective of this case study is to reconstruct the neural circuitry in the hippocampus involved in memory formation, to gain insights into the underlying mechanisms.

- *Brain Imaging:* Researchers use advanced brain imaging techniques such as functional magnetic resonance imaging (fMRI) and positron emission tomography (PET) to observe brain activity during memory-related tasks.
- *Electrophysiology:* In addition to brain imaging, researchers conduct electrophysiological experiments using electrodes to record the electrical activity of neurons in the hippocampus while subjects perform memory tasks.
- *Genetic Markers:* Genetic markers are used to label specific types of neurons in the hippocampus to identify and trace their connections.
- *Optogenetics:* Researchers employ optogenetic techniques to selectively activate or inhibit specific neurons within the hippocampus to observe their impact on memory formation.

Findings of the proposed model:

- *Hippocampal Subregions:* Researchers discover distinct subregions within the hippocampus, each playing a unique role in memory processing.

- *Neural Pathways:* They trace neural pathways connecting different hippocampal subregions with other brain regions involved in memory consolidation and retrieval.
- *Synaptic Plasticity:* The study reveals that synaptic plasticity, the ability of synapses to strengthen or weaken over time, is a fundamental mechanism underlying memory formation.

The results of this domain provides a combination of brain imaging, electrophysiology, genetic labeling, and optogenetics; researchers map out the neural circuitry involved in memory formation in the hippocampus. They identify specific regions and pathways that are crucial for encoding, storing, and retrieving memories.

The neural circuit reconstruction in the hippocampus provides valuable insights into the neural basis of memory formation. Understanding the precise mechanisms and interactions of neural circuits involved in memory could pave the way for developing new therapies for memory-related disorders and cognitive enhancement.

5.12 RECENT STUDIES AND FUTURE SCOPE

IoT and ML being a leading technology in today's world have made many groundbreaking contributions to the field of medical science. This will have a significant impact on healthcare and medical field in coming days. To understand the significance of this salient technology, let's look at a few of its practical applications in today's time.

5.12.1 Cardiac care

These days heart-related diseases have become one of the major killers of life. Hence, it is the need of the hour to ensure that such conditions and diseases are detected early to avoid catastrophe. Wearable devices are one most portable and compact form of technology. Hence, it is rather logical to involve them in the fight against these diseases. ML algorithms are used to detect irregular heartbeats and in case of any critical event, an alert is sent to the concerned authorities.

5.12.2 Asthma and COPD management

The rapid rise of pollution and various other environmental disturbances has led to an unprecedented rise in the number of asthma and COPD cases. These chronic diseases can lead to discomfort and even deadly conditions. The advanced ML models can be used to predict the incidence of these diseases and subsequently prevent them by detecting changes in lung function and air quality surrounding the patient. Thus, preventive and necessary steps such as avoiding the harmful environment can be initiated.

5.12.3 Telemedicine and remote consultations

With the influx in online presence, every field has prominently found itself face-to-face with modernization and existence in the online domain. Soon the online fever spread on to engulf the medical field too. These days most patient–doctor appointments take place online, decreasing the stress of traveling on the patients. It provides for a flexible environment where the patient can interact and communicate with the doctors even far away, which might not have been feasible otherwise. This has increased the quality of treatment most importantly because the ML models also help the doctors analyze images and X-rays efficiently leading to effective diagnosis of the disease and prior treatments.

5.12.4 Epidemiological surveillance

An epidemic will lead to loss of millions of precious lives. History proves that such epidemics not only disrupt the day-to-day life activities of the people but also lead to long-term chaos and panic among both the affected and unaffected people. Through real-time analysis of the hospital records, data from temperature sensors, social media, and health authorities, ML algorithms help us predict the chances for an epidemic and prepare us in advance for a catastrophe.

It is quite evident from the critical study of IoT and ML that the incorporation of these technologies in medical field bring with it a wave of unprecedented efficiency. But it is necessary to still fill the potholes in the technology. These widespread applications of IoT in the medical field are helpful and crucial but not perfect. More intelligent and complex devices are required for the efficient tracking, diagnosis, and treatment of these diseases. Though their use has been spotlighted in the recent years, it is necessary to understand that there are gaps in the technology due to insufficient expertise and resources in the medical field providing us with a huge scope and opportunity of improvement in the use of IoT and ML in the medical field.

5.13 CONCLUSION

IoT and ML have a great potential to change the course of life. They can be used as a powerful weapon in affecting the great masses in a huge number and leaving a mammoth positive impact on the mankind. One of the most influential fields for this technological advancement is the medical field which holds a great value in affecting the lives of a common man.

From developing technical algorithms for IGS to developing wearable technologies, the wide diversity of the targets that it targets gives it a upper hand in the modern-day medical facilities and it is a great time to unleash the strength of this technological advancement.

AI and ML is set to be a great combination and would bring about the next big revolution in the medical advances. Its super high accuracy and the memory development for the AI and the overall process of its invention, innovation, and the effective diffusion of the entire thought process and this sudden outburst of this technology make it exactly on point.

We have often witnessed failures in surgeries and the great disappointment behind the late detection of cancer cells in humans. The combination of IoT technology with computer-aided surgery has facilitated the existing system to communicate more effectively and has already started showing its utility in these fields. These technological advancements need more and more data from a wide variety of diversity and this process will keep on evolving over the period of time. The advances these studies will show is set to be an exponential curve. Continuous efforts would be needed over the period of time to make the system more and more sublime and the memory algorithms need to be updated continuously.

Furthermore, the synergy of AI, ML, and IoT has streamlined medical workflows and optimized resource allocation. Healthcare providers can leverage predictive analytics to anticipate patient needs, reducing wait times, and enhancing at the same time operational efficiency. Remote patient monitoring through IoT devices along with AI-powered algorithms has empowered the medical framework to proactively intervene in critical situations, and ultimately create an impact by saving a huge number of lives.

The convergence of these three big fields – AI, ML, IoT – holds immense potential for further futuristic breakthroughs. More rigorous research and development in these fields will likely lead to more sophisticated tools and advanced options and thereby advanced patient care. However, it is very important to remember that technology can only enhance medical practices in the long run, but the human touch and clinical expertise remain irreplaceable.

REFERENCES

1. Puja Gupta and Shruti Garg, "Breast cancer prediction using varying parameters of machine learning models." *Procedia Computer Science*, vol. 171, pp. 593–601, 2020.
2. Sumaiya Dabeer, Maha Mohammed Khan and Saiful Islam, "Cancer diagnosis in histopathological image: CNN based approach." *Informatics in Medicine Unlocked*, vol. 16, p. 100231, 2019.
3. Yawei Li, Xin Wu, Ping Yang, Guoqian Jiang and Yuan Luo, "Machine learning for lung cancer diagnosis, treatment, and prognosis." *Genomics Proteomics Bioinformatics*, vol. 20, pp. 850–866, 2020.
4. M. C. Yip, D. G. Lowe, S. E. Salcudean, R. N. Rohling and C. Y. Nguan, "Tissue tracking and registration for image-guided surgery." *IEEE Transactions on Medical Imaging.* vol. 31, no. 11, pp. 2169–2182, 2012.
5. H. G. Kenngott, J. Neuhaus, B. P. Müller-Stich, I. Wolf, M. Vetter, H. P. Meinzer, J. Köninger, M. W. Büchler and C. N. Gutt. "Development of a navigation system for minimally invasive esophagectomy," *Surgical Endoscopy.* vol. 22, no. 8, pp. 1858–1865, 2008. doi: 10.1007/s00464-007-9723-9.
6. J. B. West and C. R. Maurer, "Designing optically tracked instruments for image-guided surgery." *IEEE Transactions on Medical Imaging.* vol. 23, no. 5, pp. 533–545, 2004.

7. Qinyong Lin, Rongqian Yang, Zhiyu Dai, Huazhou Chen and Ken Cai, "Automatic registration method using EM sensors in the IoT operating room." *EURASIP Journal on Wireless Communications and Networking*, vol. 2020, 2020. doi: 10.1186/s13638-020-01754-w.

8. B. Pradhan, D. Bharti, S. Chakravarty, S. S. Ray, V. V. Voinova, A. P. Bonartsev and K. Pal, "Internet of Things and robotics in transforming current-day health-care services." *Journal of Healthcare Engineering*, vol. 2021, p. 9999504, 2021. doi: 10.1155/2021/9999504.

9. M. K. Ishak and N. M. Kit, "Design and implementation of robot assisted surgery based on Internet of Things (IoT)," *2017 International Conference on Advanced Computing and Applications (ACOMP)*, Ho Chi Minh City, Vietnam, 2017, pp. 65–70. doi: 10.1109/ACOMP.2017.20.

10. H. Su et al., "Internet of Things (IoT)-based Collaborative Control of a Redundant Manipulator for Teleoperated Minimally Invasive Surgeries." *2020 IEEE International Conference on Robotics and Automation (ICRA)*, Paris, France, 2020, pp. 9737–9742. doi: 10.1109/ICRA40945.2020.9197321.

11. S. Tanabe et al., "Designing a robotic smart home for everyone, especially the elderly and people with disabilities." *Fujita Medical Journal*, vol. 5, no. 2, pp. 31–35, 2019. doi: 10.20407/fmj.2018-009.

12. Md. Rahman, F. M. Shamrat, Mohammod Kashem, Most Akter, Sovon Chakraborty, Marzia Ahmed and Shobnom Mustary, "Internet of Things based electrocardiogram monitoring system using machine learning algo-rithm." *International Journal of Electrical and Computer Engineering*, vol. 12, pp. 3739–3751, 2022. 10.11591/ijece.v12i4.

13. S. Hiremath, G. Yang and K. Mankodiya, "Wearable Internet of Things: Concept architectural components and promises for person-centered health-care." *2014 4th International Conference on Wireless Mobile Communication and Healthcare-Transforming Healthcare through Innovations in Mobile and Wireless Technologies (MOBIHEALTH)*, 2014, pp. 304–307.

14. Yogesh Kumar Sharma and S. Khatal Sunil. "Health care patient monitoring using IoT and machine learning," IOSR Journal of Engineering (IOSR JEN), pp. 2278–8719, 2019.

Chapter 6

Ovarian cancer detection using IoT-based intelligent assistant and blockchain technology

Mohsen Ghorbian and Saeid Ghorbian

6.1 INTRODUCTION

Ovarian cancer is women's most common and dangerous disease and may appear without specific symptoms. Ovarian cancer generally has two forms, including epithelial and squamous cells. In this disease, diagnosis in the early stages of the disease formation is more likely for the patient to recover fully. However, in the advanced stages of the disease, the treatment process becomes more complicated, and the possibility of complete recovery decreases. Despite the importance of accurately diagnosing ovarian cancer recurrences, unfortunately, there is no way to prevent the recurrence of this disease after a patient has recovered. As a result, it is essential to understand the symptoms of ovarian cancer, to receive early diagnosis, and to receive timely treatment to reduce the chances of its recurrence and increase the chances of recovery (Stewart et al., 2019). New technologies, such as the IoT, permit the exchange of information and data between different objects and systems. This technology allows communication between objects and systems in various fields such as transportation, energy, health, environment, and agriculture. In healthcare, the IoT can be used as a new and advanced method to improve the efficiency and effectiveness of care. Therefore, this technology provides unique features to improve users' quality of life. It can provide better healthcare, prevent diseases, and reduce health costs. Wearable or nonwearable devices such as blood pressure gauges, blood sugar meters, weight scales, and thermometers can investigate health and submit personal health information to healthcare systems online. Therefore, the recurrence of diseases such as ovarian cancer can be monitored and diagnosed in time using the data sent from the patient's condition. IoT in healthcare can improve the care process, prevent diseases, and reduce health costs (Hamza et al., 2020). With the help of machine learning (ML), healthcare systems can obtain more and more accurate information about diseases, their diagnosis, and the effects of their treatments. ML is one of the most advanced and new technologies in various health fields. Hence, ML in healthcare can improve the diagnosis, treatment, and prevention of diseases such as ovarian cancer recurrence. By analyzing big data and applying unique algorithms, care and treatment systems can achieve greater

DOI: 10.1201/9781003487647-6

accuracy in diagnosing diseases, determining appropriate treatments, and enhancing patient health monitoring (Chen et al., 2021). Blockchain technology is a new technology that enables the encryption and verification of information through distributed networks to store and transmit it. It is also used in healthcare due to its high level of security and transparency. Hence, patients' medical information, disease histories, and other medical information can be securely stored using blockchain technology. Through this process, the doctors who will be treating the patient in the future will have easy access to all of the patient's medical information, allowing them to provide the best possible treatment. Additionally, they can assess the quality of treatment provided to the patient (Hölbl et al., 2018). In this chapter, an attempt has been made to integrate three technologies – Internet of Things (IoT), ML, and blockchain – to provide an intelligent assistant. Hence, the proposed intelligent assistant used in a scenario involves analysis of the state of ovarian cancer patients who have relapsed and prioritizes them based on their status.

The structure of this chapter is as follows: As a starting point, the first part examines the necessary prerequisites such as ovarian cancer, IoT in healthcare, ML in healthcare, and blockchain in healthcare. The second section examines blockchain and ML in healthcare through subsets such as a review of ML classification mechanisms, HLF blockchain structure as a permission-based blockchain, and ovarian cancer detection techniques. The third section comprehensively examines integrating blockchain and ML in IoT healthcare. In the fourth section, a hybrid framework is proposed to provide an intelligent assistant mechanism in IoT healthcare. Finally, the fifth section concludes this discussion.

6.2 PRELIMINARIES

This section presents information and terminology regarding ovarian cancer, IoT, ML, and blockchain technology. Furthermore, IoT technology can provide a means to monitor patients with ovarian cancer posttreatment to detect disease recurrence likelihood more quickly and increase survival rates. Also, using ML technology, referred to as an AI subset technology, provides an intelligent assistant capable of analyzing and evaluating data obtained from IoT devices concerning patients' health status. Additionally, to ensure the secure implementation of IoT and ML technologies in the form of intelligent assistants for use in the healthcare domain, other technologies, such as blockchain, can also be used to ensure the secure implementation of information exchange processes.

6.2.1 Ovarian cancer

Ovarian cancer is one of the most dangerous forms of cancer in women. In the early stages of this disease, symptoms may include abdominal pain, swelling, weight loss, anorexia, and fatigue. Due to the lack of specific symptoms in the early stages of the disease, these symptoms tend to make it difficult to diagnose (Saeedi and Ghorbian, 2020). Several risk factors are associated with ovarian cancer, including age, family history of ovarian cancer, and history of never being pregnant, and using synthetic sex hormones. Generally, the probability of infection of ovarian cancer increases after age 40 but can occur anytime during a woman's life. Women over 50 (postmenopausal women) are most likely to suffer from ovarian cancer, but it has also been a likelihood in women under 40. This disease can be diagnosed with imaging methods such as ultrasound, CT scan, and MRI. In addition to imaging techniques, tests that detect the presence of a specific type of protein called CA-125 must also be performed to confirm the presence of this disease. The most effective treatment option for ovarian cancer includes surgery to remove the ovary, chemotherapy, radiotherapy, or a combination of the two, to reduce the tumor's size, control the symptoms, and prevent its spread. Hence, patients with early diagnosis are more likely to be successful in undergoing treatment (Guo et al., 2019).

6.2.2 IoT in healthcare

IoT technology is one of the most important tools for improving individuals' and society's quality of life and health. With the help of this technology, medical devices, wearable devices, smart devices, and other objects can communicate with one another, as well as the Internet. Through these connections, it is possible to check on a person's body condition and health regularly, prevent diseases, diagnose diseases early, and follow up on their treatment. IoT technology has a wide range of applications in healthcare. Some of these applications include the following:

- Utilizing the Internet to periodically monitor the status of diseases and follow up on treatment with medical devices.
- Monitoring a person's health status by wearing wearable devices, such as measuring heart rate, blood pressure, and activity level.
- Using wearable devices to detect cardiovascular diseases like atrial fibrillation can significantly improve the process and speed of diagnosis.

It is also possible to improve healthcare services at home through IoT technology. People can, for instance, monitor their health status automatically with wearable devices and IoT systems without needing physical presence from their doctor, and they can automatically alert their doctor if any problems occur. Therefore, using IoT technology in healthcare as an effective tool can significantly improve the quality of life and health of individuals, society, and the environment. Additionally, advancing this technology by providing more capability will make it more valuable and efficient (Saji et al., 2021). Figure 6.1 depicts the mechanism and structure of using IoT

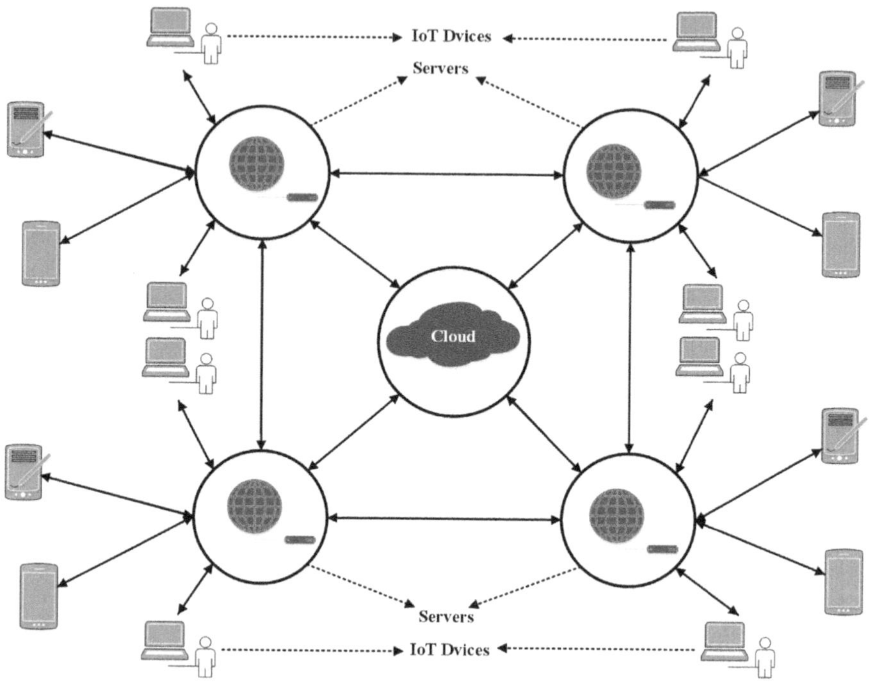

Figure 6.1 The IoT architecture. (*Source:* Author's own.)

technology. The IoT devices can send the information they collect to servers. On the other hand, servers can share information among themselves to exchange data. The servers are capable of storing the data received in the cloud environment. By storing data in a cloud environment, other servers can access the data.

6.2.3 ML in healthcare

ML is one of the subsets of AI technology that has played an essential and prominent role in healthcare. Implementing ML in healthcare makes it possible to improve healthcare quality, reduce treatment costs, and improve society's general well-being, thus contributing to a better quality of life. Due to the ever-increasing growth of medical data, ML can help improve the accuracy and speed of disease diagnosis, predict disease outcomes, improve chronic disease management, and prevent new diseases from arising. Hence, it is possible to achieve future health system improvement plans by integrating medical data and ML methods. To ensure the successful use of these methods, accuracy and exactness must be stressed in data collection and processing, as well as collaboration between medical professionals and physicians. Several applications of ML in the domain of healthcare are as follows – disease diagnosis, prediction of disease outcomes, prediction of blood sugar levels, and diagnosis of medical images. In general, due to the large amount of data in the healthcare field, ML can be used to improve efficiency and accuracy in diagnosing diseases, predicting disease outcomes, predicting drug combinations, analyzing medical images, and many other health-related tasks. Considering the ever-growing collection of medical data and the advancement of technology, ML is likely to play a significant role in improving healthcare (Manickam et al., 2022).

6.2.4 Blockchain in healthcare

Blockchain technology has been recognized as an essential and effective tool in healthcare due to its capabilities. Hence, blockchain technology can store medical information in encrypted blocks and make it available to relevant audiences. In addition to improving access to medical information, this mechanism can reduce medical errors and solve data security issues and privacy protection. A blockchain system, for instance, can allow any doctor with access to the patient's medical data to access it very quickly and safely without contacting the patient's previous physician. Additionally, the ability to track changes in a patient's medical record using blockchain blocks reduces medical errors and prevents unauthorized people from misusing patients' data and privacy (Alhadhrami et al., 2017). Using blockchain technology in tracking drugs can also help ensure that the drugs are authentic and of high quality. A blockchain-based system, for instance, allows for tracking information about the manufacturer, the production date, the production location, the distribution route, and the drug's expiration date (Bell et al., 2018). Blockchain technology can be used as an effective tool for preventing fraud in medical research, which can also be used in healthcare. Blockchain technology can ensure the authenticity and traceability of medical research by encrypting data and information used in research and storing them in encrypted blocks. (Park and Ryu, 2019). Generally, blockchain technology has been recognized as an invaluable tool in health and healthcare because it facilitates access to medical information, reduces medical errors, prevents medical research fraud, and manages health systems. Moreover, it helps prevent and deal with epidemics.

6.3 BLOCKCHAIN AND ML IN HEALTHCARE DOMAIN

Using ML and blockchain in healthcare could be viewed as a new approach to solving health-related problems due to the characteristics of these two technologies. In ML, powerful algorithms employ various approaches, which analyze data and then present the results as patterns that can be used. This technology can be highly beneficial and effective in various fields such as healthcare. One of the applications that this technology can have in the healthcare field is to use its capabilities to provide the basis for early diagnosis of diseases. Due to the nature of some diseases, any delay in the diagnosis process of these diseases can have irreparable consequences, as they are known to be difficult to diagnose. The use of ML technology in healthcare can be associated with challenges. To analyze the condition of patients using ML techniques, patients and medical centers need to share their data with researchers; however, since data and information in healthcare are so sensitive and vital, few patients and medical centers are willing to share their data. Researchers can implement ML algorithms on these datasets. However, using ML technology in medical centers is not routine and is primarily a research tool for researcher's use. Blockchain technology has the potential to be applied widely to healthcare due to its powerful encryption algorithms and mechanisms. Blockchains can be classified into various types. Public blockchains are commonly known as cryptocurrencies, such as Bitcoin and Ethereum, and are used by the general public. Permission-based blockchains are another type of these blockchains. Due to their customization ability, these blockchains provide exceptional strength and flexibility. Organizations and companies can customize this type of blockchain to meet their specific needs. HLF is one of these permission-based blockchains. The customization capabilities offered by this blockchain allow it to be applied to a wide variety of fields, particularly in healthcare. A blockchain of this type can be used in a field such as healthcare to ensure that any data-sharing process is conducted safely and securely, thanks to the security-presented mechanisms it provides. Consequently, the concerns related to disclosing the identity and information of individuals or patients and medical centers are removed to a very high degree. In other words, by implementing this technology, there are fewer concerns about unauthorized individuals misusing patient information (Mantey et al., 2022).

6.3.1 ML classification mechanisms

ML technology enables computers to learn from their input data and make predictions, recognize patterns, and make decisions based on the knowledge gained from the input data. To accomplish this, ML algorithms such as NN, DT, and SVM are utilized, depending on the application and goals being addressed. It is possible to analyze big data automatically and optimally using this technology, helping to make accurate predictions and decisions in various fields. Healthcare experts can use ML to diagnose diseases and predict future diseases, and financial professionals can use it to forecast stock returns and assess investment risks. Further, the industry can also use ML to optimize production processes and maintain product quality. In the field of smart cars, this technology can be used to improve the performance of self-driving cars and prevent road accidents. ML is used in numerous fields, including medicine, finance, industry, computer games, smart cars, etc., due to its high processing capacity and ability to analyze and learn from data. Hence, ML approaches are used to accomplish this, which vary depending on the type of data and problem to be solved. Examples of ML approaches include the following:

- *Supervised Learning:* In this type of learning, input data is provided to the algorithm along with examples of them, referred to as labels, classes, or features, and the algorithm learns how to respond to new inputs based upon these labels. Instances of this type of learning include image recognition, speech recognition, and gender recognition.
- *Unsupervised Learning:* By using this type of learning, the algorithm only uses the input data without any labels and attempts to identify patterns and relationships within the data without any labels. Text topic categorization, Internet forum exploration, and data clustering are examples of this type of learning.
- *Reinforcement Learning:* During this type of learning, the agent interacts with its environment and attempts to learn the path that leads to more rewards by receiving rewards or penalties from the environment at various stages. In addition to computer games and intelligent robots, resource management, such as communication networks, can also be used to demonstrate the application of this type of learning.
- *Deep Learning:* This type of learning involves employing deep neural networks to learn complex patterns and identify visual and audio patterns. Many artificial intelligence applications utilize this method, including face recognition, machine translation, music playback, and self-driving vehicles.

It is important to note that various ML techniques can be used to solve different problems, depending on the type of data and the problem to be solved. Recent developments in this field allow researchers to solve more complex problems with ML in the future (Janiesch et al., 2021). The architecture of ML technology is illustrated in Figure 6.2. The first step of the ML process involves converting collected data into a standard format. This data can include data collected from the environment by the IoT devices and storing them on servers. The database object stores the appropriate data in the defined format in the next step. It is crucial to perform a critical pre-processing stage on the database data before implementing ML algorithms and techniques to prepare the data according to the selected algorithm. After the data preparation stage, ML algorithms will be implemented on the data to obtain patterns. The final step involves analyzing and interpreting patterns, which will result in knowledge creation.

6.3.2 HLF blockchain structure

The HLF platform is an open-source blockchain platform designed for commercial applications. This platform provides security, transparency, and reliability for financial and non-financial transactions through blockchain technology. The use of HLF in various industries such as banking, insurance,

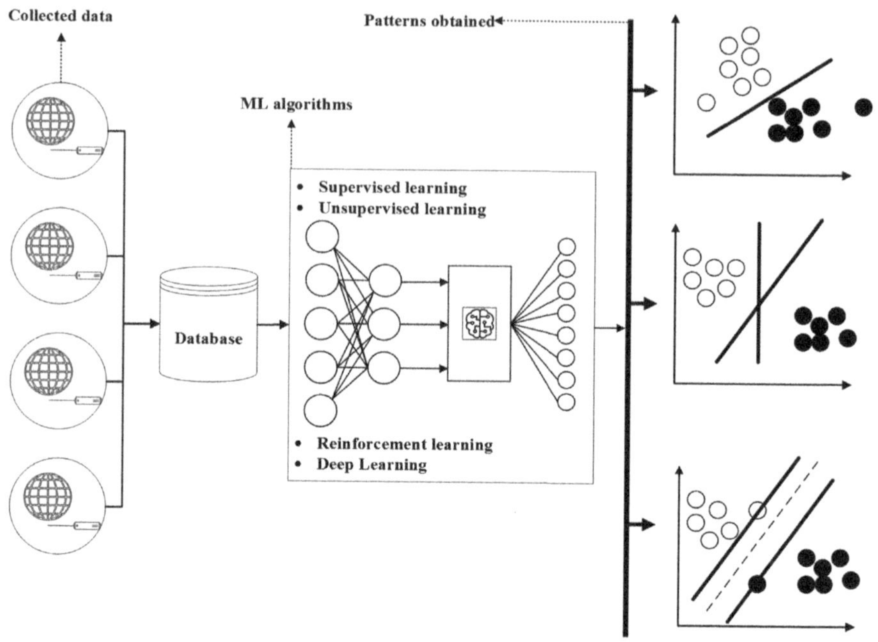

Figure 6.2 The ML architecture. (*Source:* Author's own.)

logistics, and supply chain increases the security of financial transactions, reduces transaction costs, increases speed and efficiency in processing transactions, and improves transparency in transactions and reviews. A modular architecture is employed by HLF, which includes various components, including a blockchain network, a chain of blocks, planning nodes, ordering nodes, and validation nodes. In the HLF blockchain network, several nodes run independently and communicate with each other. These nodes can include peer nodes, ordering nodes, and validation nodes. Each block in a chain of blocks contains a confirmation of a transaction by the network nodes. On the other hand, each block contains information such as a unique identifier, a time stamp, transaction information, and a digital signature. HLF utilizes set consensus algorithms such as practical Byzantine fault tolerance (PBFT) to verify the transactions. The consensus algorithms employ a combination of collective voting and digital verification to prove confirmations sent by the network nodes. The HLF platform utilizes smart contracts known as chaincode to perform transactions. With smart contracts, conditions are determined for transactions. Blockchain data is stored in NoSQL databases such as LevelDB and CouchDB by default in HLF. This platform also uses the access control list (ACL) structure to manage access to blockchain data, allowing different users and nodes to access different types of blockchain data. In addition to the ability to execute private transactions, HLF also supports various programming languages such as Java, JavaScript, Python, and Go, private and cloud networks, tools for network management,

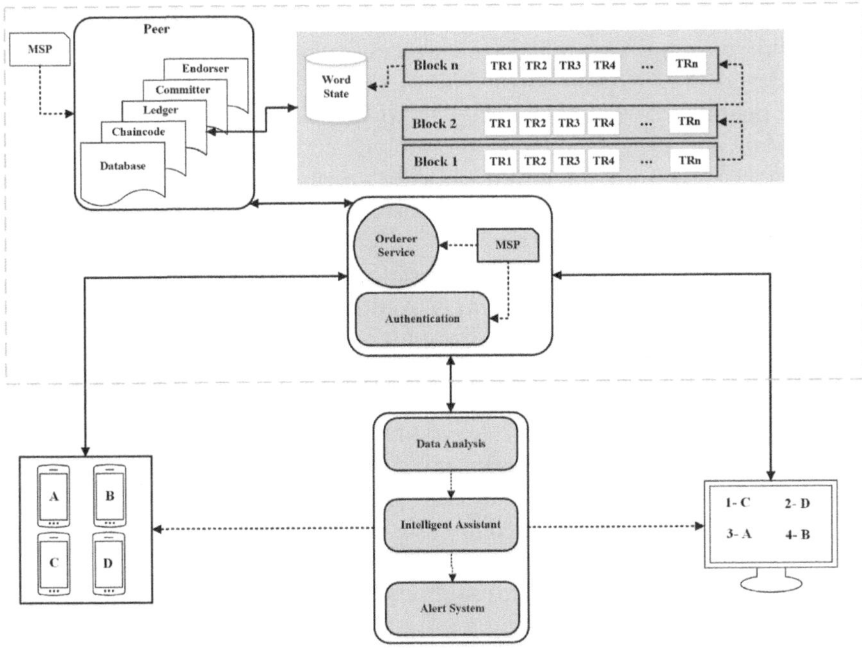

Figure 6.3 The HLF blockchain structure. (*Source:* Author's own.)

and data transfer between different networks (Uddin et al., 2021). The HLF blockchain structure is demonstrated in Figure 6.3. The following is a description of the primary features of this structure:

- *Orderer Service:* In HLF, the Orderer Service is one of the main components of the blockchain, responsible for facilitating the creation and verification of transactions within the network. In addition, this component serves as the primary authority for verifying transactions on the network. The Orderer Service maintains the order of transactions in new blocks, resulting in different transactions being placed in different blocks in their chronological order, which prevents problems such as the loss of transactions or changing their order in blocks from occurring.
- *Membership Service Provider (MSP):* The MSP in HLF is one of the most critical components of the blockchain and is responsible for managing users' identity and access to the network. In addition to verifying the identity of users, managing permissions and access, implementing security policies, and protecting sensitive network information are the responsibility of this component. As part of MSP's responsibilities, digital certificates are also generated and managed to identify individuals and devices in the network. Hence, this is accomplished using ECDSA and SHA-256 encryption and digital signature algorithms (Goswami et al., 2020).

- *Peers (Peer Node, Committer, and Endorser):* In HLF, peer nodes, endorsers, and committers all are essential components in executing and verifying transactions. One of the critical components of HLF is the peer node, which stores blockchain blocks and executes transactions sent on the network. One or more blockchain databases can be on each Peer Node, endorsing and anchoring peers. Peers that endorse transactions validate the transactions sent to the network. Endorsers ensure that transactions sent to the network are valid and digitally signed. This signature is then sent to the Orderer Service, which creates new blocks containing the transactions approved by the Endorsing Peers. A committer is a peer responsible for applying verified transactions to blockchain blocks. The Endorsing Peers receive new blocks from the Orderer Service, insert their transactions into the blocks, and then store them in the blockchain database after confirming their transactions.

- *Ledger:* HLF Ledger component stores and manages the blockchain database, comprising two key components. The State Database provides information about the current state of the network's data. As a result, this database contains data information available on the HLF network and can be used for new transactions. Each type of data in this database can be easily accessed using a unique key. In addition, the Transaction Log contains all the transactions carried out on the HLF network. For each transaction in the HLF network, the log contains information such as the transaction ID, execution time, operator specifications, and the result. The log is organized chronologically from the first transaction to the last transaction (Androulaki et al., 2018).

6.3.3 Ovarian cancer detection techniques

Ovarian cancer is one type of cancer in women that starts in the ovaries, the tissue where the ovaries' production occurs. Although ovarian cancer can occur in any age group, it is more common among women over 50. Women with a family history of ovarian cancer should also undergo genetic counseling and periodic examinations by a specialist physician. There are several early symptoms of ovarian cancer, including headaches, abdominal pain, vaginal discharge, bloating, weight changes, and periods. As the disease progresses, symptoms may include severe abdominal pain, abdominal swelling, shortness of breath, fever, general weakness, and bleeding from the vaginal area. Several methods of diagnosing ovarian cancer include blood tests, ultrasounds, mammography, and clinical examinations. The diagnosis of ovarian cancer can be accomplished in a variety of ways:

- *Blood Tests:* In this method, they seek to find disease markers. Disease markers are markers produced by cancer that blood tests can detect. In ovarian cancer, CA-125, HE4, and CEACAM are commonly detected disease markers.

- *Ultrasound:* In this method, ultrasound waves are used to produce images of the internal structure of the ovary. In addition to diagnosing the disease, ultrasound can also be used to monitor the growth of small tumors.
- *Mammography:* In this method, a diagnostic image is taken from the ovaries using X-rays and then examined by a physician. This method is commonly used in cases of ovarian cancer in women with a family history of the disease.

The treatment for ovarian cancer will depend on the stage of the disease, the type of cells, the size and characteristics of the tumor, and other factors. Treatment for ovarian cancer is determined by factors such as the stage of the disease, tumor size, cell type, and the patient's age and general health. It is sometimes necessary to remove the cancerous ovaries and fallopian tubes through surgery. Additionally, chemotherapy and radiotherapy are effective treatments (Elezaby et al., 2019).

6.4 INTEGRATING BLOCKCHAIN AND ML IN IoT HEALTHCARE

Using and implementing new technologies has always been more challenging and complex in healthcare than in other fields. During the past few years, IoT technology has been one of the novel technologies in the healthcare field that have been welcomed to some extent. As a result of its unique features and facilities, IoT technology has been able to address a significant portion of healthcare challenges. However, many challenges are generally related to lacking facilities, equipment, and specialists. Since healthcare has always faced challenges and shortages in the sectors related to facilities, equipment, and specialists, such challenges and problems can adversely affect the health of many patients. People suffering from serious diseases usually must be supervised by doctors and specialists after treatment. Therefore, performing the care process after treatment is very important (Ghorbian and Ghobaei-Arani, 2023). Some of the most important reasons for combining technologies in healthcare systems are discussed below.

- *Declining Healthcare Field Issues with IoT Technology:* Patients suffering from serious diseases such as cancer will require more posttreatment care than other patients. Because the disease can recur in people who are infected with this disease, these patients must be constantly under the supervision and control of specialists and doctors. Since healthcare is facing many issues, continuous patient care and control are proving to be challenging, and not all patients can benefit from this benefit. The IoT technology can address some of the issues raised, but significant and troubling issues remain. The use of the IoT, in turn, can solve the issue of the lack of equipment to control and monitor the condition of patients. However, doctors and specialists need to examine the condition of patients to determine their condition. As a result, the issue in this sector can be attributed to the shortage of healthcare doctors and specialists. Specialists must examine and evaluate those whose condition is dangerous as soon as possible. Hence, any delay in examining the dangerous condition of patients can cause irreparable damage. On the other hand, the condition of patients who are not dangerous can be checked with a little delay because it will not be very effective to delay checking their condition.

- *Reducing Healthcare Field Challenges with ML Technology:* One of the challenges patients generally face is waiting long to access their doctors and specialists. This challenge is more about appointment systems traditionally for patients. This mechanism allows patients to access doctors regardless of their health condition, which may pose a challenge for patients with poor health. Hence, patients' access to doctors and specialists should be determined by their condition, so those in a bad and serious state should have priority access. In light of the lack of traditional doctors and specialists and access mechanisms, it is also necessary to have a modern mechanism to determine patient access based on patients' conditions, which will solve many of the challenges associated with this field. ML technology can be highly beneficial and efficient in this case. With its powerful algorithms, ML technology can achieve patterns by examining the data and information received from patients, which can determine the condition of patients using these patterns. By checking the condition of patients, ML technology can determine the level of their condition. Consequently, this technology will be able to diagnose dangerous patients and place them on the priority list for specialist examination.

- *Overcoming IoT Challenges by Using HLF Technology:* IoT technology always faces the challenge of insecure connections between devices, which allows abusive individuals to access the data exchanged between them. One challenge in this field is that healthcare and treatment centers and patients are generally unwilling to share their data and information due to privacy protection and misuse concerns. As a result, these two issues have always been raised as barriers to the application and use of new technologies in healthcare. Due to their unique features in the data encryption process, blockchain technology, especially permission-based blockchains, provides the opportunity to overcome these challenges. Blockchain technology based on permissions, such as Hyperledger Fabric, allows companies to customize blockchains based on their corporate policies. Therefore, this technology can completely secure the data exchange process between IoT devices. Due to its powerful and complex cryptographic mechanisms, this technology can alleviate concerns regarding the lack of patient privacy protection and abuse of patient identity and information to a great extent. Therefore, integrating IoT, ML, and blockchain technologies can solve many healthcare challenges (Shahbazi and Byun, 2021).

6.5 INTELLIGENT ASSISTANT MECHANISM IN IoT HEALTHCARE

Using new technologies in sensitive areas such as healthcare can bring unique advantages and challenges. Hence, using IoT technology in healthcare, besides presenting unique advantages, can also present challenges. Therefore, other technologies can also be employed to overcome these challenges and concerns. New technologies such as blockchain and ML can significantly reduce the challenges and concerns of this technology.

This section uses AI to propose an automated decision-making mechanism. Hence, a scenario in healthcare is utilized to illustrate the automatic decision-making mechanism performance known as an intelligent assistant by using ML technology as one of the subbranches of AI and other novel technologies such as the IoT and blockchain. The proposed scenario focuses on patients who have recovered from ovarian cancer. Due to the possibility of the disease recurrence, these people must be controlled and cared for even after partial recovery. It is, therefore, essential to monitor their health status after recovery to diagnose and treat recurrences faster in case of a likelihood of ill recurrence, dramatically increasing these patients' chances of recovery and survival. Various methods are available to check the health status of people who have recovered from ovarian cancer. One of these methods is checking the amount of particular proteins in the patient's body. Recurrences of ovarian cancer are characterized by a high level of specific cancer antigens in the blood. Known as CA-125, this antigen is a glycoprotein produced by many ovarian cancer cells. It is possible to monitor the recurrence of ovarian cancer and the effect of various treatment options by measuring the levels of CA-125 in the blood. Several factors determine the amount of CA-125 in the blood, including age, gender, pregnancy, menstruation period, and other diseases associated with ovarian cancer. An increase in CA-125 in the blood may indicate cancer recurrence, as a normal level of CA-125 is less than 35 units per million (U/mL). The presence of CA-125 in patients with ovarian cancer is two to three times higher than the upper limit of normal (i.e., over 100 U/mL), and this amount of CA-125 can be considered a sign of ovarian cancer recurrence. However, it is essential to note that an increase in CA-125 in the blood can be considered a factor in ovarian cancer recurrence. Therefore, a combination of clinical symptoms, imaging tests, and blood tests should be considered when diagnosing ovarian cancer. In this scenario, the size and amount of CA-125 protein in the blood will determine the state of the patient's health. The person's condition is described as dangerous when the CA-125 protein level exceeds a certain threshold, such as 80 U/mL.

In the proposed mechanism, the patient will measure the amount of CA-125 protein in his blood using instruments such as a little blood test machine at several stages and time intervals. The measured values as data are then sent to the proposed system using IoT technology. Patients must first authenticate themselves in the system before sending their data. Next, patients can send their data after their identity is verified. With access to patients' data, the intelligent assistant analyzes the increasing trend of CA-125 protein in their blood and predicts the amount and speed of this protein increase (Matsuhashi et al., 2017). Therefore, the system estimates the patient's future condition based on the predictions it has made. As a result of this situation being recognized as dangerous, the patient will have a higher priority for accessing specialists. Therefore, in this scenario, individuals whose health status is actually in danger can receive higher priority for access to specialists. A mechanism of this nature can cause a decrease in delay in the access process of patients with dangerous conditions to specialists, which can lead to better and more effective treatment for the patient. As shown in Figure 6.4, all steps of the proposed mechanism are depicted as sequence diagrams. The following are the detailed explanations of each step. In addition, Figure 6.5 illustrates the proposed mechanism's structure and architecture.

In the first stage, clients attempt to communicate with the proposed system using embedded IoT devices after receiving information about the dose and

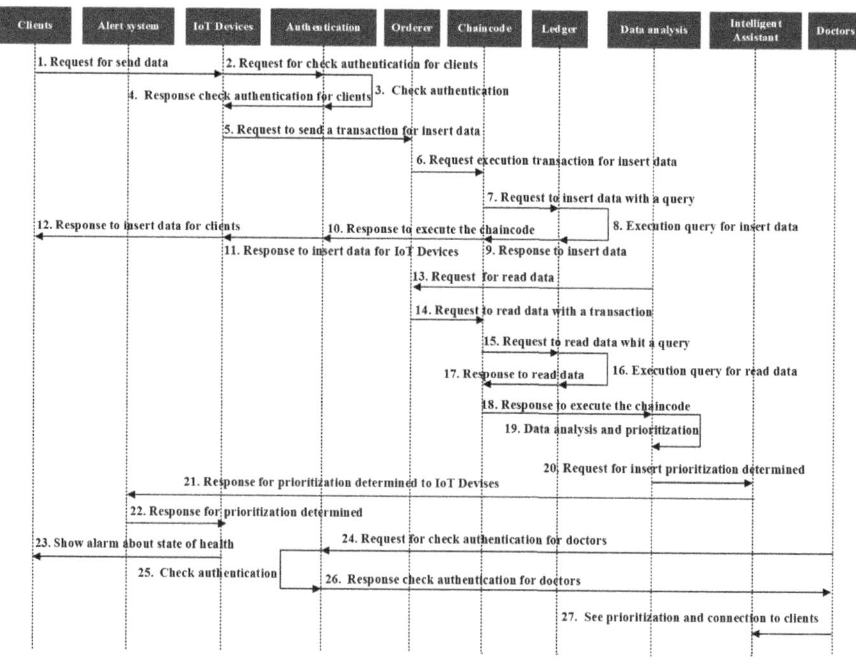

Figure 6.4 Implementation of an intelligent assistant based on IoT, blockchain technology, and ML. (*Source:* Author's own.)

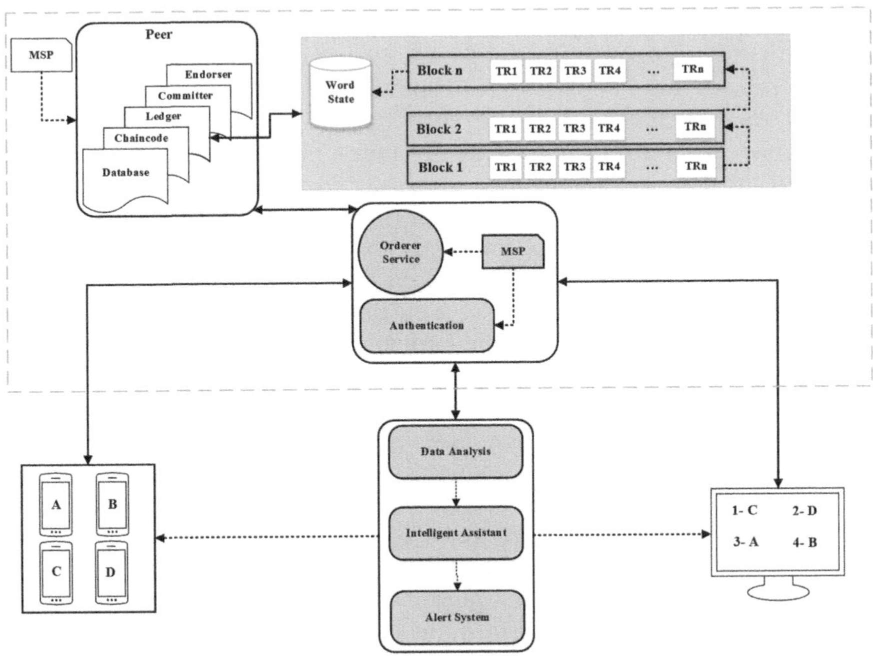

Figure 6.5 Propose an intelligent assistant mechanism for IoT healthcare applications to diagnose ovarian cancer recurrences. (*Source:* Author's owner.)

quantity of CA-125 protein (step 1). Next, to access the embedded system and prevent unauthorized devices from accessing it, IoT devices must authenticate first, so they send a request to the embedded authentication mechanism (step 2). The authentication mechanism attempts to check and verify the identity of requesting IoT devices (step 3). As soon as the authentication mechanism check result has been determined, the IoT devices get the result of the check process in the form of a response from the authentication mechanism (step 4). Next, to record the information received from clients, IoT devices attempt to send requests as transactions to the Orderer Service component after their identity has been confirmed. IoT device requests are placed in the Orderer Service queue after being approved by the Endorsers and will be executed in the order in the next step (step 5). Orderer Service requests are sent in a request format to Chaincode for processing and execution (step 6). Following the completion of processing the submitted requests in Chaincode, the submitted requests or transactions are sent in the form of a query to the Ledger so that they can perform the data storage process (step 7). As soon as Ledger receives a request from Chaincode, it attempts to execute the sent transactions containing patient data by executing a query and storing them in its database (step 8). Upon recording the information, the ledger attempts to inform Chaincode about the successful data storage in the database (step 9). The next step is for Chaincode to submit a response to the authentication mechanism informing it of the successful data storage (step 10). When the authentication mechanism receives the response of successful data insertion into the blockchain-enabled database, it attempts to prepare a response and send it to the IoT devices (step 11). As soon as the IoT device receives the response from the authentication mechanism, it attempts to send a response informing the user about the success of the data-sending process (step 12). The process can be repeated by each patient who is a client here several times, and each time the user measures the amount of CA-125 protein in his blood and stores the results in the system. ML technology is used in the second phase to implement the proposed mechanism. During this phase, a section titled Data Analysis is responsible for investigating and analyzing the patient-provided data. Hence, the Data Analysis section submits requests to the Orderer Service to obtain patient data. Following this, the request is placed in the queue to be executed by the Orderer Service (step 13). In the following step, Orderer Service attempts to send a request to Chaincode and requests that it executes the requests for read data (step 14). When Chaincode receives the sent request, it attempts to create a query and send it to the Ledger for read data (step 15). In response to the request to read the information, the Ledger attempts to prepare the information requested by Chaincode in a query (step 16). After reading and preparing the data, the Ledger informs Chaincode that the requested data is ready (step 17). As soon as Chaincode receives the response regarding the readiness of the data, it attempts to prepare an appropriate response and then sends the requested data in the form of a response to the Data Analysis section (step 18). Following receipt of the required information, the Data Analysis department uses powerful algorithms to analyze the data. It is appropriate to analyze the data received from the patients to prioritize the patient's conditions based on existing patterns and the results of the data analysis. The purpose of this section is to diagnose patients who are in bad condition from the viewpoint of the system, and then, based on the score assigned to their condition, these patients are prioritized (step 19). Next, it is necessary to send the results obtained from the Data Analysis section to the Intelligent Assistant section by requesting to record the results and priority (step 20). In this section, the Intelligent Assistant tries to identify patients with a dangerous condition and higher priority by checking the information received from the Data Analysis section and the prioritized patients and sending a response to the Alert System mechanism. The patients may be in the first stages of recurrence based on the increasing trend of CA-125 protein levels in the blood and the predictions made. As a result, the patient must communicate immediately with the appropriate specialist (step 21). The Alert System mechanism generates a response and attempts to send it to the IoT devices (step 22). Next, the IoT devices display an alert to the users indicating their predicted health status (step 23). In the third phase, doctors and specialists must connect to the system. Therefore, they must send an authentication request to the authentication mechanism (step 24). In the next step, the identity of the requesting doctors is checked and verified (step 25). As soon as the identity of the doctors has been confirmed, a response will be sent to them (step 26). By connecting to the system, doctors can see the status of their patients based on the priority set. Consequently, the Intelligent Assistant system aims to communicate with doctors and specialists for high-priority high-risk patients based on the priorities determined by the patient's condition (step 27). As a result of the proposed mechanism and the use of Intelligent Assistant, it is possible to prioritize patients according to their health status in the first stage so that patients with dangerous conditions are prioritized for control and monitoring by the doctors. Hence, by reducing the time spent handling and examining the condition of patients, the treatment process can be started in much less time if necessary, increasing the chance of survival and the effectiveness of the treatment process. As a result, the proposed mechanism has attempted to address all concerns concerning using new technologies.

One of the items that can be considered for future trends is using cloud computing technologies, such as serverless computing. By implementing functions, such technology can optimize energy consumption processes, increase program efficiency, and reduce the financial burden on patients. In addition to providing significant ease of storing patient data, cloud computing may also incur costs for the patient. Serverless computing technology uses a pay-per-use model to reduce the amount of money that users, or in other words, patients, have to pay for the storage of their data on a server.

6.6 CONCLUSION

The expansion of new technologies provides the basis for solving challenges and concerns in sensitive areas such as healthcare. Due to its attractive features and low cost, the IoT technology can be used to control and care for patients. This technology will always raise concerns about the leakage of information and the use of this information by unauthorized individuals. However, patients can communicate with their doctors and specialists by transferring their information using this technology, allowing them to consult about their health status. The lack of specialists and the large number of patients make it challenging to provide access to specialists and doctors to all patients. Hence, in the meantime, people with dangerous health conditions must communicate with specialists and physicians as soon as possible. This chapter has attempted to resolve the challenges and concerns related to the application of IoT technology in healthcare as much as possible by using technologies such as ML and blockchain. Toward this end, a mechanism called the intelligent assistant has been proposed. The proposed intelligent assistant mechanism utilizes ML technology to analyze patient status data in the system. As a next step, the intelligent assistant will attempt to receive data from the data analysis department and prioritize the patient's condition based on data analysis. The communication between patients and specialists will be based on the priority assigned to the patient's status. The prioritization of treatment according to a patient's health condition enables patients with dangerous conditions and those whose condition is continually deteriorating to access specialists earlier, thereby preventing the possibility that a recurrence will occur. Hence, this mechanism can be the treatment of ovarian cancer process but it should be more rapid and effective. In the proposed mechanism, it has been attempted to secure the information exchange process and the access of patients and specialists to the system by utilizing permission-based blockchain technology called HLF. In the proposed mechanism, HLF requires patients, doctors, and specialists to perform first the authentication process to access the system and exchange data. Hence, all communication in the system is entirely secure and encrypted.

In the future, the proposed approach will be investigated by reducing existing complexities and increasing system performance by optimizing connecting to the system and exchanging information to simplify the process. On the other side, by employing new technologies such as cloud computing, the proposed mechanism can be made accessible more extensively and provide the context for the use of more patients.

REFERENCES

Alhadhrami, Z., Alghfeli, S., Alghfeli, M., Abedlla, J. A., & Shuaib, K. Introducing blockchains for healthcare. In 2017 International Conference on Electrical and Computing Technologies and Applications (ICECTA) (pp. 1–4). IEEE, (2017). https://doi.org/10.1109/ICECTA.2017.8252043

Androulaki, E., Barger, A., Bortnikov, V., Cachin, C., Christidis, K., De Caro, A., & Yellick, J. Hyperledger fabric: A distributed operating system for permissioned blockchains. In Proceedings of the Thirteenth EuroSys Conference. ACM, (2018). https://doi.org/10.1145/3190508.3190538

Bell, L., Buchanan, W. J., Cameron, J., & Lo, O. Applications of blockchain within healthcare. Blockchain in Healthcare Today, (2018). https://doi.org/10.30953/bhty.v1.8

Chen, I. Y., Pierson, E., Rose, S., Joshi, S., Ferryman, K., & Ghassemi, M. Ethical machine learning in healthcare. Annual Review of Biomedical Data Science, (2021). https://doi.org/10.1146/annurev-biodatasci-092820-114757

Elezaby, M., Lees, B., Maturen, K. E., Barroilhet, L., Wisinski, K. B., Schrager, S., & Sadowski, E. BRCA mutation carriers: Breast and ovarian cancer screening guidelines and imaging considerations. Radiology, (2019). https://doi.org/10.1148/radiol.2019181814

Ghorbian, M., & Ghobaei-Arani, M. A blockchain-enabled serverless approach for IoT healthcare applications. In Serverless Computing: Principles and Paradigms (pp. 193–218). Cham: Springer International Publishing, (2023). https://doi.org/10.1007/978-3-031-26633-1_8

Goswami, Y., Agrawal, A., & Bhatia, A. E-governance: A tendering framework using blockchain with active participation of citizens. In 2020 IEEE International Conference on Advanced Networks and Telecommunications Systems (ANTS) (pp. 1–4). IEEE, (2020). https://doi.org/10.1109/ANTS50601.2020.9342816

Guo, B., Lian, W., Liu, S., Cao, Y., & Liu, J. Comparison of diagnostic values between CA125 combined with CA199 and ultrasound combined with CT in ovarian cancer. Oncology Letters, (2019).

Hamza, R., Yan, Z., Muhammad, K., Bellavista, P., & Titouna, F. A privacy-preserving cryptosystem for IoT E-healthcare. Information Sciences, (2020). https://doi.org/10.1016/j.ins.2019.01.070

Hölbl, M., Kompara, M., Kamišalić, A., & Nemec Zlatolas, L. A systematic review of the use of blockchain in healthcare. Symmetry, (2018). https://doi.org/10.3390/sym10100470

Janiesch, C., Zschech, P., & Heinrich, K. Machine learning and deep learning. Electronic Markets, (2021). https://doi.org/10.1007/s12525-021-00475-2

Manickam, P., Mariappan, S. A., Murugesan, S. M., Hansda, S., Kaushik, A., Shinde, R., & Thipperudraswamy, S. P. Artificial intelligence (AI) and Internet of Medical Things (IoMT) assisted biomedical systems for intelligent healthcare. Biosensors, (2022). https://doi.org/10.3390/bios12080562

Mantey, E. A., Zhou, C., Srividhya, S. R., Jain, S. K., & Sundaravadivazhagan, B. Integrated blockchain-deep learning approach for analyzing the electronic health records recommender system. Frontiers in Public Health, (2022). https://doi.org/10.3389/fpubh.2022.905265

Matsuhashi, T., Takeshita, T., Yamamoto, A., Kawase, R., Yamada, T., Kurose, K., & Kato, H. Serum CA 125 level after neoadjuvant chemotherapy is predictive of prognosis and debulking surgery outcomes in advanced epithelial ovarian cancer. Journal of Nippon Medical School, (2017). https://doi.org/10.1272/jnms.84.170

Park, D., & Ryu, D. Blockchain in health insurance: Sharing medical information and preventing insurance fraud. Korean Journal of Financial Studies, (2019). https://doi.org/10.26845/KJFS.2019.08.48.4.417

Saeedi, N., & Ghorbian, S. Analysis of clinical important of LncRNA-HOTAIR gene variations and ovarian cancer susceptibility. Molecular Biology Reports, (2020). https://doi.org/10.1007/s11033-020-05797-6

Saji, M., Sridhar, M., Rajasekaran, A., Kumar, R. A., Suyampulingam, A., & Krishna Prakash, N. IoT-based intelligent healthcare module. In Advances in Smart System Technologies: Select Proceedings of ICFSST 2019 (pp. 765–774). Singapore: Springer, (2021). https://doi.org/10.1007/978-981-15-5029-4_66

Shahbazi, Z., & Byun, Y. C. Integration of blockchain, IoT and machine learning for multistage quality control and enhancing security in smart manufacturing. Sensors, (2021). https://doi.org/10.3390/s21041467

Stewart, C., Ralyea, C., & Lockwood, S. Ovarian cancer: An integrated review. Seminars in Oncology Nursing, (2019). https://doi.org/10.1016/j.soncn.2019.02.001

Uddin, M., Memon, M. S., Memon, I., Ali, I., Memon, J., Abdelhaq, M., & Alsaqour, R. Hyperledger fabric blockchain: Secure and efficient solution for electronic health records. Computers, Materials and Continua, (2021). https://doi.org/10.32604/cmc.2021.015354

Blood oxygen level and pulse rate measurement using hemodialysis using IoT and computational intelligence

N. Vigneshwari, C. Sivamani, S. Selvi, and G. Revathy

7.1 INTRODUCTION

Dialysis is a crucial medical procedure used when the kidneys fail to perform their normal functions. It serves as a substitute for the natural filtration and waste removal processes of the kidneys, also known as renal replacement therapy (RRT). The primary role of healthy kidneys is to regulate the body's water and mineral levels and eliminate waste products. However, dialysis does not contribute to the production of certain vital fluids involved in metabolism.

While dialysis helps individuals with dysfunctional kidneys maintain their well-being, it cannot fully replace the kidneys' functions. Patients undergoing regular dialysis treatment need to adhere to strict dietary and fluid intake guidelines, as well as follow prescribed medication regimens. Unless any other health conditions restrict them, patients receiving dialysis can lead a relatively normal life and travel. However, it is essential to continue dialysis treatment according to the recommended schedule.

During hemodialysis (HD), the patient's blood is directed through a filter, known as a dialyzer or "artificial kidney", located outside the body. At the beginning of a HD session, a dialysis nanny or expert inserts two indicators into the patient's arm. With appropriate training, patients may choose to insert the needles themselves. Numbing cream or spray can be used to minimize discomfort during needle insertion. Each needle is connected to a soft tube that is attached to the dialysis machine. The machine pumps the blood through the filter, monitoring blood pressure and controlling the rate of blood flow and fluid removal from the body.

In HD, blood enters one end of the filter and is forced into numerous thin, hollow fibers. Simultaneously, dialysis solution flows in the opposite direction outside the fibers. Waste products from the blood move across the fibers into the dialysis solution, while filtered blood remains within the fibers and returns to the patient's body.

Overall, dialysis plays a vital role in maintaining the health of individuals with kidney failure. Although it does not fully replicate the functions of healthy kidneys, dialysis allows patients to continue their daily activities while adhering to the prescribed treatment schedule and medical guidelines.

DOI: 10.1201/9781003487647-7

HD is a crucial medical treatment for affected role with end-stage renal disease (ESRD). It acknowledges the premature challenges in establishing this groundbreaking therapy but credits pioneers like Dr. Scribner for successfully developing and spreading modern HD techniques worldwide in the 1960s.

While HD has seen substantial advancements in technology and drugs over time, the passage suggests that there are still unresolved issues and lesser-known problems associated with HD. Various researchers have identified and discussed these problems from different perspectives, including urogenital, cardiac, muscular, gerontological issues, as well as complications related to anemia, multiple myeloma, blood access, erythropoietin, and anticoagulant therapy. The passage also mentions the inclusion of findings on treatment through exercise and a new method called hemodiafiltration (HDF).

Although the newly published findings may not provide perfect solutions to the HD-associated problems in nephrology, the hope is that they will contribute to useful resolutions and novel developments in overcoming these challenges in the future. The passage also expresses a desire for future issues of the journal to cover additional important topics such as CKD-mineral bone disease (MBD), HD gathering occurrence and duration, and the usage of herbal or alternative medicines, which remain controversial and require active discussion.

The foremost unbiased of the project is to progress an automated urine sample analyzer kit that can determine the presence of specific substances in urine samples. The substances targeted for analysis in this project are albumin, urea, and bile salt.

The automation of the urine sample analysis process aims to simplify and streamline the testing procedure. By developing an automated analyzer kit, the project seeks to eliminate or minimize the need for manual handling and interpretation of urine samples, reducing the potential for human error and improving the accuracy and efficiency of the analysis. The presence of albumin, urea, and bile salt in urine samples can provide valuable information about a person's health and the functioning of their kidneys and liver. Detecting abnormal levels of these substances can help diagnose and monitor various medical conditions, such as kidney disease, liver dysfunction, or urinary tract infections.

The automated urine sample analyzer kit would likely involve a combination of hardware and software components. The hardware may include a device for sample processing, measurement, and analysis, while the software would be responsible for data interpretation, presentation, and potentially providing automated diagnostic results.

- The main objective is to identify the risk of hypoxemia using pulse oximetry.
- To monitor the oxygen saturation using the sensor technology.
- To evaluate the data for accurate diagnosis using AI-based methods.

Overall, the development of an automated urine sample analyzer kit for the detection of albumin, urea, and bile salt would provide a valuable tool for medical professionals in diagnosing and monitoring certain health conditions. It could improve the efficiency and reliability of urine sample analysis, ultimately benefiting patient care and treatment.

7.2 LITERATURE SURVEY

N.M. Banach and Priefer (2018) had presented the development of a transportable spectrophotometer-based breathalyzer for point-of-care difficult of diabetic patients. It addresses the issue of therapy nonadherence in diabetic patients, which can lead to complications such as diabetic ketoacidosis. The embarrassment allied with the member hole method of glucose monitoring is identified as a potential factor contributing to therapy nonadherence. To overcome this issue, the paper proposes a less invasive method for monitoring diabetes by analyzing the levels of acetone in the breath of diabetic patients. Acetone is a volatile organic compound that can be detected in the breath and has been found to correlate with elevated glucose levels, particularly in the context of diabetic ketoacidosis. The portable breathalyzer device being developed aims to provide an abridged tactic for monitoring acetone levels, which can serve as an indicator of the onset of diabetic ketoacidosis. By eliminating the need for frequent finger pricks, this device may improve patient comfort and adherence to therapy. However, without access to the specific details of the paper, it is not possible to provide a comprehensive analysis of the proposed technique or discuss its advantages and limitations in detail. If you require further information or have specific questions about the development of this portable breathalyzer, please provide additional details or specific points of interest.

Chen Chong (2020) had presented a theory of automatic detection in the context of a handheld urine analyzer system founded on photoelectric technology and the STM32F103 embedded system. The goal is to achieve integration between the photoelectric detection part and the micro-appliance to develop an efficient optical, mechanical, and electronic system. The hardware and software of the system are designed to enable the measurement of urine components. The system utilizes the transformation sorter procedure for developing image data and ensuring accurate measurement results. The means employed in this system are atraumatic and non-intrusive, allowing for rapid, convenient, and automated detection of urine components. Additionally, the system is equipped with various output and display options such as an LCD touchscreen, RS485, and Ethernet, enabling the presentation of results in a user-friendly manner.

Diabetic ketoacidosis is a severe complication of diabetes, and monitoring urine ketone levels can be helpful in diagnosing this condition. A portable electronic nose (E-nose) was built in the study employing five metal oxide (MOX) gas sensors arranged and controlled by an 8-bit microprocessor. A 10-bit analogy-to-digital converter (ADC) incorporated into the microcontroller was used to convert the analogy signals from the gas sensors to digital signals. Dimethyl ketone was dissolved in synthetic urine samples at quantities 1–100 mg/dL in the studies. The findings showed that the approach could properly identify the concentration of dimethyl ketone with a rate of more than 85% accuracy. This indicates the potential of using this method for detecting ketoacidosis in real urine samples. It's important to note that this study focuses on synthetic urine samples, and further research and validation would be needed to assess the effectiveness of this method in detecting ketoacidosis in real-world clinical settings with actual urine samples from diabetic patients.

YA study aimed at developing a process for envisaging the urine volume in the bladder without the need for attaching sensors to the body and also it focuses on elderly individuals living in nursing homes who may experience urinary incontinence and rely on caregivers to change their diapers after each episode. The objective is to enable caregivers to anticipate the need for toileting by predicting the urine volume in the bladder, thus potentially avoiding incontinence episodes and eliminating the need for diapers. This is particularly important for individuals who may have cognitive issues or feel embarrassed about informing caregivers about their incontinence episodes. To that end, the study proposes a macroscopic model for urine accumulation in the bladder as well as a technique for forecasting urine volume based on the absorption spectrum of urine acquired shortly after urination. Significantly, the suggested approach does not need the attachment of a sensor to the skin. The researchers conducted a series of experiments to evaluate the suggested approach and compared its error rate to that of an ultrasonic sensor applied to the skin above the bladder. The error rate represents the method's ability to forecast urine volume accurately.

The use of complex event processing (CEP) technology, enables the processing and correlation of huge dimensions of data by leveraging occurrence patterns. The primary objective is to detect explicit circumstances promptly that may require superior handling. In order to implement event categories and event decorations for a specific submission domain, an event processing language (EPL) is utilized. However, when generating the code automatically from the EPL, the created code is only syntactically validated and not semantically validated. This poses a challenge in ensuring the correctness and accuracy of the generated code. To address this problem, the paper proposes the use of a prioritized colored Petri net (PCPN) model for CEP. The PCPN model is a well-known graphical formalism that, when combined with CPNTools, allows for the modeling, simulation, analysis, and semantic validation of complex event-based systems. By utilizing the PCPN model and CPNTools, the proposed approach provides a means to validate the generated code and ensure the correct functioning of complex event-based systems.

7.3 EXISTING SYSTEM

Various methodologies such as dipstick test (based on PH levels), visual examination (based on physical parameters), and microscopic examination (based on the macroscopic view of sample) are available.

7.3.1 Dipstick test

Urine dipstick testing is a rapid and convenient method used to analyze urine samples. Normally, urine is sterile and contains waste chemicals from various metabolic processes in the body. However, in certain conditions, abnormal substances may pass through the kidney's filtration system and appear in the urine.

During a urine dipstick test, a specially treated paper strip, known as a dipstick, is dipped into a sample of urine. This can be done during a medical appointment with a doctor, midwife, or other healthcare professional. The dipstick contains chemical reagents that react to specific substances in the urine, such as glucose, protein, blood, nitrites, leukocytes, and pH levels. The results of a urine dipstick test are usually available within a short period, typically 60–120 seconds. Unlike other tests, a urine dipstick test does not require the sample to be sent to a laboratory for analysis. However, if the test yields abnormal results, additional samples may be collected and sent to a laboratory for further testing.

Urine dipstick testing provides a quick and initial assessment of the presence of certain substances in the urine. It can help healthcare professionals screen for various conditions, such as urinary tract infections, kidney disease, diabetes, and other metabolic disorders. Further diagnostic tests and investigations may be necessary based on the results of the dipstick test.

It's important to note that while urine dipstick testing is a valuable tool, it has limitations. It cannot provide a definitive diagnosis and may yield false-positive or false-negative results in certain situations. Therefore, if the test indicates an abnormal result, further evaluation and confirmatory tests may be required to establish a diagnosis.

7.3.2 Visual examination

In areas where kidney disease is prevalent, but diagnostic facilities are limited and expensive, examining the urine becomes a valuable and cost-effective method for enhancing the diagnosis of kidney disease. Urine analysis can provide important insights into the underlying pathology of the kidneys and can also help identify evidence of systemic disorders such as diabetes mellitus.

In the field of nephrology, one of the advantages is that urine, the "substrate" of the kidneys, is generally easily accessible for examination. It can be readily collected from patients and provides valuable information about the underlying condition of the kidneys. Therefore, all patients with suspected kidney disease should be asked to submit a urine sample for examination.

Moreover, it is essential for physicians to actively inquire about the characteristics of the urine being passed by patients. This aspect of patient history-taking is sometimes overlooked but can be equally important as physically examining the urine sample itself. Changes in urine color, volume, frequency, presence of foam, or other unusual features can provide valuable clues about kidney function and potential abnormalities. By incorporating urine examination and thorough questioning about urine characteristics into the diagnostic process, healthcare professionals can gain valuable insights into kidney health and associated systemic conditions. This approach can help optimize the diagnosis and management of kidney disease, particularly in resource-limited settings where other diagnostic options may be limited or costly.

7.3.3 Microscopic examination

The description provided accurately explains the process of urine microscopy. This test involves examining a sample of urine under a microscope to observe various components and detect any abnormalities. The microscope allows for the visualization of cells from the urinary tract, blood cells, crystals, bacteria, parasites, and even cells from tumors. Urine microscopy is often used as a complementary test to confirm or provide additional information to a diagnosis made through other tests. It provides insights into the appearance, concentration, and content of the urine sample, helping healthcare professionals assess the health of the urinary system and identify potential issues.

During the test, a urine sample is typically centrifuged, a process that separates the solid particles from the liquid portion. The sediment obtained from the centrifugation is then examined under a microscope. This sediment contains various elements that can be visually identified, such as crystals (indicative of certain conditions or metabolic disorders), casts (abnormal protein structures indicating kidney disease), white and/or red blood cells (suggesting infection or inflammation), and bacteria or yeast (indicating an infection).

By analyzing the microscopic characteristics of the urine sample, healthcare professionals can gain important diagnostic information and guide appropriate treatment decisions. Urine microscopy is a valuable tool in the evaluation of urinary tract disorders, kidney diseases, urinary tract infections, and other related conditions.

7.4 PROPOSED SYSTEM

The proposed model of urine auto analyzer is explained in detail. Till today, the lab technicians test urine samples by a manual method. This model is going to simplify and eliminate the manual method, it consumes less time. Because of the hardware cost, digital method is better than the manual method. It will detect the albumin (Heller's test), urea (hypobromite test), bile salt (Smith's test), and sugar (benedict test). The database is collected from the website physionet.org. The dataset is separated for training and testing. The training dataset is applied to the AI algorithm. After training, the testing data is used.

7.4.1 Block diagram of proposed system

The proposed block diagram consists of various blocks such as input module, motor, microcontroller, LDR, relay, and output module; these are explained in the following sections (Figure 7.1).

7.4.1.1 Power supply

The input to the circuit is applied from the regulator power supply. About 9–12 V of current supply is given to the mask cleaner aid. Current is supplied to the microcontroller and pass through the other circuits.

7.4.1.2 Microcontroller

The Arduino Uno is a popular open-source microcontroller board based on the Microchip ATmega328P microprocessor. It was created by Arduino.cc and has grown in popularity owing to its ease of use and adaptability. The board has both digital and analog input/output (I/O) pins that may be linked to various expansion boards (shields) and circuits for additional functionality. Arduino is recognized for its open-source nature, which means that both the hardware and software are freely available for modification and customization. The Arduino boards can interface with a wide range of sensors and devices, allowing users to read inputs such as light levels, button presses, or other sensor data, and convert them into outputs that control motors, LEDs, or even connect to the internet for data communication.

In terms of memory, the Arduino Uno has 32 kb of flash memory for storing the program code. It also has 2 kb of SRAM, which is used for temporary data storage during program execution. Additionally, it has 1 kb of EEPROM memory, which is non-volatile memory used for storing data that needs to be retained even when the power is disconnected. The Arduino Uno is widely used in various fields, including embedded systems, control

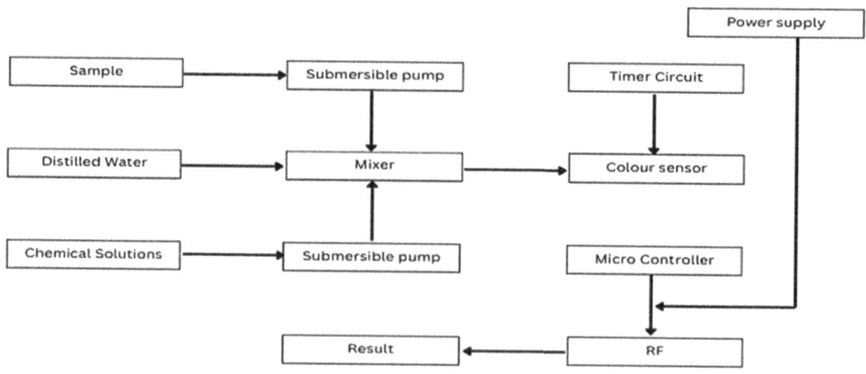

Figure 7.1 Block diagram.

systems, robotics, instrumentation, and condition monitoring. It can be programmed to control functions such as motor control, measurement devices like electrostatic meters, activating UV LEDs, controlling heaters, and managing recharge processes.

Overall, the Arduino Uno offers a flexible and accessible platform for building and prototyping electronics projects, making it popular among hobbyists, students, and professionals in the field of electronics and programming.

7.4.1.3 LDR

An LDR is a type of resistor whose resistance changes based on the amount of light that falls on its surface. It is also referred to as a photoresistor, photocell, or photoconductor. The resistance of an LDR decreases when exposed to light and increases when in darkness. This property makes it suitable for various applications where light sensing is required. When the light intensity increases, the resistance of the LDR decreases, and when the light intensity decreases, the resistance increases. One common use of LDRs is in light-sensitive circuits. For example, in a circuit controlling a light source, an LDR can be used to automatically turn on the light when it becomes dark (low resistance) and turn it off when it becomes light (high resistance). This makes LDRs useful in applications such as automatic streetlights, security systems, and outdoor lighting control. LDRs come in different types and have a range of resistance values. The specific resistance characteristics of an LDR can vary based on factors such as the material composition and construction.

Overall, LDRs provide a simple and effective way to incorporate light-sensing capabilities into electronic circuits, allowing them to respond and adapt to changes in ambient light conditions (Figure 7.2).

As light strikes the surface of an LDR, the conductivity of the material diminishes, and electrons in the valence band of the semiconductor material are stimulated to the conduction band. This phenomenon happens in semiconductor materials due to the absorption of photons with energies larger than the bandgap of the material. In a semiconductor, there is an energy gap between the valence band (which includes bound electrons) and the conduction band (which allows electrons to move freely). To migrate from the valence band to

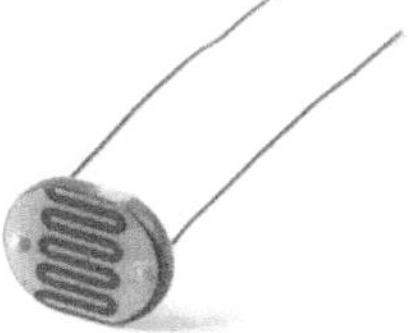

Figure 7.2 Light-dependent resistor.

the conduction band, an electron must gain energy equal to or higher than the bandgap energy.

When photons with energies larger than the bandgap collide with the LDR's surface, their energy is transferred to electrons in the valence band. This energy absorption raises the electrons' energy level in the conduction band, allowing them to flow freely and enhancing the material's conductivity. The change in conductivity of the LDR due to the absorption of light allows it to act as a light sensor, as its resistance varies with the amount of incident light. When exposed to light, the LDR's resistance decreases due to the increased conductivity, and when in darkness, the resistance increases.

7.4.1.4 Relay

A relay is an electrically functioned adjustment that consists of input terminals for control signals and operating contact terminals (Figure 7.3). The relay switch can have multiple contacts, including make contacts (normally open) and break contacts (normally closed).

Relays are widely employed when a circuit must be controlled by a separate, low-power signal or when numerous circuits must be controlled by a single signal. They let you to electrically separate distinct circuits while controlling the flow of current between them.

Relays can operate both electronically and electromechanically. In an electronic relay, the switching action is performed by solid-state components such as transistors or thyristors. In an electromechanical relay, the switching action is achieved through the movement of mechanical parts, typically an electromagnetic coil that controls the position of the contacts. The state of the relay contacts determines whether the circuit connected to the relay is open or closed. When the relay contact is in the open state (normally open or NO), the circuit is not energized and no current flows through it. Conversely, when the relay contact is closed (normally closed or NC), the circuit is energized, and current can flow through it.

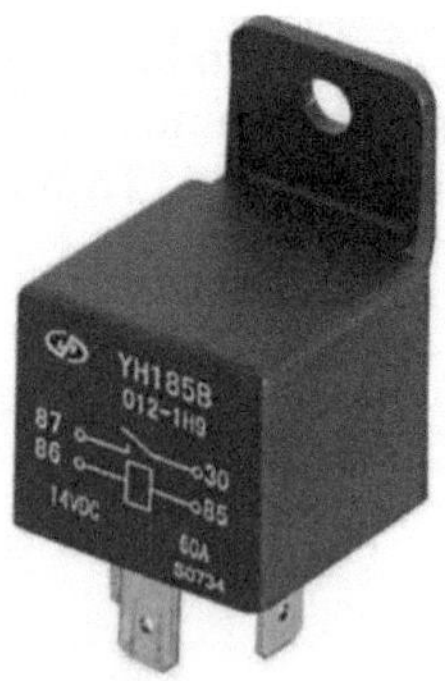

Figure 7.3 Relay.

The state of the relay contacts can be changed by applying energy, such as electricity or a charge, to the relay coil. When the coil is energized, it creates a magnetic field that attracts or repels the mechanical parts, causing the contacts to change their position Relays are widely used in various applications, including control systems, automation, power distribution, telecommunications, and automotive electronics. They provide a reliable means of controlling circuits and isolating different electrical components or systems.

7.4.2 Test tubes

Test tubes are commonly used in chemistry and biology laboratories for various purposes. Chemists use them to mix, heat, and hold small quantities of chemicals during experiments and assays. Biologists use test tubes for culturing and handling organisms, fluids, and samples. Test tubes are handheld tubes that are open at the top and have a rounded bottom. They are typically made of glass or plastic materials. Glass test tubes are often preferred for their transparency, chemical resistance, and ability to withstand high temperatures. Plastic test tubes, on the other hand, are lighter, less breakable, and can be disposed of after use. Some test tubes are designed to be reusable, while others are disposable and meant for single use. Reusable test tubes can be cleaned and sterilized for repeated use, whereas disposable test tubes are convenient for certain applications and eliminate the need for cleaning and sterilization.

In addition to test tubes, there are variations in labware called culture tubes or sample tubes, which serve specific purposes. Culture tubes are similar to test tubes but typically do not have a lip at the top. They are commonly used in microbiology for culturing microorganisms or in tissue culture experiments. Overall, test tubes are essential tools in laboratory settings and play a crucial role in conducting experiments, mixing chemicals, and handling various samples and cultures.

7.4.3 Parameters to be found

- Albumin
- Bile salt
- Urea

7.4.3.1 Albumin

Albumin is a protein present in the blood that helps maintain the balance of fluid between blood vessels and body tissues. Normally, the kidneys filter waste products from the blood, allowing them to be excreted in urine while retaining albumin and other proteins in the bloodstream. However, if albumin appears in urine, it may indicate kidney damage or dysfunction.

To determine the extent of kidney damage, healthcare providers often assess the amount of albumin lost in a 24-hour urine collection. In this type of test, you need to collect all the urine you produce over a 24-hour period. The first urine voided in the morning is usually discarded, and subsequent urine samples are collected throughout the day. The healthcare provider may also use a test strip to analyze a urine sample for albumin.

7.4.3.2 Bile salt

The bile salt test is used to detect the level of bile salts in the urine or blood. Bile is a yellow-green fluid that contains water and organic molecules such as cholesterol, bile acids, and bilirubin. In humans, the two main functions of bile are digestion and absorption of fats and elimination of bile salts from the body by secretion into bile. Adult humans produce around 400–800 ml of bile daily. The bile is produced by the liver, and the gall bladder holds the bile produced in the liver. The bile salt test is used to measure the level of bile salts in blood/urine. The test is performed to confirm liver disorder and pruritus in pregnancy. It can be concluded from the test reports that the normal result for bile salts is <10 μmol/L for unisex gender and for all age groups. If the test shows positive, it could be a case of obstructive jaundice. A minimum of 5 ml of blood is required for the test. The test with the urine sample includes the following procedure: Urine sample is collected in a vessel. Sulfur powder is sprinkled over the surface of urine. The sulfur powder sinks if bile salts are present. The sulfur powder remains over the surface of urine if bile salts are absent.

The normal amount of albumin in urine is typically less than 30 mg/day. Additionally, the normal total protein amount in urine is usually less than 150 mg/day. Higher levels of albumin or total protein may indicate kidney disease.

For individuals with diabetes, increased urine albumin levels may suggest diabetic nephropathy, a type of kidney disease associated with diabetes. An albumin-to-creatinine ratio (ACR) test is commonly used to detect albumin in urine. A normal ACR value is typically less than 30 mg/g. If the ACR is higher than 30 mg/g, it may indicate kidney disease, even if the glomerular filtration rate (GFR) is above 60.

7.4.3.3 Urea

Urea levels are typically measured in blood, not urine. Urea is a waste product that forms when the liver breaks down proteins, and it is excreted from the body through urine. The normal range for blood urea levels is generally around 7–20 mg/dl in adults, but reference ranges can vary slightly depending on the laboratory and the specific population being tested. In contrast, urine urea levels are not commonly measured as a routine test. The focus is usually on measuring urea levels in blood to assess kidney function and overall health. Urine tests may be performed to assess other components such as albumin, creatinine, and electrolytes, which can provide valuable information about kidney function and various metabolic processes.

7.5 RESULTS AND DISCUSSIONS

Software results of proposed urine auto analyzer using embedded system are discussed. The software tools Arduino UNO and ATmega328P are used for simulation and layout purposes. The data is trained with random forest, and highest accuracy is achieved compared with other state-of-the-art models.

7.5.1 Prototype model

A sample is collected in a test tube and placed in a tray with slider mechanism. It is then inserted and the power supply is given to the Arduino. The motor then starts to suck the chemical solution from three different containers for which three different tests to be taken. The chemical solution is delivered to the test tube via pipeline and after this process the LED gets turned on one side of the slider where the light oases through the sample solution and reflects on the LDR which is placed on the other slider. For each tests, there is a different nanometer and the result is finally shown in the LCD display (Figures 7.4 and 7.5).

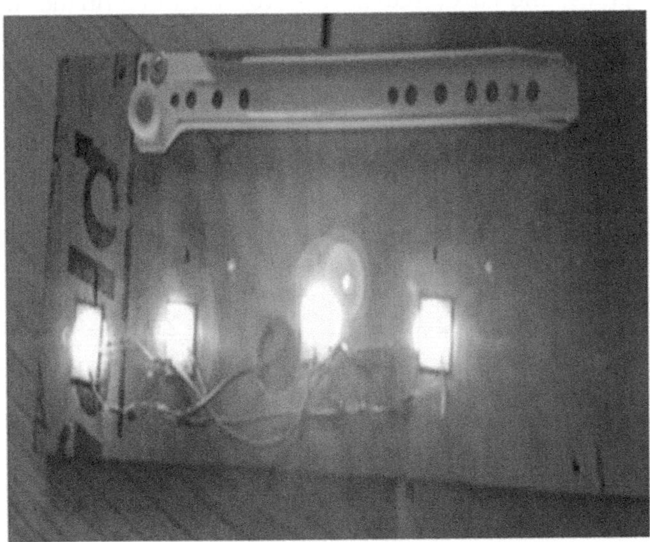

Figure 7.4 The placement of LED on one slider.

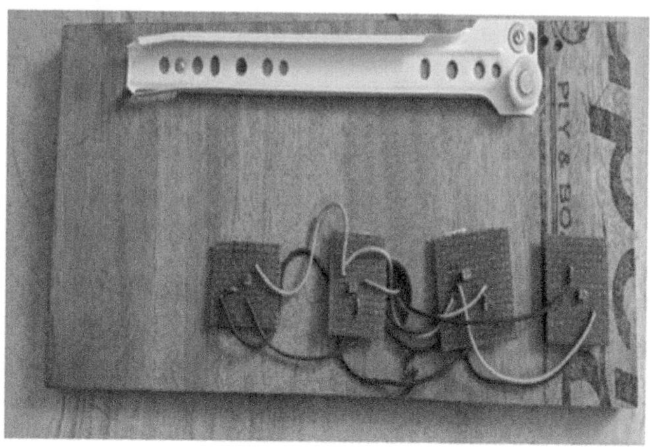

Figure 7.5 The placement of LDR on another slider.

7.5.2 Support vector machine (SVM) result

SVM outpowers all other machine learning algorithms and has a highest accuracy. Figure 7.6 exposes that SVM shows an extraordinary result when compared with other state-of-the-art models.

7.5.3 Future work

It can be manufactured at very low cost and can be installed in diagnostic centers, hospitals, and labs (Figures 7.7–7.10). It can be further implemented

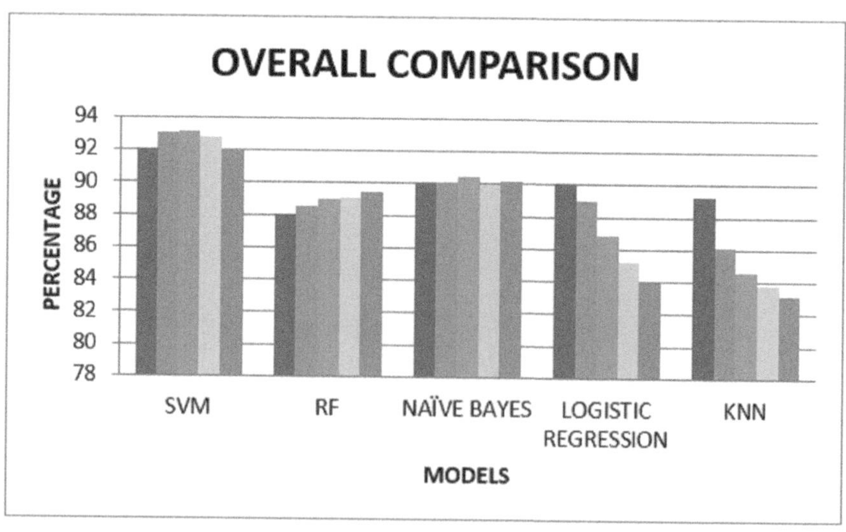

Figure 7.6 Overall comparison of RF with other ML models.

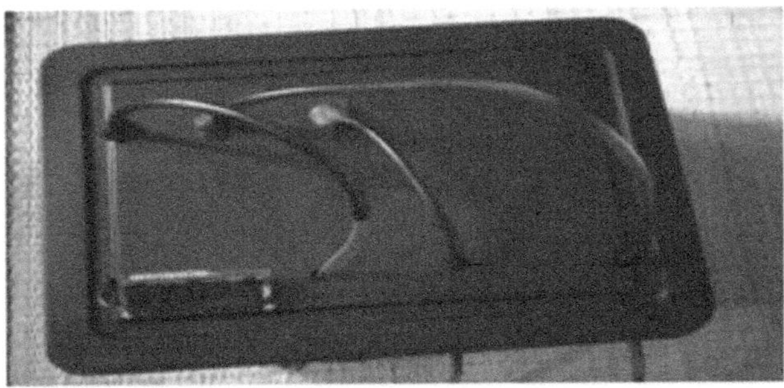

Figure 7.7 Whole setup of the hardware.

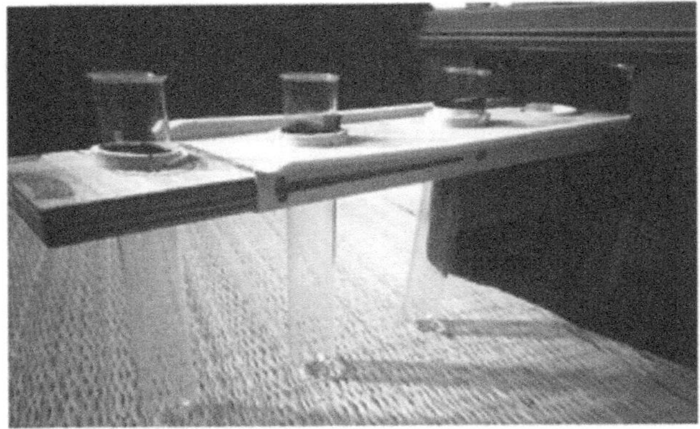

Figure 7.8 Slider setup for sample placing.

in thermal printers and patient details storing application. It has the following advantages:

1. More cost-effective
2. Increases accuracy in output
3. Accurate output
4. Consumes less time

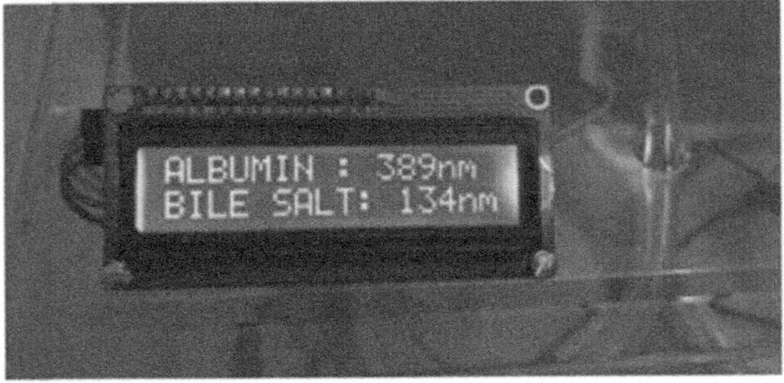

Figure 7.9 Albumin and bile salt wavelength values.

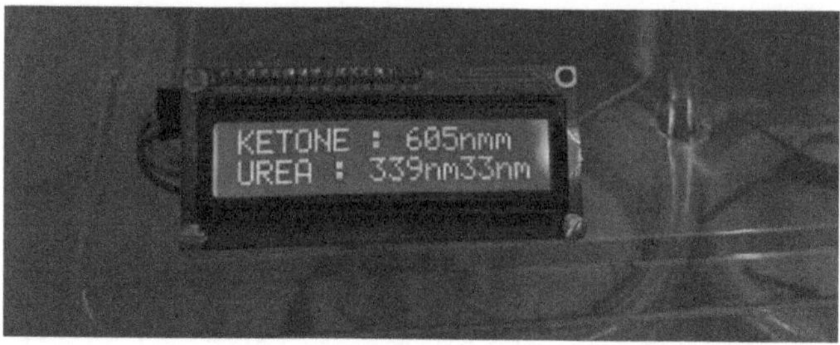

Figure 7.10 Ketone and urea wavelength values.

7.6 CONCLUSION

Pulse oximetry is used to identify patients at risk of hypoxemia, monitor them during HD, and administer oxygen to those whose SpO_2 falls below 90%, especially if they have anemia or cardiovascular disease. SVM is used to evaluate the data and the accuracy is 91%, and it is comparatively higher than the state-of-the-art models.

REFERENCES

1. N.M. Banach and R. Priefer, (2018) "A Portable spectrophotometer breath analyser for point care testing for diabetic patient Digital Object Identifier". 10.1109.
2. Chen Chong and Chen Shangting (2020) "Research on hand-held urine analyser based on photoelectric technology". International Conference on Computational and Information Sciences, IEEE.
3. Jorge Javier, (2021) "Monitoring diabetic ketoacidosis by urine ketones tracing using an E-Nose". 2020 IEEE International Instrumentation and Measurement Technology Conference (I2MTC), IEEE.
4. Hermanedlida and Macia (2016) "Complex event processing modelling by prioritized coloured petri nets". IEEE Access, vol. 4, pp. 7425–7439.
5. Y. Kurihara and T. Yamsaki, (2018) "Model of urine accumulation in bladder and method or predicting urine". IEEE Access, vol. 27, No 1, pp. 81–94.
6. Y. Kurihara and T. Yamsaki, (2018) "Model of urine accumulation in bladder and method or predicting urine volume". IEEE Instrumentation and Measurement Society, 2018.21785.
7. Araba Afenyi-Annan and Monte S. Willis, (2019) "Thomas Albumin management of sickle cell patients at comprehensive sickle cell centers". 39th Annual Bioengineering conference, 2019.76890.
8. A. Tapanan and Yeophanton, (2019) "in Calculation of urine parameters." Vol.42, TENCON 2019 Conference 92652.

Chapter 8

Dental shade matching using machine learning models

Shishira R., S. Deepthi Nayak, M. N. Suma, and Geetishree Mishra

8.1 INTRODUCTION

Dental procedures, such as tooth-colored fillings, dental veneers, crowns, and bridges, aim to restore or enhance a patient's smile. To achieve a natural and appealing appearance, it's crucial to match the shade of the dental material to the patient's existing teeth [1, 3]. Patients seeking cosmetic or restorative dental treatments have specific expectations about the outcome [3, 5] Hence, in dentistry, shade matching is a critical aspect of restorative and cosmetic dental procedures, as it directly affects the appearance of a patient's teeth. Achieving a natural and aesthetically pleasing result is paramount, and shade matching plays a significant role in this process. Tooth shade matching in dentistry often relies on a trial and error approach, which can be influenced by the clinician's skill level, visual fatigue, and the surrounding light source. Achieving accurate color reproduction with restorative materials poses a significant challenge. In dental practice, shade selection can be accomplished through visual methods, such as shade guides, or instrumental methods, including spectrophotometers, colorimeters, and the recent intraoral digital scanners [1, 9, 13]. While the human vision is adept at detecting minor variances in tooth color, effectively communicating these differences to dental technicians can be complex. The extensive range of tones, translucency, opacities, and characterizations in natural teeth may go unnoticed during visual shade matching. Additionally, visual shade matching is subject to various variables, such as age, experience, sex, type of scale used, light exposure, eye fatigue, and physiological factors like color deficiency, which can lead to inconsistencies [10].

To ensure practical applicability, when the color difference between the real tooth color and the shade tab falls within the identical range, it becomes indistinguishable to the human eye, thereby meeting the criteria for practical applications. Currently, the VITA classical color cards serve as the standard in the dental market, providing a reference for shade selection [9–11]. Figure 8.1 illustrates the VITA classical color guide and the VITA 3D-Master, which are widely utilized in dental practice.

DOI: 10.1201/9781003487647-8

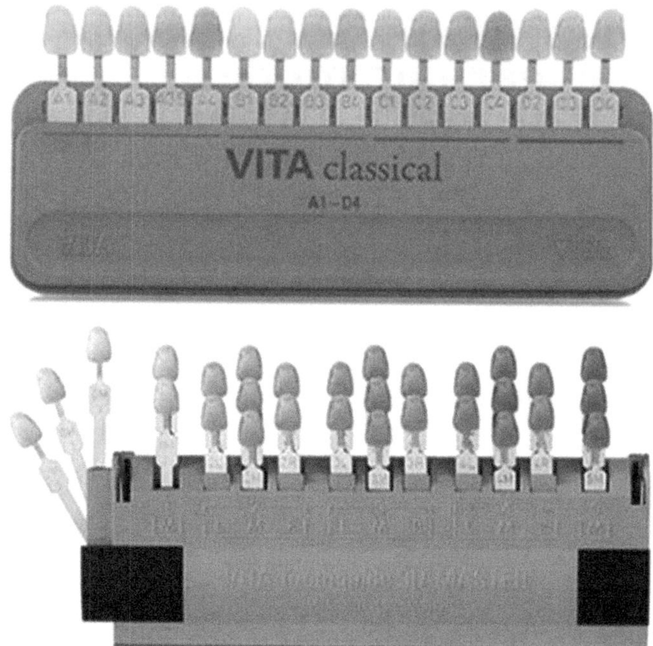

Figure 8.1 VITA classical (a) and (b) VITA Master shade tab.

The VITA classical A1–D4 shade guide is widely used for determining tooth shade in dentistry. The shades in the VITA classical family are arranged in the following manner: A1–A4 represent reddish-brownish shades, B1–B4 represent reddish-yellowish shades, C1–C4 represent grayish shades, and D2–D4 represent reddish-gray shades. This standardized arrangement of shades provides dental professionals with a consistent and reliable reference for matching tooth color accurately. The process of selecting a visual shade using various commercial or customized shade guides is impacted by several external factors, including surrounding lighting, environment, attributes of the teeth (such as textures, layers, and vitality), the dentist's professional judgment, and patient-specific considerations. This subjective assessment poses challenges for clinicians seeking consistent and reliable shade matching. To aid in tooth color selection and improve aesthetic outcomes, several measurement devices have been developed. However, these devices still struggle to provide highly accurate results [10, 12].

Artificial intelligence (AI) is rapidly emerging as a transformative field in dentistry, offering numerous advantages over traditional methods. In the dental clinic, AI technology can efficiently carry out various tasks with enhanced precision, reduced staffing requirements, and minimized errors compared to human counterparts [2, 4, 6, 7, 8]. One specific application where AI proves beneficial is dental shade matching. By leveraging machine learning (ML) models, a subset of AI, the limitations associated with visual shade matching can be overcome. AI has revolutionized dental shade matching by offering precision, consistency, efficiency, and the ability to process large datasets. It ensures that dental restorations closely match a patient's natural tooth color, contributing to better treatment outcomes, increased patient satisfaction, and the overall success of restorative and cosmetic dental procedures [1, 3]. This chapter explains how ML models can be trained on datasets of dental images for various tooth shades and provide an objective assessment of tooth color without human bias and subjective judgments.

8.2 LITERATURE REVIEW

A comprehensive analysis to compare color matching systems for dental recognition have been proposed in References [17–26]. In References [14, 15, 16], mobile phones were employed as instruments to reduce errors in color assessment. The primary goal was to utilize smartphone-captured photographs to assist dental surgeons in selecting the correct color for oral rehabilitation procedures. In a publication from 2017, researchers introduced an AI system called DentShadeAI. This framework is designed to predict the most accurate dental shade within the VITA classical A1–D4 range for a given tooth based on an image captured using a mobile phone camera. DentShadeAI comprises two main components: an image capture process and a ML algorithm. Remarkably, the image can be taken using a standard mobile phone camera, eliminating the need for controlled lighting conditions. The researchers assessed the performance of three ML models, namely, random forests (RF), support vector machine (SVM), and XGBoost, in the DentShadeAI system. In Reference [19], the authors discuss the application of a computer vision system that facilitates automatic color matching. The primary objective is to guarantee precise color accuracy in all processed images. The paper introduces two interrelated techniques: (i) one that uses a camera characterization algorithm enabling the device to produce photos with colorimetric responses and (ii) another that utilizes the computed CIE L*a*b values to conduct the matching process over shade guide color samples to identify the optimal match.

Based on the fundamental components of color analysis, which include the red, green, and blue (RGB) model, the hue, saturation, and value (HSV) model, and the International Commission on Illumination (CIELAB), these parameters are commonly employed in color analysis systems [18, 21, 22, 26, 27]. Nevertheless, the color characteristics of teeth exhibit nonuniformity and involve intricate layering within the tooth structure. Therefore, additional techniques are necessary to accurately determine specific features of each tooth. Various ML algorithms have been suggested for automating the process of teeth color matching using image processing.

The study explored the performance of various algorithms including K-nearest neighbors (KNN), neural network (NN), and decision tree (DT) in References [23, 24, 26]. Simulation results demonstrated that the RGB color model coupled with the KNN algorithm classifier yielded the best performance under stable lighting conditions. Conversely, in situations with unstable lighting conditions, a combination of the HSV color model and DT algorithm or the Lab color model with the KNN algorithm classifier can be utilized. In References [23, 24], the authors have established the efficiency of KNN algorithm for tooth shade prediction.

In Reference [22], researchers developed a digital device for dental color assessment using the SVM algorithm. The SVM algorithm's classification performance was compared to other algorithms, including RF, logistic regression, and KNN. The leave-pair-out cross-validation method was employed to evaluate and validate the performance of SVM algorithm's classification, whereas "leave-one-out" strategy was employed for SVM training and classification in Reference [22]. The CIELAB color features of teeth images are utilized as training features for the ML models. Subsequently, classification algorithms such as KNN, RF, DT, AdaBoost, XGBoost, gradient boost, and SVM are employed to classify different shades. This approach enables more standardized and accurate color matching compared to conventional techniques.

In References [21, 26], a dental shade matching method based on the hue, saturation, value (HSV) color model was proposed. Performance evaluation of the proposed method included metrics such as structural similarity index (SSIM), peak signal-to-noise ratio (PSNR), composite peak signal-to-noise ratio (CPSNR), and S-CIELAB (Special International Commission on Illumination, L* for lightness, a* from green to red, and b* from blue to yellow). The fuzzy decision method, which incorporated the HSV color model, PSNR(H), PSNR(S), and SSIM details, demonstrated superior performance. Reference [20] discusses the significance of color matching in the context of dental shade selection for prosthesis fabrication. The method proposed in the paper involves several steps. First, digital images are analyzed to separate their color features into RGB and HSV color spaces. To determine the appropriate shade for teeth, the system employs classifier algorithms such as NN, DT, and KNN algorithms. These algorithms are applied to the color histogram feature spaces to facilitate accurate dental shade selection.

In this chapter, the CIELAB color features extracted from teeth images serve as the training features for the learning models proposed. CIELAB is device-independent, which means that it is not tied to any specific hardware or software [28, 29]. This is important in dental applications where various dental clinics may use different imaging devices, such as cameras or spectrophotometers, to capture tooth colors. Hence CIELAB color space model ensures consistency in color representation across different devices. Subsequently, classification to different shades is carried out using various classification algorithms, including KNN, RF, DT, AdaBoost, XGBoost, gradient boost, and SVM. This approach enables more precise and standardized color matching compared to traditional techniques.

8.3 METHODOLOGY

The CIELAB color space is based on the concept of human vision and models the entire range of perceivable colors. It consists of three components: L*, a*, and b*. The L* component represents the lightness of a color, ranging from 0 (black) to 100 (white). The a* and b* components represent the color's position on the chromaticity axes. The a* axis spans from green (−a*) to red (+a*), while the b* axis ranges from blue (−b*) to yellow (+b*), as shown in Figure 8.2. One of the key advantages of the CIELAB color space is its device independence [28]. By using standardized color profiles and transformations, colors represented in Lab values can be accurately reproduced across different devices and color spaces. This property makes it useful for applications such as color difference calculations, color matching, and color correction.

Figure 8.3 depicts the flowchart of the proposed tooth color matching algorithm. There are four main stages – data collection and preprocessing, data augmentation, EDA, and data modeling using ML models.

8.3.1 Data collection

The dataset used in this study comprises two distinct sets of data. The first set encompasses the CIELAB values of the VITA Classical dental shades, collected from multiple research papers (Datasets). These values were obtained through measurements conducted under diverse lighting conditions and with various spectroscopic devices. The second set comprises the CIELAB values

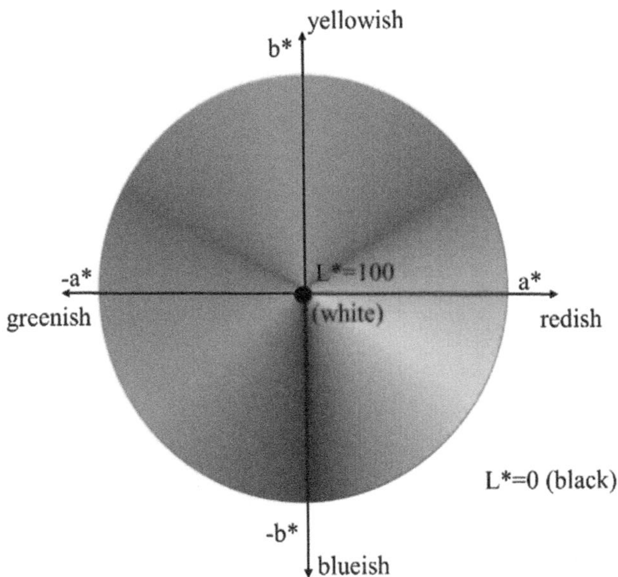

Figure 8.2 CIELAB color model.

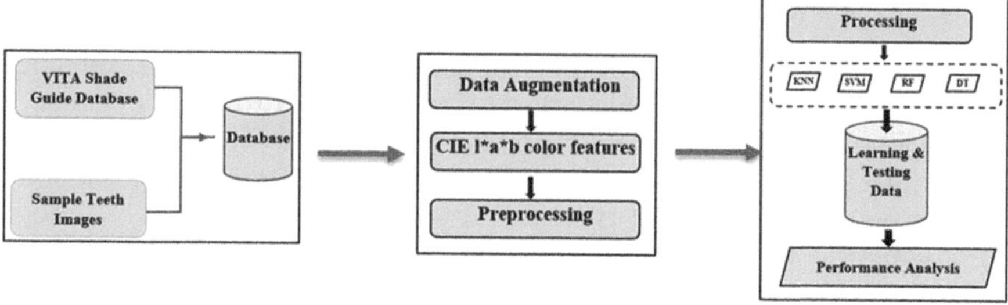

Figure 8.3 Flowchart depicting various steps.

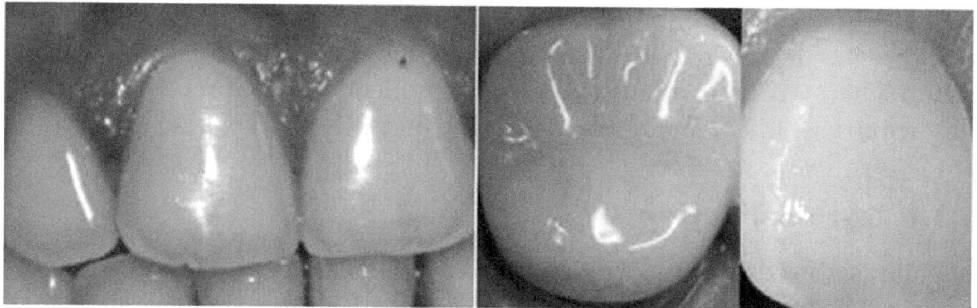

Figure 8.4 Sample images collected from the dentist.

derived from sample tooth images obtained from Dental Clinic. The shades for these images were determined under the supervision of a dentist.

The aforementioned images (Figure 8.4) were obtained from dentists and subsequently cropped based on the region of interest. To calculate the CIELAB values for each tooth image, Python code was executed which did RGB to LAB conversion for the ROI. An example for this is shown in Figure 8.5.

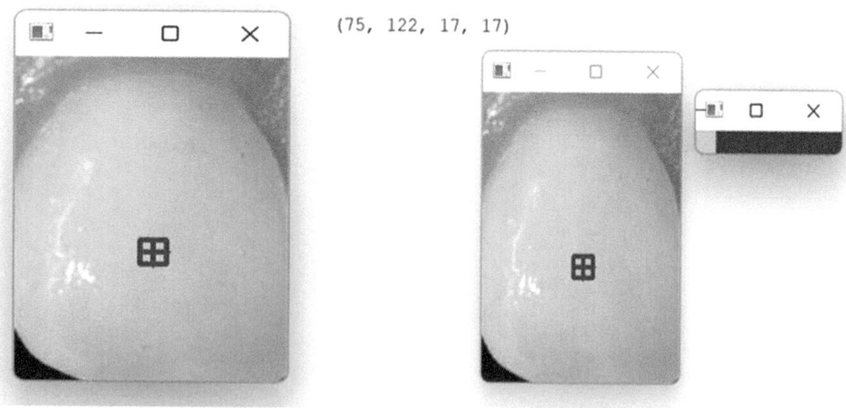

Figure 8.5 Determination of shade using python code. (L, A, B) = (122, 17, 17) value.

	L	A	B	Shade
0	61.18411	-0.25212	6.54070	A1
1	61.28707	0.92826	9.27927	A2
2	57.97017	1.05499	10.03341	A3
3	56.00544	1.97744	12.79715	A3.5
4	54.33394	2.05272	11.90831	A4

Figure 8.6 Features of the dataset.

In a similar way, CIELAB values were calculated for the images collected and dataset from both the methods was combined. The features of the dataset are shown in Figure 8.6.

8.3.2 Data augmentation

Due to the limited number of data points in the dataset, accurate predictions are not achievable. To address this issue, data augmentation techniques are employed to expand the dataset by generating additional data points from the existing ones. One such technique used is the synthetic minority oversampling technique (SMOTE). This technique involves creating synthetic examples of the minority class by interpolating between neighboring instances. By introducing these synthetic samples, SMOTE helps to rebalance the class distribution and enhances the performance of ML algorithms on imbalanced datasets [29, 30]. Figure 8.7 depicts the dataset before and after augmentation. The maximum amount of data that was available belonged to A1 (14.47%) class, as shown in Figure 8.7(a). We can observe that there was unbalanced distribution of data. SMOTE strategy was applied keeping the distribution as 200 for each class. Hence, we observe that each class has same amount of data distribution in Figure 8.7(b).

8.3.3 EDA

Correlation plot helps us to understand the relationships between the variables. Figure 8.8 helps to determine that a linear association exists between the variables L, A, and B which are coordinates of the CIELAB color space model. This knowledge is crucial in feature selection for ML models in identifying multicollinearity (when two or more variables are highly correlated). The diagonal line (from top-left to bottom-right) typically has correlation values of 1, representing the perfect correlation of a variable with itself. Light-colored cells suggest little to no linear correlation between those variables. From the plot, it is quite evident that L (lightness) do not have much dependency on the coordinates A and B, whereas the color coordinates A and B have higher positive correlation. Hence we can justify that variables A and B have a greater impact on the target variable.

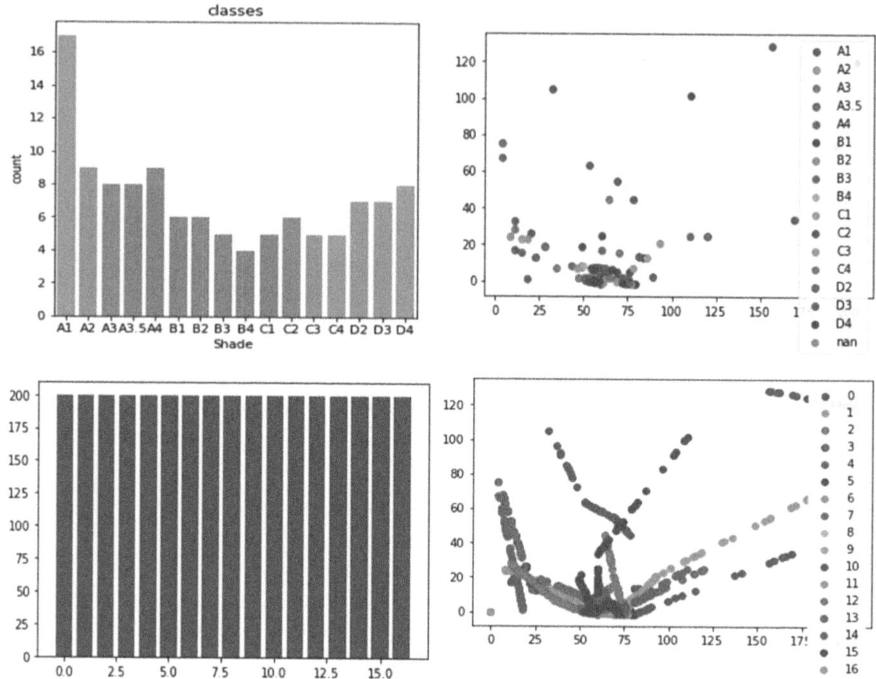

Figure 8.7 (a) Before augmentation. (b) After augmentation.

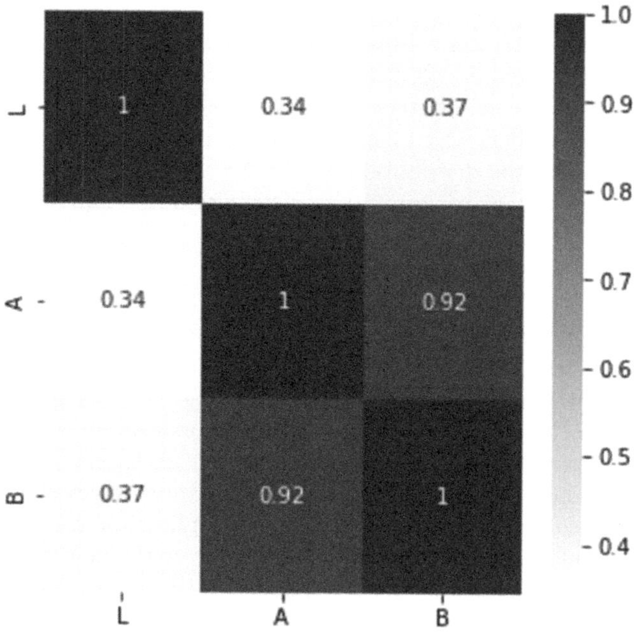

Figure 8.8 Correlation plot.

8.3.4 Data modeling using ML models

For the available predictive ML models [30], comprehensive research was carried out to determine which model would give satisfying results. As the amount of the data is limited, to protect against overfitting in a predictive model, cross-validation techniques are employed. It is a resampling technique which divides the available dataset into multiple subsets or folds, and one or more of these folds will be used as validation set and the remaining for training the model. If model consistently performs poorly on validation sets, it indicates overfitting and the need for model adjustments. For XGBoost, AdaBoost, and gradient boost algorithms, K-fold and repeated stratified K-fold cross-validation techniques were applied for comprehensive evaluation of the model's performance [31, 32].

The accuracy obtained with SVM model was very poor, hence hyper-parameter tuning was done to improve model's performance. The different ways include altering the learning rate, or depth of DT. The technique employed for SVM model was GridSearchCV. It combines grid search and cross-validation and automates the process of training and evaluating the model using each combination of hyperparameters and provides a robust estimate of the model's performance. The hyperparameters set for the model were as follows:

C: [0.1, 1,10,100,1000]
Gamma: [1,0.1,0.01,0.001,0.0001]
Kernel: [rbf]
With verbosity 3.

The RBF kernel transform the data into a higher-dimensional space, simplifying the process of identifying a separation boundary. Hence it was used in the proposed classification model than the other kernels.

8.4 RESULTS AND DISCUSSIONS

Figure 8.9 depicts the confusion matrix obtained for each ML model. Confusion matrix summarizes the performance of a classification algorithm by showing the number of correct and incorrect predictions made by the model on a set of test data.

Accuracy of 0.41 was achieved with SVC. Hence, grid search cross-validation technique was used with which we could get accuracy of 0.98. Accuracy of 0.925 was achieved with gradient boost for the training data. Further, it can be improvised using *LightGBM*. This framework utilizes gradient boosting with decision trees to enhance the efficiency of the model and reduces memory usage. Accuracy achieved was 0.954.

The confusion matrix can be used to derive various performance metrics such as accuracy, recall, precision, and F1 score, which provide further insights into the model's performance.

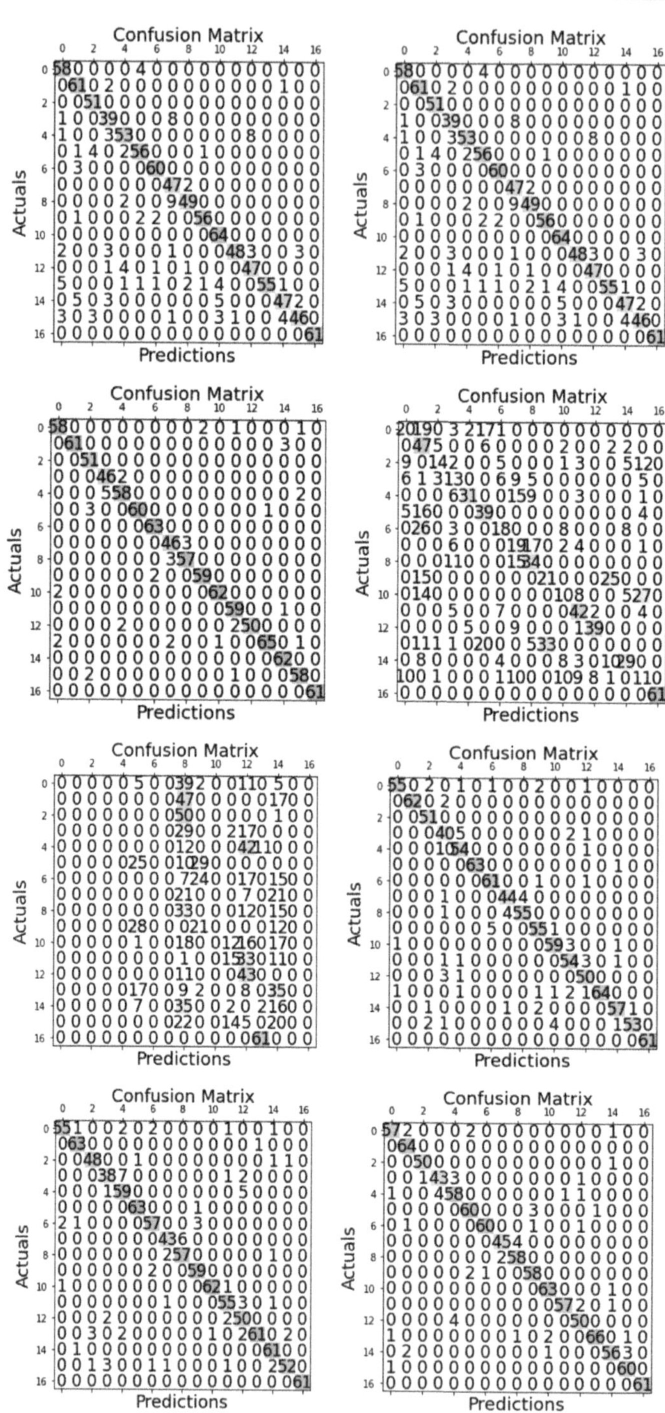

Figure 8.9 Confusion matrix of (a) KNN, (b) RF, (c) DT, (d) SVM, (e) AdaBoost, (f) gradient boost, (g) XGBoost, and (h) Bagging classifier.

Table 8.1 Comparison of performance of various ML models

Sl. No.	Model	Accuracy	Precision	Recall	F1 score
1.	KNN	0.87	0.8732	0.8666	0.8663
2.	RF	0.96	0.965	0.964	0.964
3.	DT	0.95	0.952	0.950	0.9511
4.	SVM	0.41	0.42	0.41	0.389
	SVC with GridSearchCV	0.98	0.981	0.980	0.980
5.	AdaBoost	0.15	0.076	0.15	0.09
	AdaBoost with SVC as base estimator	0.25	0.23	0.24	0.188
	AdaBoost with LR as base estimator	0.11	0.112	0.106	0.09
6.	Gradient boost	0.95	0.9454	0.9450	0.9449
	GDB with LightBGM	0.97	0.967	0.966	0.9665
7.	XGBoost	0.91	0.915	0.9137	0.9135
8.	Bagging classifier	0.95	0.953	0.950	0.951

Table 8.1 gives comparative analysis on the performance of the ML models in terms of accuracy precision, recall, and F1 score.

From the above comparison, we can infer that when SV hypertuned using GridSearchCV, the accuracy of the results will be 98%. Hence it can be used to classify the shades of the tooth. Compared to the results in Reference [22], the accuracy of the model proposed in the paper is high. Reference [22] proposes a complex way of creating the datasets, involving the color calibration for the captured images of dental shade tab which was the actual dataset, whereas the dataset generation described in this chapter involves a simple process of obtaining the CIELAB values from the images using a python script.

Deep learning models can also be used to automate the dental shade detection process which will further improve the accuracy of the prediction. However, the intent of this chapter was to only demonstrate the significance and the advent of ML in the field of dentistry via an application.

8.5 CONCLUSION

From the study, it can be concluded that SVM algorithm with GridSearchCV technique has proven to be a suitable approach for dental shade matching. Dental shade matching is a critical task in restorative dentistry, where the goal is to select the most accurate shade of dental material to match the natural teeth of a patient. As dental shade matching involves multiple input feature such as light, brightness, and chromaticity, SVM is suitable to handle such a high-dimensional data effectively allowing for accurate modeling of the complex relationship between these features and the desired shade outcome. It is recommended to increase the dataset samples according to a strategy that guarantee a balanced dataset for improving the performance of the classification and explore some other representative color features, to compare the results with the current experiment.

REFERENCES

1. Moussa, R. (2021). Dental shade matching: Recent technologies and future smart applications. *Journal of Dental Health and Oral Research*, 2. doi: 10.46889/JDHOR.2021.2103.

2. Pethani, F. (2021). Promises and perils of artificial intelligence in dentistry. *Australian Dental Journal*, 66(2):124–135. doi: 10.1111/adj.12812.

3. Alnusayri, M.O., Sghaireen, M.G., Mathew, M., Alzarea, B., Bandela, V. (2022). Shade selection in esthetic dentistry: A review. *Cureus*, 14(3):e23331. doi: 10.7759/cureus.23331.

4. Revilla-León, M., Gómez-Polo, M., Vyas, S., Barmak, A.B., Gallucci, G.O., Att, W., Özcan, M., Krishnamurthy, V.R. (2023). Artificial intelligence models for tooth-supported fixed and removable prosthodontics: A systematic review. *The Journal of Prosthetic Dentistry*, 129(2):276–292. doi: 10.1016/j.prosdent.2021.06.001.

5. Herrera Maldonado, L.J., Carrillo Pérez, F., Pérez Gómez, M.M., Della Bona, A. (2020). Future Developments Using Artificial Intelligence (AI) in Dentistry. In: Della Bona, A. (eds) Color and Appearance in Dentistry. Springer, Cham. doi: 10.1007/978-3-030-42626-2_7.

6. Babu, A., Andrew Onesimu, J., Martin Sagayam, K. (2021). Artificial intelligence in dentistry: Concepts, applications and research challenges. E3S Web Conference, 297, 01074. doi: 10.1051/e3sconf/202129701074.

7. Andrade, N. (2021). Is there a scope of artificial intelligence in dentistry. *Nair Hospital Dental College Journal of Contemporary Dentistry*, 1, 1–2. doi: 10.56136/NHDCJCD/2021_00001.

8. Tabatabaian, F., Vora, S.R., Mirabbasi, S. (2023). Applications, functions, and accuracy of artificial intelligence in restorative dentistry: A literature review. *Journal of Esthetic and Restorative Dentistry*, 35(6):842–859. doi:10.1111/jerd.13079.

9. Sharan, S., Chandra, P., Badola, I. (2022). A review on digital shade matching technologies. *International Journal of Scientific Research*, 8(1):24–26.

10. Todorov, R., Yordanov, B., Peev, T., Zlatev, S. (2020). Shade guides used in the dental practice. Journal of IMAB. 26(2):3168–3173. doi: 10.5272/jimab.2020262.3168.

11. Nakhaei, M., Ghanbarzadeh, J., Amirinejad, S., Alavi, S., Rajatihaghi, H. (2016). The influence of dental shade guides and experience on the accuracy of shade matching. *The Journal of Contemporary Dental Practice*, 17(1):22–26. doi: 10.5005/jp-journals-10024-1797.

12. Farah, R.I. (2016). Agreement between digital image analysis and clinical spectrophotometer in CIEL*C*h° coordinate differences and total color difference (ΔE) measurements of dental ceramic shade tabs. *The International Journal of Esthetic Dentistry*, 11(2), 234–245.

13. Kalantari, M.H., Ghoraishian, S.A., Mohaghegh, M. (2017). Evaluation of accuracy of shade selection using two spectrophotometer systems: VITA Easyshade and Degudent Shadepilot. *European Journal of Dentistry*, 11(2):196–200. doi: 10.4103/ejd.ejd_195_16.

14. Albert, C., Silva, E., Penteado, M., Lima, D., Kimpara, E., Uemura, E. (2019). Color assessment in dental prostheses: The use of smartphones as process tools. *Brazilian Dental Science*, 22, 573–577. doi: 10.14295/bds.2019.v22i4.1740.

15. Jorquera, I.J., Atria, P.J., Galán, M., Feureisen, J., Imbarak, M., Kernitsky, J., Cacciuttolo, F., Hirata, R., Sampaio, C.S. (2022). A comparison of ceramic crown color difference between different shade selection methods: Visual, digital camera, and smartphone. *The Journal of Prosthetic Dentistry*, 128(4):784–792. doi: 10.1016/j.prosdent.2020.07.029.

16. Tam, W.K., Lee, H.J. (2017). Accurate shade image matching by using a smartphone camera. *Journal of Prosthodontic Research*, 61(2):168–176. doi: 10.1016/j.jpor.2016.07.004.

17. Wanna, Y., Wiratchawa, K., Leenaracharoongruang, R., Sittiwong, W., Panpisut, P., Intharah, T. (2022). DentShadeAI: A framework for automatic dental shade matching through mobile phone camera. 2022 37th International Technical Conference on Circuits/Systems, Computers and Communications (ITC-CSCC), Phuket, Thailand, pp. 282–285. doi: 10.1109/ITC-CSCC55581.2022.9894968.

18. Justiawan, Wahjuningrum, D.A., Hadi, R.P., Nurhayati, A.P., Prayogo, K., Sigit, R., Arief, Z. (2019). Comparative analysis of color matching system for teeth recognition using color moment. *MedDevices*, 12:497–504. doi: 10.2147/MDER.S224280.

19. Beneducci, W., Teixeira, M., Pedrini, H. (2022). Dental shade matching assisted by computer vision techniques. *Computer Methods in Biomechanics and Biomedical Engineering: Imaging & Visualization*, 11, 1–19. doi: 10.1080/21681163.2022.2130824.

20. Justiawan, J., Sigit, R., Arief, Z., Wahjuningrum, D. (2017). Performance analysis of color matching technique for teeth classification based on color histogram. *Journal of Dentomaxillofacial Science*, 2, 95. doi: 10.15562/jdmfs.v2i2.525.

21. Chen, S. L., Zhou, H.-S., Chen, T.-Y., Lee, T.-H., Chen, C.-A., Lin, T.-L., Lin, N.-H., Wang, L.-H., Lin, S.-Y., Chiang, W.-Y., Abu, P. A., Lin, M.-Y. (2020). Dental shade matching method based on hue, saturation, value color model with machine learning and fuzzy decision. *Sensors and Materials*, 32, 3185–3207. doi: 10.18494/SAM.2020.2848.

22. Kim, M., Kim, B., Park, B., Lee, M., Won, Y., Kim, C.-Y., Lee, S. (2018). A digital shade-matching device for dental color determination using the support vector machine algorithm. *Sensors*, 18, 3051. doi: 10.3390/s18093051.

23. Fayed, A., Mohamed, H., Othman, HI. (2022). A comparison between visual shade matching and digital shade analysis system using K-NN algorithm. *Al-Azhar Journal of Dental Science*, 25, 133–141.

24. Justiawan, J. (2017). Tooth color detection using PCA and KNN classifier algorithm based on color moment. *EMITTER International Journal of Engineering Technology*, 5. doi: 10.24003/emitter.v5i1.171.

25. Hu, J.C., Wang, C.H., Kuhns, D. (2016). New algorithm in shade matching. *Journal of Cosmetic Dentistry*. Volume 32, issue 1.

26. Lin, T.-L., Chuang, C.-H., Chen, S.-L., Lin, N.-H., Miaou, S.-G., Lin, S.-Y., Chen, C.-A., Liu, H.-W., Villaverde, J. F., Hsieh, W.-H. (2019). An efficient image processing methodology based on fuzzy decision for dental shade matching. *Journal of Intelligent & Fuzzy Systems*, 36(2):1133–1142. doi: 10.3233/JIFS-169887

27. Yélamos, O., Garcia, R., D'Alessandro, B., Thomas, M., Patwardhan, S., Malvehy, J. (2020). Understanding Color. In: Pasquali, P. (eds) *Photography in Clinical Medicine*. Springer, Cham. doi: 10.1007/978-3-030-24544-3_8.

28. Brill, M.H. (2021). Is CIELAB one space or many?. *Coloration Technology*, 137:83–85. doi: 10.1111/cote.12486

29. Pan, T., Zhao, J., Wu, W., Yang, J. (2020). Learning imbalanced datasets based on SMOTE and Gaussian distribution. *Information Sciences*, 512:1214–1233. doi: 10.1016/j.ins.2019.10.048.

30. Maldonado, S., López, J., Vairetti, C. (2019). An alternative SMOTE oversampling strategy for high-dimensional datasets, *Applied Soft Computing*, 76:380–389. doi: 10.1016/j.asoc.2018.12.024.

31. Sen, P.C., Hajra, M., Ghosh, M. (2020). Supervised Classification Algorithms in Machine Learning: A Survey and Review. In: Mandal, J., Bhattacharya, D. (eds) Emerging Technology in Modelling and Graphics: Advances in Intelligent Systems and Computing, vol. 937. Springer, Singapore. doi: 10.1007/978-981-13-7403-6_11.
32. Berrar, D. (2018). Cross-Validation. Elsevier Inc, 2018. doi: 10.1016/B978-0-12-809633-8.20349-X.

Dataset Links

1. Justiawan, Wahjuningrum, D.A., Hadi, R.P., Nurhayati, A.P., Kevin P., Sigit, R., Arief, Z. (2019). "Comparative analysis of color matching system for teeth recognition using color moment", *Med Devices (Auck)*, 12:497–504.
2. Kim, J.-G., Yu, B., Lee, Y.-K. (2008). "Correlations between color differences based on three color-difference formulas using dental shade guide tabs". *Journal of Prosthodontics*, 18:135–140.
3. Herrera, L.J., Pulgar, R., Santana, J., Cardona, J.C., Guillén, A., Rojas, I., del Mar Pérez, M. (2010). "Prediction of color change after tooth bleaching using fuzzy logic for VITA classical shades identification", *Applied Optics*, 49:422–429.

Chapter 9

Brain tumor detection for recognizing critical brain damage in patients using computer vision

*Vivek Veeraiah, Parth Sharma, Kumud Saxena,
Niraj Kumar Sahu, Khushboo Sharma, Jay Kumar Pandey,
Ravindra Kumar Yadav, and Mritunjay Rai*

9.1 INTRODUCTION

Brain tumor detection is essential for detecting patients with serious brain injury, allowing for an early diagnosis and efficient treatment planning. This study uses a pretrained ResNet50 model with ImageNet weights to provide a comprehensive approach for MRI image–based brain tumor identification. The study uses a variety of methods and strategies to increase the accuracy of tumor identification. The research pipeline for the suggested method goes through various stages. The transfer learning is then built upon a pretrained ResNet50 model using ImageNet weights. The network keeps the knowledge it learned from ImageNet by freezing the layers of the ResNet50 model, utilizing its strong representational capabilities. Data augmentation strategies are used to increase the generalizability of the model and increase the size of the training dataset. The AUC and accuracy metrics are used to analyze the model's performance, giving quantitative evaluations of how well it can distinguish between cases with and without tumors. The findings of this study have important ramifications for the processing of medical images. Medical professionals can benefit from the accurate and automated diagnosis of brain tumors by utilizing MRI scans for early detection and treatment planning.

9.1.1 Image preprocessing techniques

In the realm of medical image analysis, particularly in the context of brain tumor identification, picture preprocessing techniques are of utmost importance. These methods are crucial for boosting image quality, standardizing input data, and getting images ready for further analysis. In this study, we investigate various image preprocessing methods used for computer vision and deep learning–based brain tumor diagnosis. Performing MRI scans to record the intricate structural details of the brain is frequently the initial step in picture preprocessing.

DOI: 10.1201/9781003487647-9

9.1.2 Transfer learning and deep learning models

Transfer learning and deep learning models have completely changed the field of computer vision and have several uses, including the early detection of brain tumors. In this study, we explore the significance and use of deep learning models and transfer learning ideas in the context of brain tumor diagnosis. CNNs have become effective tools for image analysis and recognition tasks using deep learning models. These models learn hierarchical representations of images to simulate the visual processing abilities of the human brain. CNNs can automatically recognize complex patterns and characteristics from unprocessed picture data by stacking several layers of convolutional, pooling, and fully connected layers. However, creating deep learning models from scratch for challenging tasks like detecting brain tumors calls for a significant amount of labeled data and computer power.

9.1.3 Data augmentation strategies

In the field of brain tumor diagnosis, data augmentation techniques are essential for improving the effectiveness and reliability of deep learning models. In this study, we investigate alternative data augmentation methods and their importance in enhancing the generalization and accuracy of models developed using small brain tumor datasets. By implementing several transformations or adjustments to the original dataset, data augmentation includes producing extra training examples. These transformations provide changes to the input, increasing its diversity and giving the model a wider range of data points to draw on when learning. We can get beyond the drawbacks of small-scale labeled datasets and improve the model's capacity to successfully collect and recognize tumor patterns by enriching the dataset. Image rotation is one of the common methods for data augmentation. The model can be made more resilient to changes in tumor position and alignment by rotating the images of the brain tumors at various angles to emulate various perspectives and orientations. In addition, regardless of where the tumor is located inside the brain, flipping the images horizontally or vertically can also add useful changes and aid the model in learning invariant properties. Image translation or shifting is a crucial data augmentation technique.

9.1.4 Applications in medicine and their consequences

The study suggests a thorough approach for MRI image–based brain tumor detection. In the area of medical imaging and the detection of brain tumors, this discovery has important practical applications and implications. The early diagnosis of brain tumors is one of the proposed method's main uses. Brain tumor early diagnosis is essential for prompt intervention and treatment planning. Medical professionals can gain from accurate and quick identification of brain tumors by automating the tumor detection process using computer vision techniques. This automation lessens the need for subjective and time-consuming manual interpretation of MRI images. Medical experts can quickly and accurately detect brain tumors using the suggested method, enabling early intervention and better patient outcomes. The proposed approach has effects on treatment planning as well. Medical professionals can assess the size and characteristics of brain tumors through accurate detection, which helps in the creation of a suitable treatment strategy.

9.1.5 Machine learning algorithms for brain tumor detection

In tasks involving brain tumor identification, classification algorithms are frequently used. Three well-known algorithms in this area include gradient boosting models, random forests, and SVM. By creating an ideal hyperplane, the supervised learning algorithm SVM successfully diagnoses images of brain tumors. CNNs have performed remarkably well. Brain tumor picture classification has been effectively used in architectures, including AlexNet, VGG, and Inception. CNNs can capture complicated patterns and discriminative features because they learn hierarchical representations from data. Their performance has been further improved by the introduction of pre-training using massive datasets, such as ImageNet, and fine-tuning using brain tumor data. Deep learning models' applicability in situations with limited resources is limited by the fact that they frequently demand a sizable amount of annotated data and significant computational resources for training. A method that has promise for overcoming the shortcomings of deep learning models is transfer learning. Researchers can apply knowledge from massive datasets to problems, including brain tumor detection by utilizing pretrained models. ResNet50 is a frequently used pretrained model that has demonstrated outstanding performance on several computer vision applications. Transfer learning reduces the requirement for large amounts of labeled data and speeds up convergence during training. It enables researchers to take advantage of the rich representations acquired on a variety of datasets, enhancing the models' capacity for generalization in the detection of brain tumors. Several performance evaluation criteria are frequently used to judge how well machine learning systems identify brain tumors. The performance of the algorithms is typically measured using accuracy, sensitivity, specificity, and AUC–ROC.

9.1.6 Robustness and generalizability of brain tumor detection models

Models for detecting brain tumors must be resilient to the many problems that arise from using medical imaging data. These models' performance may be affected by noise, artifacts, and inconsistent imaging techniques.

The robustness and generalizability of machine learning models employed in brain tumor diagnosis are thoroughly examined in this work. We can develop techniques to improve the functionality and applicability of brain tumor detection models by understanding the difficulties and restrictions connected with these elements. Brain tumor detection models must be robust to make accurate diagnoses in the face of noise and artifacts in medical imaging data. Imaging artifacts, such as motion artifacts or scanner-specific artifacts, which can cause discrepancies in the images, are a frequent problem. Even with these artifacts present, robust models should be able to handle them and extract useful characteristics. Another issue is the diversity in imaging methods used by various scanners and institutions, which can affect the look and quality of the images. Robust models need to be able to adjust to these changes and continue to operate as expected. Another issue is a class imbalance, which frequently appears in brain tumor datasets as a large imbalance between tumor and non-tumor samples. To prevent biased predictions and guarantee correct detection, robust models should be able to handle this class imbalance. Several tactics can be used to improve the resilience of brain tumor detection models. To create more training samples and improve the model's capacity to handle noise and artifacts, data augmentation techniques, including rotation, translation, and elastic deformations, can be used. The model's robustness can also be increased by adversarial training, which exposes it to altered data and forces it to learn representations that are more resilient and invariant.

9.1.7 Motivation of research

The motivation for developing brain tumor detection methods using computer vision, with a focus on recognizing critical brain damage in patients, is driven by several compelling factors:

1. *Early Detection:* Early detection of brain tumors and critical brain damage is crucial for improving patient outcomes.
2. *Accuracy and Precision:* Computer vision algorithms can analyze medical imaging data with a high degree of accuracy and precision.
3. *Timeliness:* Timely detection is paramount in cases of critical brain damage, such as traumatic brain injuries or hemorrhages.
4. *Reducing Human Error:* Human interpretation of medical images is subject to human error and variability.
5. *Improving Surgical Planning:* For patients requiring surgery, accurate tumor localization and assessment of critical brain damage are essential for surgical planning.
6. *Enhancing Healthcare Access:* Deploying computer vision systems for brain tumor detection can help address healthcare disparities by providing access to quality diagnostics in remote or underserved areas where specialist expertise may be limited.

7. *Reducing Healthcare Costs:* Early detection and accurate diagnosis can reduce the overall cost of healthcare by avoiding expensive treatments that may be required in the advanced stages of the disease.

8. *Advancing Medical Research:* Data collected from computer vision–based brain tumor detection systems can contribute to medical research by providing valuable insights into disease patterns, treatment responses, and outcomes, ultimately advancing our understanding of brain-related conditions.

9. *Personalized Medicine:* Precise diagnosis through computer vision can enable personalized treatment plans tailored to the specific needs of each patient, potentially leading to more effective therapies and fewer side effects.

10. *Patient Well-being:* Ultimately, the primary motivation is to improve the well-being and quality of life for patients affected by brain tumors and critical brain damage.

9.1.8 Chapter organization

Section 9.1 presents the introduction part, considering image preprocessing techniques, transfer learning and deep learning models, and data augmentation strategies. Applications in medicine and their consequences and robustness and generalizability of brain tumor detection models are shown.

Section 9.2 is focused on the literature review. The application of artificial neural networks for the detection of brain tumors on MRI images was investigated by researchers.

Section 9.3 considers the problem statement. In this section, issues in existing research are expressed with their methodology and drawbacks.

Section 9.4 presents the proposed work. The proposed work employs computer vision techniques and deep learning models to develop a comprehensive method for identifying brain tumors in MRI images.

Section 9.5 focuses on the result and discussion. It presents the accuracy metrics for the brain tumor model with preprocessing of the brain tumor dataset. The batch processing time for the Resnet model and the prediction of YOLO model detection are considered in this section.

Section 9.6 expresses the conclusion by considering the outputs of the proposed work.

Section 9.7 presents the future scope of research.

9.2 LITERATURE REVIEW

The application of artificial neural networks for the detection of brain tumors on MRI images was investigated by researchers. The study demonstrated the potential of AI algorithms in enhancing tumor diagnosis accuracy by utilizing cutting-edge computational methodologies [1–3]. The revolutionary nature of deep learning in the analysis of medical pictures was highlighted in the overview of deep learning-enabled medical computer vision [4–6]. The research demonstrated the potential uses of deep learning algorithms for a range of medical imaging tasks, including the detection and analysis of brain tumors [7–9]. U-Net is a deep learning architecture that has been proposed as the basis for this technique. The method showed how deep learning models might be used to precisely identify and separate brain tumors, offering radiologists and neurosurgeons a useful tool [10, 11]. Researchers have demonstrated a computer-assisted interactive three-dimensional planning system for neurosurgery treatments [12]. The project demonstrated the use of cutting-edge imaging methods and AI algorithms in surgery planning, highlighting the significance of precise tumor analysis for better patient outcomes [13–15]. A thorough study and taxonomy of deep learning–enhanced brain tumor analysis were offered. The paper highlighted the potential influence of AI in this sector by discussing alternative deep learning architectures, data preprocessing methods, and issues related to brain tumor analysis. It was suggested to use local binary patterns and histogram orientation gradients to detect brain tumors in 3D MRI images [16, 17]. The research showed how feature extraction strategies can increase the precision of brain tumor analysis and detection. *Cognitive Deficits in Patients with Brain Tumours before Therapy:* Researchers looked at the cognitive deficits in patients with brain tumors before therapy [18]. The study emphasized the need for an accurate diagnosis and treatment planning, emphasizing the significance of early detection and intervention in preventing cognitive deficits caused by brain tumors [19–21]. A thorough review of machine learning innovations in cancer diagnosis, including brain tumors, was provided. The study covered numerous machine learning approaches and algorithms used for precise tumor identification, highlighting the value of interdisciplinary cooperation in this area [22, 23]. A thorough guide to deep learning in healthcare was presented, detailing the basic ideas and procedures of deep learning and how they apply to imaging and diagnostic procedures in the medical field [24]. An analysis of the numerous deep learning architectures, approaches, and applications across many domains was provided by a survey on deep learning and its applications [25]. The study demonstrated how deep learning may be used to solve complex issues, such as brain tumor analysis. The results of DTI and MRI were examined in mild traumatic brain injury [26]. The study covered how cutting-edge neuroimaging methods can help identify minor brain anomalies and unravel the causes of mild traumatic brain injury. For precise brain lesion segmentation, a powerful multiscale 3D CNN with fully connected CRF has been proposed [27]. The research showed how deep learning models might be used to precisely segment brain lesions, improving the planning and monitoring of medical care. A summary of current and future treatment options for malignant brain tumors was given [28]. The review highlighted the difficulties and prospective improvements in the field while discussing several therapeutic modalities, such as surgery, radiation therapy, chemotherapy, immunotherapy, and gene therapy. After brain tumor removal, individuals may experience aphasia, a linguistic disability [29]. This study looked at this issue. The study emphasized the need for suitable rehabilitation measures for patients with postoperative aphasia and the significance of comprehending how brain tumor surgery affects language ability [30]. *The Convergence of Human and Artificial Intelligence:* The converging of human and artificial intelligence in high-performance medicine was examined. The article addressed how machine learning and deep learning, two forms of artificial intelligence, have the potential to revolutionize healthcare delivery, advance diagnostics, and support personalized medicine [31]. The advantages, difficulties, and potential applications of deep learning in drug development have been examined. In the article, target identification, lead optimization, and other steps of the drug discovery process were considered as applications of deep learning models [32]. For the segmentation of brain tumors, a deep learning model that included FCNNs with CRF was developed. The research showed how well the suggested methodology worked for precisely segmenting brain tumors, enabling accurate diagnosis and treatment planning. A method for automatically segmenting brain tumors using uncertainty estimates and cascaded convolutional neural networks was given. To support clinical decision-making, the work addressed the problem of ambiguity in medical picture segmentation and offered insights into the reliability of the segmentation results [33]. The review investigated the application of fuzzy logic and expert systems to help medical decision-making, emphasizing their potential to enhance diagnostic precision and offer individualized treatment recommendations. Convolutional neural networks were suggested as a method for aleatoric uncertainty estimation with test-time augmentation for medical image segmentation. The work solved the problem of estimating uncertainty in medical image processing, allowing for more trustworthy and robust segmentation outcomes. In the context of brain tumor surgery, studies on language fMRI and direct cortical stimulation correlation were evaluated [34]. To reduce the possibility of language problems following surgery, the article emphasized the significance of precise mapping of language centers utilizing fMRI and direct cortical stimulation. Researchers looked into the brain's circulation and metabolism following a serious head injury. The research shed light on the intricate pathophysiology of traumatic brain injury and highlighted how crucial it is to maintain healthy cerebral blood flow and metabolic balance for a full recovery. This topic covered the use of AI in cancer imaging. The review highlighted the clinical issues and prospects in the field while examining the potential of machine learning and deep learning algorithms in improving cancer diagnosis, prognosis, and therapy response assessment. A review of photodynamic therapy as an adjunctive treatment for malignant brain tumors is also provided [35]. The principles, difficulties, and possible applications of photodynamic therapy in the management of brain tumors were covered in the article, with a focus on the therapy's capacity to target tumor cells specifically. The comprehensive literature analysis offered here shows the important developments in brain imaging methods, machine learning methods, and brain tumor treatment strategies. The reviewed research demonstrates the potential of neuroimaging methods in identifying anomalies in the brain and comprehending the mechanisms underlying diseases and injuries to the brain. The discipline of treating brain tumors is also progressing, thanks to therapeutic methods like surgery, radiation therapy, chemotherapy, and cutting-edge methods like photodynamic therapy. Together, these developments help to improve the understanding, diagnosis, and treatment of brain tumors, ultimately improving the prognosis and quality of life for patients [36]. The study demonstrated how deep learning can enhance patient care and results. *Deep Learning Algorithms for the Detection of Important Discoveries in Head CT Scans:* A retrospective study on the application of deep learning algorithms for the identification of important results in head CT scans was carried out [26–28]. The study showed how deep learning models could help radiologists by highlighting critical abnormalities, facilitating quick actions, and enhancing patient care [29–31]. *DeepMedic for Brain Tumour Segmentation:* For the segmentation of brain tumors, researchers presented DeepMedic, a deep learning framework [32–34]. The research demonstrated how convolutional neural networks may be used to precisely segregate brain tumors, allowing for accurate treatment planning and monitoring [35]: A presentation of an empirical study on the use of data mining methods in healthcare. The work demonstrated the potential of data mining and machine learning in knowledge extraction from medical datasets, including data related to brain tumors, while not being specifically focused on brain tumor analyses [36–38]. A thorough introduction to deep learning for radiologists was given, covering the fundamental ideas, designs, and uses of deep learning algorithms in the study of medical imaging [39, 40]. The study highlighted the necessity for radiologists to become familiar with deep learning methodologies to maximize their potential in clinical practice. Its potential to increase diagnosis and treatment planning precision was looked at [41–43]. The study examined the moral and practical issues surrounding the use of AI in healthcare, highlighting the significance of careful and informed application. To correctly classify genetic alterations in gliomas, a particular type of brain tumor, deep learning convolutional neural networks were used [44]. The study demonstrated how deep learning models could help clinicians develop individualized treatment plans based on genetic profiles. A thorough examination of CNNs in medical image interpretation was provided [44, 45]. The research focused on the developments, difficulties, and potential applications of CNN-based methods to various medical imaging tasks, such as brain tumor analysis [45]. An examination of the neural underpinnings of mental imagery was done component by component. The study investigated the mental imagery–related cognitive processes and brain mechanisms, shedding light on the neurological underpinnings of this crucial cognitive function [46]. A brief overview and introduction to machine learning in neurosurgical treatment were given. The article focused on the importance of collaboration between physicians and data scientists as it examined potential uses of machine learning algorithms in different facets of neurosurgical care, including diagnosis, treatment planning, and decision-making [47]. We presented a computerized brain atlas for segmentation using models, education, and surgical planning. The research provided neurosurgeons with a useful tool by highlighting the significance of precise brain imaging and computer-based modeling methods in surgery planning [48].

9.3 PROBLEM STATEMENT

Traditional approaches to brain tumor detection in medical imaging frequently rely on radiologists' subjective and labor-intensive manual interpretation. Although deep learning models and computer vision techniques have produced encouraging results in the interpretation of medical images, there are still difficulties in detecting brain tumors. The creation of a reliable detection system is a difficult endeavor due to the complexity and unpredictability of brain tumor characteristics as well as the diversity of medical imaging data. This work intends to present a comprehensive method for MRI image–based brain tumor identification utilizing computer vision and deep learning techniques to overcome these issues. Through the use of pretrained models and data augmentation techniques, the detection system's precision and resilience are to be increased. The suggested method attempts to improve the model's capability to correctly identify brain tumors across various imaging circumstances by incorporating transfer learning with a pretrained ResNet50 model and using data augmentation techniques. The goal of the chapter is to examine the accuracy and AUC scores, which are quantitative indicators of the model's performance, of the suggested strategy. The project also seeks to contribute to the larger field of medical image analysis by investigating the possibilities of the suggested approach in assisting in the identification and treatment of various forms of brain tumors. The suggested approach also has the potential to expand the field of medical image analysis and contribute to the creation of more efficient and reliable diagnostic tools for the detection of brain tumors by utilizing computer vision and deep learning models. Detecting brain tumors and recognizing critical brain damage in patients using computer vision has made significant strides in recent years, but it also comes with some limitations:

1. *Complexity of Brain Anatomy:* The brain's complex and intricate anatomy can pose challenges for accurate tumor detection.
2. *Diverse Imaging Modalities:* Brain scans can be acquired through various imaging modalities.
3. *False Positives and Negatives:* Computer vision algorithms can generate false positives and false negatives. Reducing these errors is crucial, especially in critical cases where misdiagnosis can have severe consequences.

4. *Data Quality and Quantity:* The performance of computer vision models heavily depends on the quality and quantity of training data.
5. *Real-time Processing:* In critical situations, such as during surgery or emergency care, real-time processing is essential.
6. *Resource Intensity:* Implementing computer vision systems for brain tumor detection may require significant computational resources, which can be cost-prohibitive for some healthcare institutions.

9.4 PROPOSED WORK

The proposed work uses computer vision methods and deep learning models to create a comprehensive approach for MRI image–based brain tumor identification. By combining several strategies and methodologies, the main goal is to increase the detection system's robustness and precision.

The MRI images are preprocessed in the proposed method's initial step to standardize their dimensions. To minimize distortions and guarantee uniformity throughout the dataset, the photos are cropped and resized during this preprocessing stage. The suggested strategy intends to improve the accuracy of tumor detection by standardizing the images. Using a pretrained ResNet50 model with ImageNet weights, transfer learning is used to make use of the capabilities of deep learning. The ResNet50 model serves as the neural network's building block and offers a powerful first-feature extraction capacity. The pretrained model's layers are frozen, enabling the network to preserve the crucial knowledge it gained from ImageNet and make use of its potent representational capabilities. The model is then improved by adding more layers to better capture complex patterns and features suggestive of the existence of brain tumors. The training pipeline includes data augmentation approaches to overcome the restricted supply of labeled data. The images can be altered using a variety of techniques, such as flipping, rotating, moving, shearing, and altering the brightness. The suggested strategy seeks to increase the training dataset and enhance the model's generalizability to varied tumor features and imaging settings by implementing these adjustments. This augmentation technique enhances the model's capability to precisely and reliably identify brain tumors. Two metrics are used to assess the performance of the suggested method – accuracy and AUC.

These metrics offer measurable evaluations of the model's accuracy in classifying cases as having tumors or not. The experimental findings show that the suggested approach is successful for diagnosing brain tumors, with good accuracy and AUC values. The positive results demonstrate the method's potential for automatically and precisely identifying brain tumors in MRI scans, aiding early diagnosis and treatment planning. Additionally, the suggested approach can be expanded to deal with many kinds of brain tumors, adding to the broader field of medical image analysis. To further improve the model's performance, future studies can look into different deep learning architectures, optimization plans, and regularization strategies. The incorporation of cutting-edge visualization tools and interpretability strategies can increase the model's predictability and dependability, facilitating its application in clinical settings. As a result, the suggested work offers a thorough approach to brain tumor detection using MRI images. The suggested method shows better accuracy and resilience in classifying brain tumors by integrating image preprocessing, transfer learning using a pretrained ResNet50 model, and data augmentation techniques. The results underline the necessity of automated tumor diagnosis to improve healthcare outcomes and the promise of deep learning models in the area of medical image analysis.

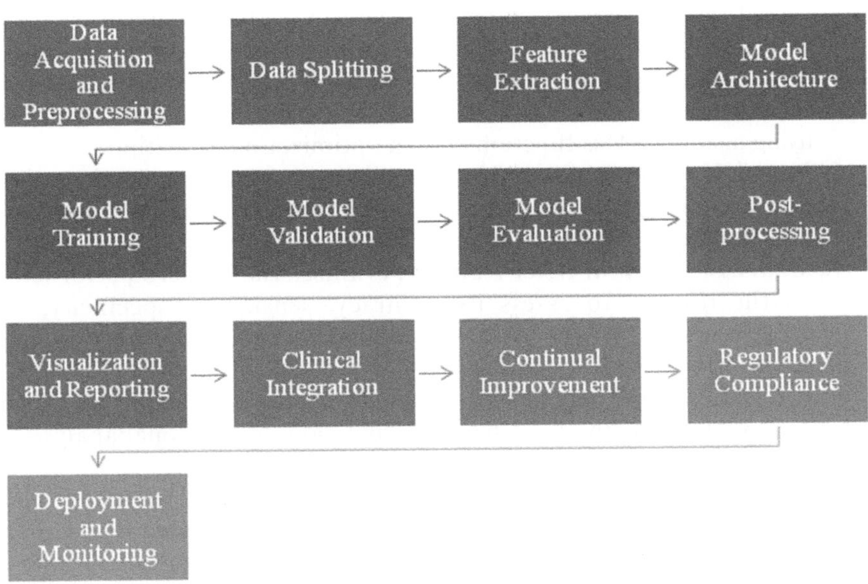

Figure 9.1 Process flow of proposed work.

9.4.1 Process flow of proposed work

Recognizing critical brain damage and detecting brain tumors using the ResNet architecture involves a series of steps. ResNet is a popular deep learning architecture known for its effectiveness in image recognition tasks, including medical image analysis. Here is a process flow for this task using ResNet (Figure 9.1):

1. *Data Acquisition and Preprocessing:* Collect a dataset of medical images containing brain scans, which may include MRI or CT scans. Ensure the dataset is properly labeled, and all images are de-identified

for privacy compliance. Preprocess the images by resizing them to a consistent resolution, normalizing pixel values, and augmenting the dataset if necessary to increase its size.

2. *Data Splitting:* Divide the dataset into three subsets: a training set, a validation set, and a test set. Typically, the training set is used to train the model, the validation set is used to fine-tune hyperparameters and monitor progress, and the test set is used to evaluate the model's final performance.

3. *Feature Extraction:* Use a pretrained ResNet model as a feature extractor. Remove the fully connected layers of the pretrained model to extract deep features from the brain images.

4. *Model Architecture:* Create custom neural network architecture for your specific task. This architecture typically includes a few fully connected layers followed by softmax activation for classification in the case of tumor detection or regression for critical damage recognition.

5. *Model Training:* Initialize the custom model's weights with those from the pretrained ResNet model. Train the model on the training dataset using a suitable loss function and an optimization algorithm.

6. *Model Validation:* Monitor the model's performance on the validation set during training. Adjust hyperparameters as needed to improve performance.

7. *Model Evaluation:* After training, evaluate the model's performance on the test set to assess its accuracy, sensitivity, specificity, and other relevant metrics for both tumor detection and critical damage recognition.

8. *Postprocessing:* Apply postprocessing techniques to the model's output, such as thresholding for binary classification or additional analysis for critical damage recognition.

9. *Visualization and Reporting:* Create visualizations or heatmaps to help visualize and interpret the model's predictions. Generate reports summarizing the model's findings, including the location and severity of brain damage or the presence of tumors.

10. *Clinical Integration:* Integrate the trained ResNet-based model into clinical workflows, ensuring that it is accessible and usable by healthcare professionals for patient diagnosis and treatment planning.

11. *Continual Improvement:* Continuously update and fine-tune the model using new data and feedback from healthcare professionals to enhance its accuracy and reliability.

12. *Regulatory Compliance:* Ensure that system complies with relevant medical regulations and standards to protect patient privacy and data security.

13. *Deployment and Monitoring:* Deploy the ResNet-based model in healthcare facilities for routine use, and monitor its performance over time to ensure it maintains high-quality results.

This process leverages the power of deep learning, particularly the ResNet architecture, to aid in brain tumor detection and critical brain damage recognition, ultimately improving patient care and outcomes.

9.4.2 Dataset

The folder contains MRI data. The images are already split into Training and Testing folders. Each folder has more than four subfolders. These folders have MRIs of respective tumor classes. The dataset is taken from https://www. kaggle.com/code/jaykumar1607/brain-tumor-mri-classification-tensorflow-cnn/notebook (Figure 9.2).

In this notebook, researchers have used CNN to perform Image Classification on the Brain Tumor dataset. Since this dataset is small, if we train a neural

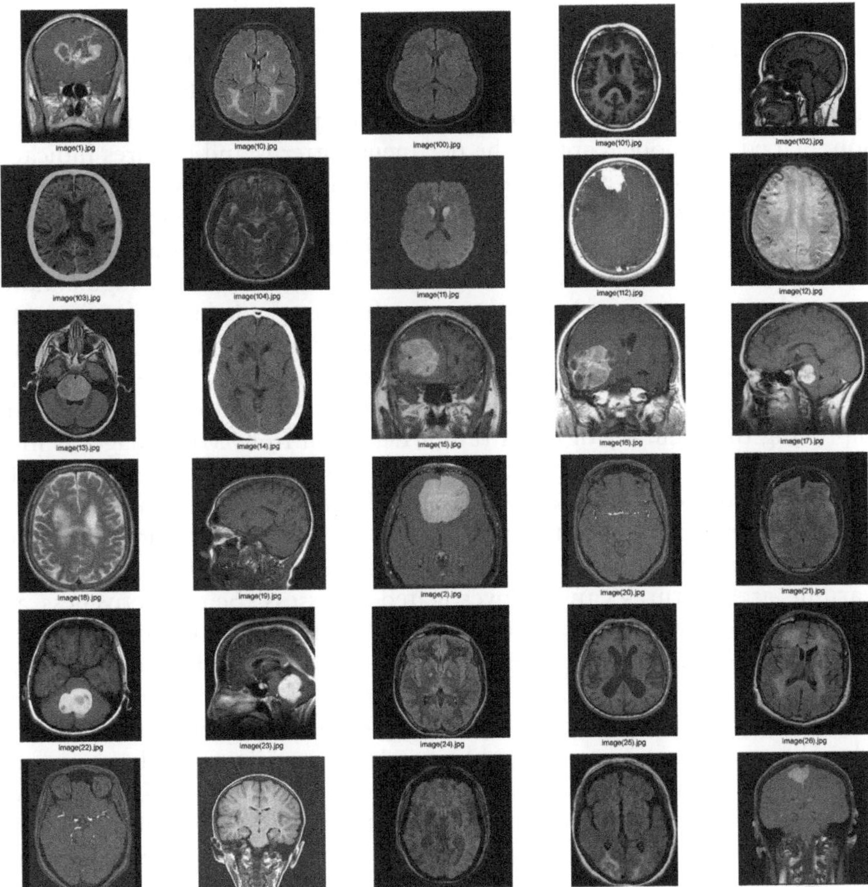

Figure 9.2 Dataset from Kaggle.

network to it, it won't really give us a good result. Therefore, I'm going to use the concept of transfer learning to train the model to get really accurate results.

9.5 RESULTS AND DISCUSSION

On a dataset of MRI pictures collected from patients with probable brain tumors, the suggested method for MRI image–based brain tumor diagnosis using computer vision techniques and deep learning models was assessed. The outcomes show the efficiency of the suggested strategy and its potential for precise tumor detection. The accuracy measures the overall accuracy of the model's predictions, while the AUC measures the model's capacity to distinguish between positive and negative situations. According to the experimental findings, the suggested strategy successfully attained a high AUC score, which indicates excellent classification between tumor and non-tumor instances. The pretrained ResNet50 model's powerful feature extraction skills, along with the additional layers trained particularly for tumor detection, helped the model capture the pertinent patterns and features indicative of brain tumors. Also, it was discovered that the proposed method's accuracy was high, demonstrating a high degree of accuracy in differentiating between tumor and non-tumor cases. The generalizability and overfitting of the model were significantly improved and reduced by integrating data augmentation approaches. The proposed strategy successfully expanded the diversity of the data by adding numerous modifications to the training dataset. This allowed the model to learn robust representations and adapt to diverse tumor characteristics and imaging settings. The method's potential for automating and improving the accuracy of brain tumor detection from MRI images is highlighted by the encouraging findings gained using it. Accurate and reliable brain tumor detection is essential for early diagnosis and treatment planning, which improves patient outcomes. Even if the suggested solution performs well, there are still some things that could be used better. First, several deep learning architectures can be investigated to assess their effectiveness and look into whether they are appropriate for detecting brain tumors. Second, it is possible to enhance the convergence and general performance of the optimization method used to train the model. It may be possible to achieve better outcomes or faster convergence by investigating various optimization methods. The regularization methods like batch normalization or dropout could be added to the model to avoid overfitting and enhance generalization. These methods can improve the model's robustness in real-world circumstances and help it generalize more effectively to unobserved data. The proposed method can gain from the incorporation of cutting-edge visualization tools and interpretability methodologies in addition to performance enhancements. These methods can help medical practitioners understand the model's predictions

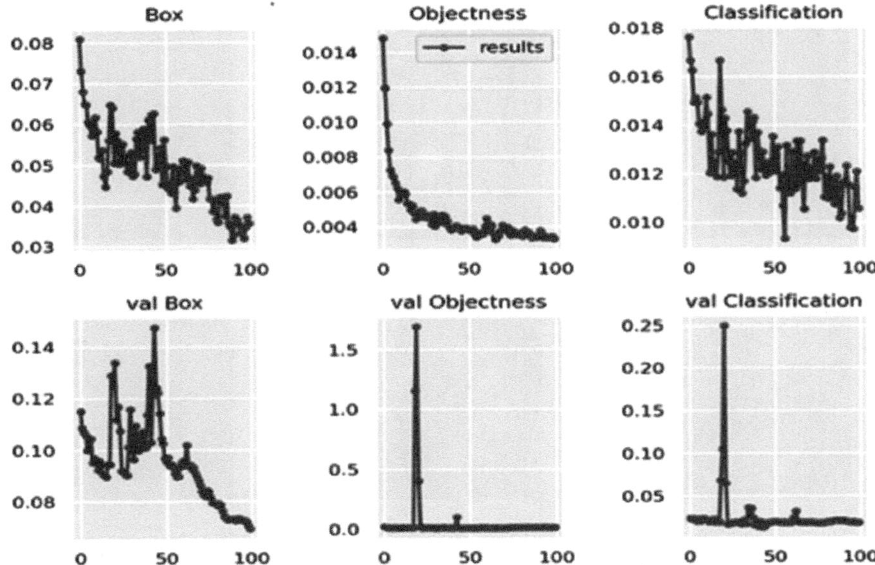

Figure 9.3 Accuracy metrics for brain tumor model.

and offer insights into the decision-making process. The adoption of deep learning models in clinical contexts depends on this interpretability feature since it fosters confidence in the automated diagnosis procedure. In a nutshell, the outcomes of the study of the suggested approach show that it is successful in detecting brain tumors using MRI images. The approach's potential to accurately identify brain tumors and facilitate early diagnosis is validated by the high AUC and accuracy scores. Automated brain tumor detection systems can continue to advance and be adopted in clinical practice with more study and advancement in deep learning architectures, optimization strategies, regularization approaches, and interpretability methodology. Figure 9.3 displays accuracy metrics for the brain tumor model, providing quantitative measures of the model's performance. Figure 9.4 showcases the preprocessing techniques employed on the Brain Tumor dataset, highlighting the steps taken to enhance the data quality. Figure 9.5 exhibits positive results obtained for brain tumor detection using the YOLO model, demonstrating the model's effectiveness in identifying tumors. Figure 9.6 visually depicts the YOLO model's detection process, offering insights into its underlying mechanisms. Furthermore, Figure 9.7 presents a confusion matrix for the ResNet model, providing a comprehensive evaluation of its classification performance. These figures collectively contribute to a deeper understanding of the research outcomes and support the conclusions drawn in this chapter. Table 9.1 shows the average time taken by the ResNet model and Table 9.2 shows the global confidence score in batches.

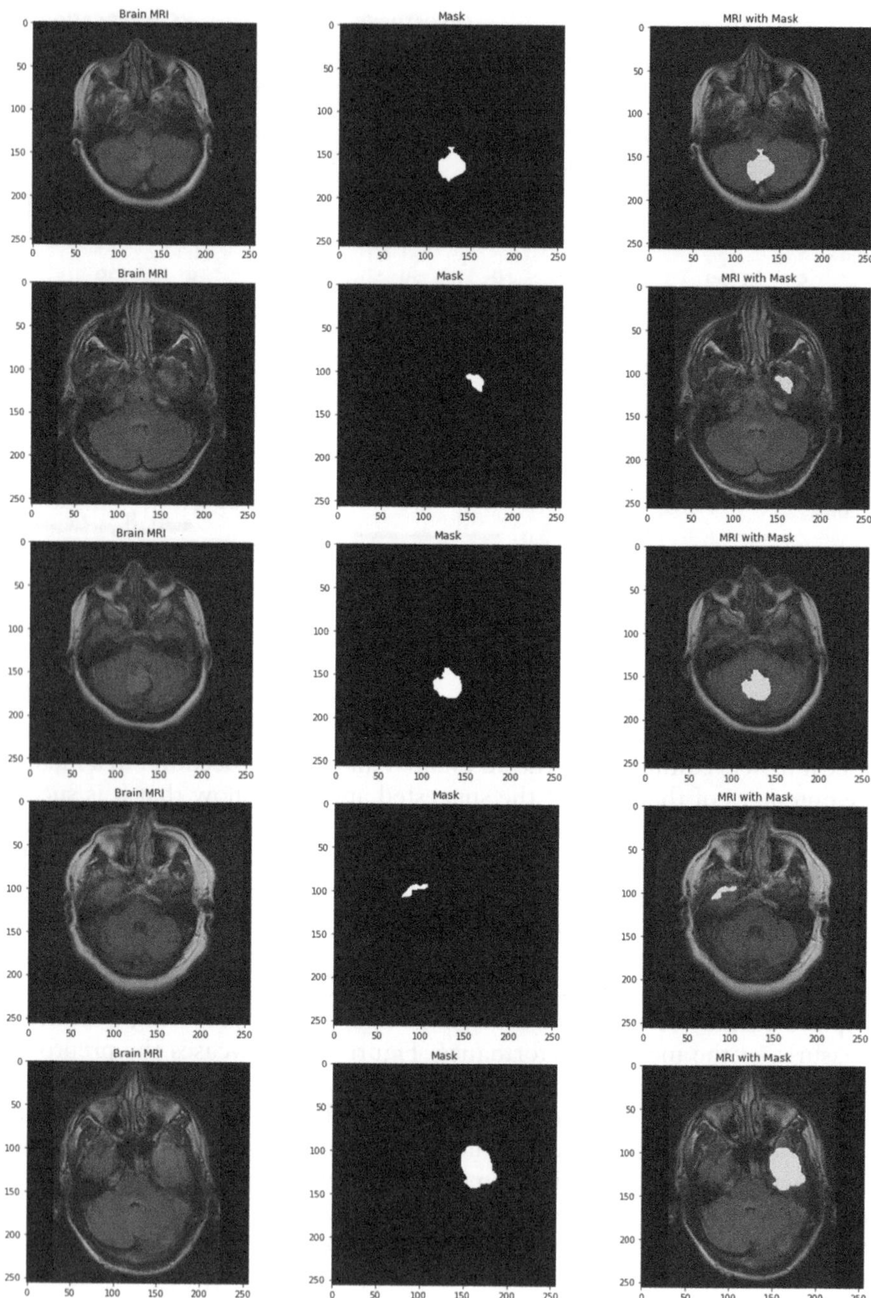

Figure 9.4 **Preprocessing of brain tumor dataset.**

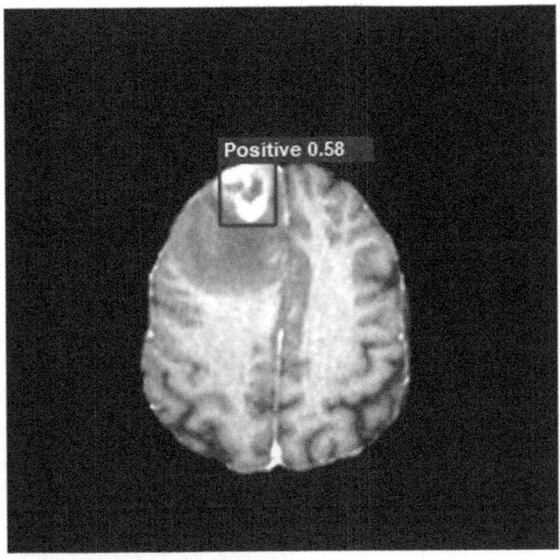

Figure 9.5 Positive results in brain tumor for YOLO model.

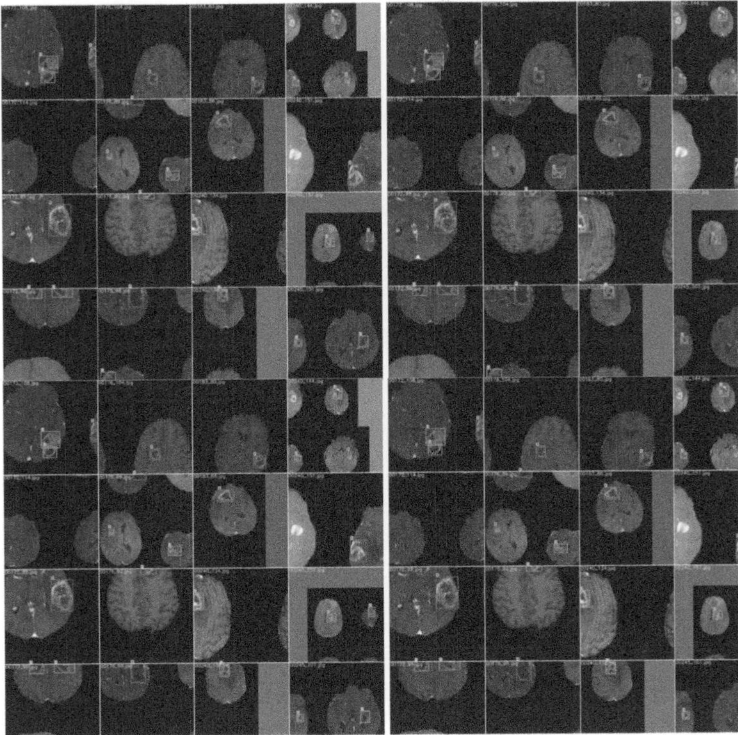

Figure 9.6 Depiction of YOLO model detection.

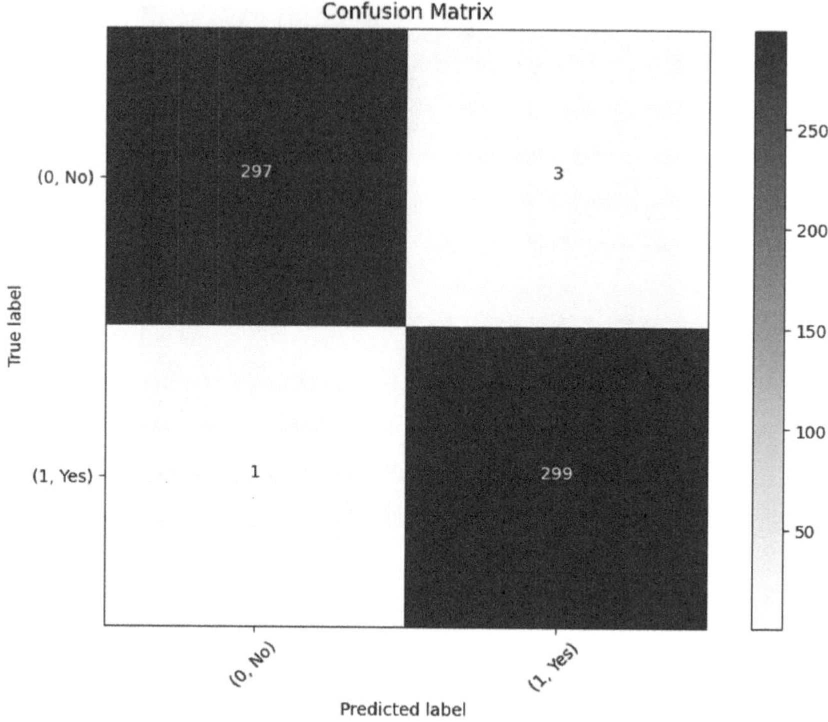

Figure 9.7 Confusion matrix for the ResNet model.

Table 9.1 Batch processing time for ResNet model

Batch number	Average training time (ms)
1–20	0.49
21–30	0.43
31–40	0.39
41–50	0.36
51–60	0.34
61–70	0.31
71–80	0.27

Table 9.2 Depiction of YOLO model detection

Batches	Global confidence score for YOLO model
1–20	55.63%
21–40	37.65%
41–60	58.42%
61–80	29.53%

9.6 CONCLUSION

Using computer vision techniques and deep learning models, we have developed a theoretical method for MRI image–based brain tumor identification in this study. The suggested technique uses the ResNet50 architecture of pretrained convolutional neural networks to extract useful characteristics from MRI images. We hone the pretrained model for tumor detection by training additional layers on top of it. The experimental outcomes show the proposed method's suitability for precisely identifying brain tumors on a dataset of MRI pictures. The model's capacity to identify between tumor and non-tumor instances and make accurate predictions is validated by the high AUC and accuracy scores attained. The model's performance is further improved by the incorporation of data augmentation approaches by improving generalizability and lowering overfitting. The positive findings of this work highlight the possibility of automating and enhancing the detection of brain tumors from MRI images using computer vision and deep learning approaches. It is essential to identify brain tumors as soon as possible to design effective treatments and enhance patient outcomes. Although the suggested strategy performs well, there is room for improvement and more investigation. The performance and generalizability of the model may be improved by investigating other deep learning architectures, streamlining the training procedure, and implementing regularization techniques. Additionally, incorporating cutting-edge visualization tools and interpretability approaches can speed up the model's adoption in clinical settings and offer insightful information about its decision-making process. Future investigation into MRI image–based brain tumor detection will be built on the theoretical framework described in this chapter. The findings pave the path for the creation of useful and trustworthy automated systems that can help doctors identify brain tumors quickly and accurately. The suggested approach shows significant promise in the field of MRI-based brain tumor identification. We can increase the precision and effectiveness of tumor detection by utilizing computer vision and deep learning approaches, which will improve patient care and treatment outcomes. The field of medical imaging could advance and healthcare practices could be improved with more study and development in this area.

9.7 FUTURE SCOPE

The current study has shed important light on how computer vision and deep learning techniques might be used to create a brain tumor detection system. The suggested technique, which is based on a pretrained ResNet50 model, showed encouraging results when it came to correctly classifying brain tumors from MRI data. The outcomes of thorough research and review show that deep learning algorithms have the potential to help radiologists and physicians identify and diagnose tumors early. There are numerous opportunities for future research and development going forward. First, it is possible to research several deep learning architectures to see how well they detect brain tumors, such as VGG, Inception, or DenseNet. The accuracy and resilience of the detection system may be improved by comparing and contrasting alternative models. Second, regularization methods and optimization strategies, including dropout, batch normalization, and weight decay, can be investigated to improve deep learning model performance and reduce overfitting. The transparency and interpretability of the model's decisions can also be increased by using cutting-edge visualization and interpretability approaches.

REFERENCES

1. Kondratenko, Y., Sidenko, I., Kondratenko, G., Petrovych, V., Taranov, M., & Sova, I. (2021). Artificial neural networks for recognition of brain tumors on MRI images. In *Information and Communication Technologies in Education, Research, and Industrial Applications: 16th International Conference, ICTERI 2020, Kharkiv, Ukraine, October 6–10, 2020,* Revised Selected Papers (pp. 119–140). Springer International Publishing.
2. Esteva, A., et al. (2021). Deep learning-enabled medical computer vision. *NPJ Digital Medicine, 4*(1), 5.
3. Dong, H., Yang, G., Liu, F., Mo, Y., & Guo, Y. (2017). Automatic brain tumor detection and segmentation using U-Net-based fully convolutional networks. In *Medical Image Understanding and Analysis: 21st Annual Conference, MIUA 2017, Edinburgh, UK, July 11–13, 2017, Proceedings 21* (pp. 506–517). Springer International Publishing.
4. Kikinis, R., et al. (1996). Computer-assisted interactive three-dimensional planning for neurosurgical procedures. *Neurosurgery, 38,* 640–651.
5. Nadeem, M. W., Ghamdi, M. A. A., Hussain, M., Khan, M. A., Khan, K. M., Almotiri, S. H., & Butt, S. A. (2020). Brain tumor analysis empowered with deep learning: A review, taxonomy, and future challenges. *Brain Sciences, 10*(2), 118.
6. Abbasi, S., & Tajeripour, F. (2017). Detection of brain tumor in 3D MRI images using local binary patterns and histogram orientation gradient. *Neurocomputing, 219,* 526–535.
7. Tucha, O., Smely, C., Preier, M., & Lange, K. W. (2000). Cognitive deficits before treatment among patients with brain tumors. *Neurosurgery, 47*(2), 324–334.
8. Saba, T. (2020). Recent advancement in cancer detection using machine learning: Systematic survey of decades, comparisons and challenges. *Journal of Infection and Public Health, 13*(9), 1274–1289.
9. Esteva, A., et al. (2019). A guide to deep learning in healthcare. *Nature Medicine, 25*(1), 24–29.
10. Chilamkurthy, S., et al. (2018). Deep learning algorithms for detection of critical findings in head CT scans: A retrospective study. *The Lancet, 392*(10162), 2388–2396.
11. Kamnitsas, K., et al. (2016). DeepMedic for brain tumor segmentation. In *Brainlesion: Glioma, Multiple Sclerosis, Stroke and Traumatic Brain Injuries: Second International Workshop, BrainLes 2016, with the Challenges on BRATS, ISLES and mTOP 2016, Held in Conjunction with MICCAI 2016, Athens, Greece, October 17, 2016,* Revised Selected Papers 2 (pp. 138–149). Springer International Publishing.
12. Bansal, R., Gupta, A., Singh, R., & Nassa, V. K. (2021, July). Role and impact of digital technologies in E-learning amidst COVID-19 pandemic. In *2021 Fourth International Conference on Computational Intelligence and Communication Technologies (CCICT)* (pp. 194–202). IEEE.

13. Jain, V., Beram, S. M., Talukdar, V., Patil, T., Dhabliya, D., & Gupta, A. (2022). Accuracy enhancement in machine learning during blockchain-based transaction classification. In *2022 Seventh International Conference on Parallel, Distributed and Grid Computing (PDGC)* (pp. 536–540). IEEE.

14. Kaur, H., & Wasan, S. K. (2006). Empirical study on applications of data mining techniques in healthcare. *Journal of Computer Science*, 2(2), 194–200.

15. Chartrand, G., et al. (2017). Deep learning: A primer for radiologists. *Radiographics*, 37(7), 2113–2131.

16. Miller, D. D., & Brown, E. W. (2018). Artificial intelligence in medical practice: The question to the answer? *The American Journal of Medicine*, 131(2), 129–133.

17. Chang, P., et al. (2018). Deep-learning convolutional neural networks accurately classify genetic mutations in gliomas. *American Journal of Neuroradiology*, 39(7), 1201–1207.

18. Talukdar, V., Dhabliya, D., Kumar, B., Talukdar, S. B., Ahamad, S., & Gupta, A. (2022). Suspicious activity detection and classification in IoT environment using machine learning approach. In *2022 Seventh International Conference on Parallel, Distributed and Grid Computing (PDGC)* (pp. 531–535). IEEE.

19. Veeraiah, V., Gangavathi, P., Ahamad, S., Talukdar, S. B., Gupta, A., & Talukdar, V. (2022). Enhancement of meta verse capabilities by IoT integration. In *2022 2nd International Conference on Advance Computing and Innovative Technologies in Engineering (ICACITE)* (pp. 1493–1498). IEEE.

20. Sarvamangala, D. R., & Kulkarni, R. V. (2022). Convolutional neural networks in medical image understanding: A survey. *Evolutionary Intelligence*, 15(1), 1–22.

21. Kosslyn, S. M. (1996). *Image and Brain: The Resolution of the Imagery Debate*. MIT Press.

22. Farah, M. J. (1984). The neurological basis of mental imagery: A componential analysis. *Cognition*, 18(1-3), 245–272.

23. Senders, J. T., et al. (2018). An introduction and overview of machine learning in neurosurgical care. *Acta Neurochirurgica*, 160, 29–38.

24. Kikinis, R, et al. (1996). A digital brain atlas for surgical planning, model-driven segmentation, and teaching. *IEEE Transactions on Visualization and Computer Graphics*, 2(3), 232–241.

25. Dong, S., Wang, P., & Abbas, K. (2021). A survey on deep learning and its applications. *Computer Science Review*, 40, 100379.

26. Pandey, B. K., Pandey, D., Gupta, A., Nassa, V. K., Dadheech, P., & George, A. S. (2023). Secret data transmission using advanced morphological component analysis and steganography. In *Role of Data-Intensive Distributed Computing Systems in Designing Data Solutions* (pp. 21–44). Cham: Springer International Publishing.

27. Wang, Q., Cheng, M., Huang, S., Cai, Z., Zhang, J., & Yuan, H. (2022). A deep learning approach incorporating YOLO v5 and attention mechanisms for field real-time detection of the invasive weed *Solanum rostratum* Dunal seedlings. *Computers and Electronics in Agriculture*, 199, 107194.

28. Kaushik, D., Garg, M., Annu, Gupta, A., & Pramanik, S. (2022). Utilizing machine learning and deep learning in cybersecurity: An innovative approach. In *Cyber Security and Digital Forensics: Challenges and Future Trends* (pp. 271–293). New York: Wiley.

29. Shenton, M. E., et al. (2012). A review of magnetic resonance imaging and diffusion tensor imaging findings in mild traumatic brain injury. *Brain Imaging and Behavior*, 6, 137–192.

30. Kamnitsas, K., et al. (2017). Efficient multi-scale 3D CNN with fully connected CRF for accurate brain lesion segmentation. *Medical Image Analysis*, 36, 61–78.

31. Castro, M. G., et al. (2003). Current and future strategies for the treatment of malignant brain tumors. *Pharmacology & Therapeutics*, 98(1), 71–108.

32. Davie, G. L., Hutcheson, K. A., Barringer, D. A., Weinberg, J. S., & Lewin, J. S. (2009). Aphasia in patients after brain tumour resection. *Aphasiology*, *23*(9), 1196–1206.

33. Topol, E. J. (2019). High-performance medicine: The convergence of human and artificial intelligence. *Nature Medicine*, *25*(1), 44–56.

34. Gupta, M., Ghatak, S., Gupta, A., & Mukherjee, A. L. (Eds.). (2022). *Artificial Intelligence on Medical Data: Proceedings of International Symposium (ISCMM 2021)* (Vol. 37). Berlin: Springer Nature.

35. Lavecchia, A. (2019). Deep learning in drug discovery: Opportunities, challenges and future prospects. *Drug Discovery Today*, *24*(10), 2017–2032.

36. Zhao, X., Wu, Y., Song, G., Li, Z., Zhang, Y., & Fan, Y. (2018). A deep learning model integrating FCNNs and CRFs for brain tumor segmentation. *Medical Image Analysis*, *43*, 98–111.

37. Wang, G., Li, W., Ourselin, S., & Vercauteren, T. (2019). Automatic brain tumor segmentation based on cascaded convolutional neural networks with uncertainty estimation. *Frontiers in Computational Neuroscience*, *13*, 56.

38. Sikchi, S. S., Sikchi, S., & Ali, M. S. (2013). Fuzzy expert systems (FES) for medical diagnosis. *International Journal of Computer Applications*, *63*(11), 7–16.

39. Wang, G., Li, W., Aertsen, M., Deprest, J., Ourselin, S., & Vercauteren, T. (2019). Aleatoric uncertainty estimation with test-time augmentation for medical image segmentation with convolutional neural networks. *Neurocomputing*, *338*, 34–45.

40. Giussani, C., Roux, F. E., Ojemann, J., Sganzerla, E. P., Pirillo, D., & Papagno, C. (2010). Is preoperative functional magnetic resonance imaging reliable for language areas mapping in brain tumor surgery? Review of language functional magnetic resonance imaging and direct cortical stimulation correlation studies. *Neurosurgery*, *66*(1), 113–120.

41. Bouma, G. J., Muizelaar, J. P., Choi, S. C., Newlon, P. G., & Young, H. F. (1991). Cerebral circulation and metabolism after severe traumatic brain injury: The elusive role of ischemia. *Journal of Neurosurgery*, *75*(5), 685–693.

42. Humphreys, G. W., & Riddoch, M. J. (1987). *To See But Not to See: A Case Study of Visual Agnosia*. Psychology Press.

43. Bi, W. L., et al. (2019). Artificial intelligence in cancer imaging: Clinical challenges and applications. *CA: A Cancer Journal for Clinicians*, *69*(2), 127–157.

44. Bechet, D., Mordon, S. R., Guillemin, F., & Barberi-Heyob, M. A. (2014). Photodynamic therapy of malignant brain tumours: A complementary approach to conventional therapies. *Cancer Treatment Reviews*, *40*(2), 229–241.

45. Bansal, B., Jenipher, V. N., Jain, R., Dilip, R., Kumbhkar, M., Pramanik, S., Roy, S., & Gupta, A. (2022). Big data architecture for network security. In *Cyber Security and Network Security* (eds S. Pramanik, D. Samanta, M. Vinay and A. Guha). Springer.

46. Gupta, A., Kaushik, D., Garg, M., & Verma, A. (2020). "Machine learning model for breast cancer prediction. In *Fourth International Conference on I-SMAC (IoT in Social, Mobile, Analytics and Cloud) (I-SMAC)* (pp. 472–477). IEEE.

47. Li, R., & Wu, Y. (2022). Improved YOLO v5 wheat ear detection algorithm based on attention mechanism. *Electronics*, *11*(11), 1673.

48. Wang, Z., Jin, L., Wang, S., & Xu, H. (2022). Apple stem/calyx real-time recognition using YOLO-v5 algorithm for fruit automatic loading system. *Postharvest Biology and Technology*, *185*, 111808.

Chapter 10

Smart therapist

The mental health detector

*Arunabha Dutt, Nizar Banu P. K., Akarshi Bansal,
and Krishna Bansal*

10.1 INTRODUCTION

Mental health is one of the global issues of great concern. Nearly 1 billion people worldwide are affected with mental disorders [1]. There has been a surge for the mental health crisis in clinical practice where the patients have difficulty in functioning effectively in the community. If not treated on time, the symptoms may aggravate leading to some adverse situations. It is observed in India that one out of seven suffers from some or the other form of mental disorder. Around 30% of Indians consider mental health as the country's biggest contributor to health problems and morbidity [2]. Therefore, identifying these vulnerable patients at risk of a mental crisis before the occurrence becomes our primary concern to improve the global health statistics.

Machine learning (ML) is gradually being adopted all across the globe by medical practitioners and neuroscientists to develop treatments and remedial therapies to combat life-threatening illness. ML-based techniques are used to identify the potential risk of mental illness by performing predictions on the patient based on their regular and recurrent activities. Previously, the diagnosis was dependent on population statistics and group average, which is now overcome by ML techniques. Further, ML assists the doctors to identify and uncover relevant patterns of illness that might have taken time without it [3]. As a prerequisite for this research work, appropriate datasets on mental health illness were explored. Mental health data being sensitive information, many datasets are not publicly available. The DASS [4] and OSMHO [5] datasets available in public repositories are considered to develop this model.

The IoT sensors that can be integrated into wristbands and smartphones has made it possible to evaluate many hallmark symptoms of depression objectively and passively track behavioural indices of poor mood. Additionally, it has been shown that longer phone screen time, more entertainment apps utilised, and overall smartphone engagement time are all inversely connected with more severe depressive symptoms and lower moods [6]. Last but not least, wearable activity sensors can monitor dysregulated sleep, a typical issue in depression. According to studies, passive smartphone feature aggregations can help forecast daily mood and the existence of depressive symptoms.

DOI: 10.1201/9781003487647-10

Digital smart watches are an effective instrument for studying a wearer's behaviour and collecting data for various projects, for instance, the average amount of time spent working out each day, daily calorie burn, and much more [7]. These days, academicians are concentrating on collecting data from smart watches to examine people's mental health. Nearly 40% of people in the population reported having experienced sadness or anxiety at some point in their lives but never seeking help. This may be because they were unsure of where to start. The smart watches and applications come into play here since they can collect data passively from the wearer.

For real-time data collection, several IoT handheld devices and embedded sensors can be used. The wrist-worn sleep sensor can be used to analyse the sleeping pattern of the user along with other biomedical parameters [8]. This chapter focuses on the dataset that is accessible from the public repository.

For the research work carried out in this chapter, two datasets are obtained. One is on DASS (depression anxiety stress scales) and the other one is on Mental Health in Workspace. DASS dataset is based on the survey which anyone can take it up to get personalised results. The research survey data was collected from 2017 to 2019 [4]. This dataset includes a questionnaire which helps in estimating the person's mental health. The second dataset, Mental Health in Workspace, primarily focuses on the well-being of the working professionals. This survey was conducted by Open Sourcing Mental Health Organisation in 2014 [5]. A ML model is developed using the datasets. The ML model tries to classify the users using this data. After performing necessary pre-processing, classification algorithms like support vector classifiers and random forest classifier are applied and their performance is measured. An AI-based chatbot is developed and integrated to the website for anyone on the internet to access this. The chatbot is used for data acquisition, where the end user will be asked to answer certain questions, their answers will be recorded, and will serve as an input to the ML model.

The ultimate motive of this research work is to create an AI therapist that will interact with the user and based on their answers, it will predict whether a person is facing some mental health issues. Based on the results, the person can decide to meet a psychiatrist, psychologist, or start regular exercise that can uplift their moods. So the advantage of this model is that it is safe on legal terms. It does not provide full advice to the users, but based on their score, options are provided. It advises you to meet the psychologist in person if he/she is classified under a severe category. In the recent post-pandemic situation, a drastic increase is seen in the rate of individuals affected from depression and anxiety. This AI-based chatbot can be instrumental in accessing an individual mental state.

The model proposed and discussed in this chapter will help people to be more aware of their mental health. It will help people to overcome the stigma and get access to the treatment. Most of the people find it difficult to get his/her mental health accessed or sometimes feel embarrassed to consult an expert when they are experiencing adverse mental health conditions. It helps family and friends to better understand their condition and connect with support networks. AI therapists will recommend all the necessary information to the user. They don't have to refer to any other external websites, which might give wrong information. This research work provides assistance to the users as well as helps them to interact with a bot so that the fear of judgement can be eliminated from their mind. Continuous availability of an assistant makes a lot of difference as it keeps its focus on the patient and pinpoints him on a regular basis. This research work addresses this issue by providing the user to self-assess his mental conditions and provide assistance to enhance their mind-set.

Woebot is a cognitive behavioural therapy (CBT) process automation solution offered through Facebook Messenger or mobile apps [9]. With the help of the smartphone software Replika, users may hold talks about themselves and learn more about their positive traits [10]. These are some of the applications that were created to keep track of the signs and handle anxiety and depressive episodes. In this chapter, we develop a more customised AI chatbot for detecting the severity of the mental disorder which can be used by both people and doctors for diagnosis purposes. The persistent global health crisis is exacerbating psychiatric symptoms, and researchers are looking into therapeutic gadgets that function over text messaging devices to help those who already have a mental health condition [11]. AI bots might lack a human counterpart's sophisticated emotional awareness and sympathetic reaction and their capability to use specific patient information to support the patient's necessary cognitive effort is constrained. They also lack the wide range of skills that a trained psychiatrist or therapist possesses. There are now no direct clinical applications accessible, and there is no national benchmark against which technological advancement can be measured.

The datasets used in the existing systems are highly confidential owing to the personal sensitive nature of the data and are not publicly available. Our proposed model combines the two available datasets that cover both the general and the employed populations. Therefore, the comparison with the existing systems will bring disparity in the research work. This chapter aims to collate the different datasets into one broader generalised model.

The remaining of the chapter is organised as follows. Section 10.2 discusses the methodology followed in this research work. Section 10.3 explains the experimental analysis followed by the results and discussion in Section 10.4. Section 10.5 concludes the chapter.

10.2 METHODOLOGY

This section gives detailed information and steps followed while building the AI therapist for mental health prediction. The block diagram describes the phases and their interaction with each other schematically. The functional and non-functional requirement specifies all the needs of the user and various constraints which are considered while constructing this model.

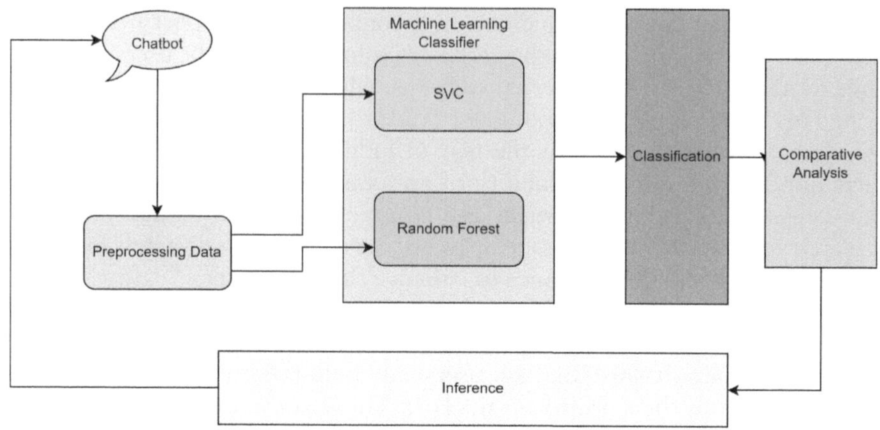

Figure 10.1 The schematic diagram of the system architecture.

The overall system architecture of the smart therapist is presented in Figure 10.1. The chatbot helps in acquiring the data from the user and it acts as an interface to the consumers. This response, after applying the necessary pre-processing, is pipelined to the ML classifier which runs the optimal classifying algorithms and categorises the data into appropriate classes.

10.2.1 Data pre-processing

The success of any ML algorithm is dependent on the quality of the data on which the model is built. In a real-world dataset, the chance that the data contains irrelevant, redundant, or inadequate extraneous data is more. These impact the accuracy and the performance of the ML algorithms [12]. Thus, data pre-processing is a vital step in developing a ML model which resolves the discrepancies such as missing values and noisy data. Data cleaning, feature extraction, transformation, and normalisation are some of the data pre-processing steps used in creating a robust ML model. The outcome of pre-processing is the final dataset which is used to train the ML model.

In both the datasets, the missing values present are refilled with the mode of the data; the outliers are identified and removed. Grouping is performed on the age attribute in the DASS dataset to smoothen the noisy data. The datasets can be too large, so data transformation is performed in which the dimensions of the dataset is reduced through feature selection [13]. In the OSMHO dataset, several misspelled words are present, which is resolved in this step. Data Normalisation is one of the crucial steps in data pre-processing. Here the data is scaled up or scaled down to fit within a particular range. This can be achieved through any of the normalisation techniques such as Min–Max normalisation and Z-score normalisation.

10.2.2 ML techniques

The ML model is deployed on a web server that can interact with the end users and help in predicting if the user is succumbed to any kind of mental disorder. This is the primary functionality of the AI therapist. This data is used by the underlying ML model to perform classification. The model provides accurate results in cross-validation using holdout datasets. The model also determines the severity of the disorder and provides a rating considering all the corner cases. ML algorithms which are used to build and experiment the AI Therapist system are random forest and support vector machine (SVM) classifier and K-nearest neighbours. In the next section, the details of the algorithm are given.

10.2.2.1 Random forest

A supervised ML algorithm, random forest, can be applied to both regression and classification. In this case, we use a random forest algorithm for classification purposes. The random forest grows and expands by combining multiple decision trees. The main objective of this algorithm is that multiple unrelated individual decision trees perform better. Every tree provides a vote classification. The majority of votes is used by the forest to determine the classification. [14].

Random forest algorithm as given in Reference [14]:

Let $D = \{(x_1,y_1), (x_2,y_2),\ldots, (x_n,y_n)\}$ denote the user responses which serves as our training dataset, with $x_i = (x_{i,1},\ldots, x_{i,p})^T$.

1. Begin by assembling every observation into a single node.
2. Until the stop requirement is met, the subsequent actions are recursively repeated for each individual node that is not divided.
   a. Determine which binary split on p predictors is the best of all the binary splits.
   b. The optimal split is applied to divide two descendant nodes (step 2a).
3. To reach a terminal node for a prediction at x, move x down the tree. Let k be a terminal node and let $y_{k1},\ldots, y_{kn}$ denote the response values of the training data in node k. The predicted values of the response variable are as follows:
   a. $h(x) = a\,'\mathrm{gmax}_y \sum_{i=1}^{n} I(y_{ki} = y)$ for classification, where $I(y_{ki} = y) = 1$ if $y_{ki} = y$ and 0 otherwise.

As an illustration, we consider a random forest with 1,000 decision trees. Let us assume that 10,000 people were involved in the original data. Then, this random forest goes through two steps for training and testing. First, a decision tree is generated based on new data with 10,000 participants using random sampling with replacement. Some original data participants being left out of the new data called out of the bag data. This procedure is performed

1,000 times, resulting in 1,000 decision trees, 1,000 new datasets, and 1,000 out-of-bag datasets. The out-of-bag error is calculated as the percentage of incorrect votes cast on all of the participants in the out-of-bag data. The 1,000 decision trees predict the dependent variable of each participant in the out-of-bag data, using their majority vote as their final prediction [15].

10.2.2.2 SVM

The primary goal of the SVM technique is to locate a hyperplane in an N-dimensional space which classifies the input points. The hyperplane's size is determined by the quantity of features. If the number of input features is equal to 2, then the hyperplane is just a line. In the event that three features are considered as inputs, the hyperplane changes into a 2D plane. It becomes more complex when the number of features is more than three. Thus, SVM helps in linearly separating related samples in a higher dimensional space which was not linearly separable in lower dimensional space [16].

In the DASS dataset, the number of features is more and the data cannot be classified using linear separability; a multidimensional hyperplane is used to classify the data. This dataset has multiple classes; one versus rest technique is used by default along with the RBF kernel in this algorithm. The OSMHO dataset has binary classification and it is possible to segregate using linear separability.

10.2.2.3 K-nearest neighbour (KNN)

KNN locates the k user response samples in the dataset that are closest to one another based on feature similarity and the distance function [17]. Euclidean, Manhattan, and Minkowski distances are used in KNN to compute the distance between the test data samples and all of the training cases so as to find the distance between unknown response and all other responses, the following equation is used:

$$dt = \sqrt{\left(\left(x_1 - x_2 \right)^2 + \left(y_1 - y_2 \right)^2 \right)} \tag{10.1}$$

Here, dt is the distance, and x_1, x_2, y_1, and y_2 are the Cartesian coordinates and the distance between x and y is calculated as shown in the Equation 10.1. Once the distance is calculated, the new data points are assigned a category such that the number of neighbours is maximum [18].

In both datasets, each individual response is considered as data points. The Minkowski distance is used to calculate the distance between data points considering all the input parameters. The value of K is determined for elbow criteria having less fluctuations in the error rate.

The optimal ML algorithm is seen to be dependent on the number of samples in the training set, the dimension of the dataset, and how the features are correlated. The random forest algorithm can be thought of as multiple decision trees combined together, It works well with large and high dimensional datasets. Similarly, SVM works well for high dimensional space but the time taken is more. The KNN algorithm is not recommended for large datasets as it requires more computation in generating the distance between a sample point and all the sample points in the dataset.

10.3 EXPERIMENTAL ANALYSIS

The ML algorithms discussed in the previous section are applied on both the datasets. The model is trained and tracked to evaluate its performance. This section describes the nature of both the datasets in detail and strategies used to develop the model such as the data preparation and system design.

10.3.1 Dataset description

The first dataset was obtained from the DASS (depression anxiety stress scale) online survey [4]. This dataset contains several questions pertaining to different segments which will help in generating accurate results related to the mental health of an individual. This dataset has generalised questions which focus on all age groups. The entire questionnaire is divided into three sections. The first set had 42 questions and a set of sample questions are listed in Table 10.1 as taken from the source [4].

Table 10.1 Questionnaire set 1

Q. No.	Question	Q. No	Question
Q1	I found myself getting upset by quite trivial things	Q10	I felt that I had nothing to look forward to
Q2	I was aware of the dryness of my mouth	Q11	I found myself getting upset rather easily.
Q3	I couldn't seem to experience any positive feeling at all	Q12	I was in a state of nervous tension
Q4	I experienced breathing difficulty (e.g. excessively rapid breathing, breathlessness in the absence of physical exertion)	Q13	I felt I was pretty worthless
Q5	I felt down-hearted and blue	Q14	I was intolerant of anything that kept me from getting on with what I was doing
Q6	I found that I was very irritable	Q15	I felt terrified
Q7	I had a feeling of shakiness (e.g. legs going to give way)	Q16	I felt that life was meaningless
Q8	I found it difficult to relax	Q17	I found myself getting agitated
Q9	I found myself in situations that made me so anxious I was most relieved when they ended		

Table 10.2 Users response description

Options	Description
1	Didn't even pertain to me
2	Applied to me partially, or occasionally
3	Applied to me a good portion of the time, or to a significant extent
4	Applied to me a lot, or the majority of the time

Each item from Questionnaire set 1 was shown to a new participant one at a time in a random order, accompanied by a 4-point rating scale that asked the user to identify how often that question had applied to them in the previous week. Table 10.2 depicts the options given.

The dataset also contains information about the time taken to answer the questions in milliseconds:

Surveyelapse: The amount of time used to complete the remaining survey and demographic questions.

Introelapse: The amount of time (in seconds) spent on the landing page and introduction.

Testelapse: How much time was spent answering every DASS question.

It includes some of the generic questions like value check, education, country, hand preference, orientation, family size, marital status, and unique network location.

The Ten Item Personality Inventory [19] was administered and included in the questionnaires referred to in Table 10.3.

The following items were presented as a checklist and subjects were instructed "In the grid below, check all the words whose definitions you are sure you know". Some of them are mentioned in Table 10.4.

If it is checked, the value is 1, else it is unchecked. We can use the words at VCL6, VCL9, and VCL12 as a validity check, but they are not actual words.

Table 10.3 Questionnaire set 2

Question	Personality traits	Question	Personality traits
TIPI1	Extraverted, enthusiastic	TIPI6	Reserved, quiet
TIPI2	Critical, quarrelsome	TIPI7	Sympathetic, warm
TIPI3	Dependable, self-disciplined	TIPI8	Disorganised, careless
TIPI4	Anxious, easily upset	TIPI9	Calm, emotionally stable
TIPI5	Open to new experiences, complex	TIPI10	Conventional, uncreative

Source: The TIPI items were rated "I see myself as:" ______ such that

1 = severe disagreement; 2 = moderate disagreement; 3 = slight disagreement; and 4 = neither agreement nor disagreement; 5 = somewhat agree; 6 = moderate agreement; 7 = strong agreement

Table 10.4 Questionnaire set 3

Questions	Words
VCL5	Audible
VCL6	Cuivocal
VCL7	Paucity
VCL8	Epistemology
VCL9	Florted
VCL10	Decide

The DASS questionnaire also included the following values as questions:

Country: The user's ISO country code upon connection.

Display Size: One is a small-screen device (phone, etc.), and two are large-screen devices (laptop, desktop, etc.).

Uniquenetworklocation: 1 refers only one survey from user's specific network in dataset, Multiple surveys submitted from this user's network equals a score of 2. This does not necessarily mean that a single person has duplicate records because it could be different students at the same school or different family members. Even if the score is 1, a single person may still have duplicate records if they took the survey on both their phone and Wi-Fi.

Source: The user's discovery of the test 1 is from the survey's home page, 2 is from Google, and 0 is from another source.

The Open Sourcing Mental Health Organization surveyed workers in 2014 to gauge attitudes toward mental health and the prevalence of mental health illnesses in the software industry [5]. This dataset focuses mostly on the working professionals. It has questions as mentioned in Table 10.5.

This dataset has a question, "Have you sought treatment for a mental health condition?" which acts as the target variable. This target variable is necessary for the supervised ML models to map the sample data to its outcome.

Table 10.5 Questionnaire from OSMHO dataset

Q. No.	Questions
Q1	If you have a mental health condition, do you feel that it interferes with your work?
Q2	How many employees does your company or organisation have?
Q3	Do you work remotely (outside of an office) at least 50% of the time?
Q4	Does your employer provide mental health benefits?
Q5	Do you know the options for mental healthcare your employer provides?
Q6	Is your employer primarily a tech company/organisation?
Q7	Do you think that discussing a mental health issue with your employer would have negative consequences?

Table 10.6 Age groups

Group	Age
1	≤ 12
2	$13 \leq \text{Age} \leq 16$
3	$17 \leq \text{Age} \leq 21$
4	$21 < \text{Age} \leq 35$
5	$35 < \text{Age} \leq 48$
6	≥ 49

10.3.2 Data preparation

Data preparation is a crucial step in any ML model to get accurate results. The dataset chosen contains some irrelevant attributes which need to be removed before proceeding with building the model.

In the DASS dataset, the attributes which are removed include source, introelapse, testelapse, surveyelapse, hand, orientation, voted, country, screensize, unique networklocation, major subject along with value check questions as these do not have any influence on determining the mental state of the user [20]. In the dataset, it is seen that the family size of certain sample points have values more than 12, which seems to be an outlier and are removed from the dataset. The age attribute in the dataset has varying values, so it is categorised into six bins, as shown in the Table 10.6.

The threshold values for each age category are chosen in such a way that the entire sample population follows a Gaussian distribution. This dataset does not have any dependent variable. The target variable (dependent variable) is added to the dataset by summing all the attributes for each row as follows:

$$\text{Target}_i = \sum_{j=1}^{n} \text{att}_j \tag{10.2}$$

where j is the attribute number.

The breakpoints for different categories are chosen randomly and then fine-tuned using several trial and error methods [21]. The threshold values chosen give the highest accuracy while training and testing ML models. This is shown in Table 10.7.

Table 10.7 Depression categories

Category	Target value
Normal	≤ 165
Mild	$165 < \text{value} \leq 184$
Moderate	$184 < \text{value} \leq 213$
Severe	$213 < \text{value} \leq 241$
Extremely Severe	$\text{value} > 241$

Table 10.8 Category definitions

Category	Definition
Normal	The person is perfect and not having any risk of mental illness
Mild	The person is mostly normal, but at times gets affected with the illness
Moderate	The person is affected and requires assistance
Severe	The person is suffering for a long period of time and needs assistance from a medical practitioner as early as possible
Extremely severe	The person is suffering from acute mental illness and advised to visit the doctor immediately without any delay

Here the different categories refer to the different mental state of the person, as shown in Table 10.8.

In the OSMHO dataset related to mental health in tech workspace, several pre-processing have been applied. Some of the attributes like country, timestamp, and comments seemed to be irrelevant in developing the model, so they were dropped. In the response, certain outliers were present in the age attribute. Since this dataset is for working professionals, records having age less than 18 or more than 75 have been set to the lower and higher limits, respectively. Here the age has not been categorised owing to less number of records and a constricted age range. The null values present in some of the attributes are replaced with its mode. The response for all the attributes are categorical and have been encoded into numerical values for better prediction. The resulting dataset has been normalised as it resulted in better accuracy.

10.3.3 Chatbot and interface design

This acts as an interface between the user and the ML model. The chatbot interacts with the user and answers all the questions which form the input attributes to the ML model. The user will be given options to choose and in the end this returns all the answers in a collated appropriate data structure such as a list or an array.

Figure 10.2 depicts the entire data flow of the proposed system. The GUI chatbot feeds the input from the user to the ML module. This ML model is deployed on a server. The ML model has been built by experimenting with several classification algorithms like KNN and SVM. The best performing algorithm is used as the classifier. The result obtained can be further used by the person to decide whether to consult a medical practitioner or start with home remedies. Sample screenshots of the implemented system is shown in Figures 10.3–10.6.

Figure 10.3 refers to the home page of the web-based chatbot system. Here the user needs to register before taking the self-assessment test on mental health. Once registered, the user is free to take the test for an unrestricted number of times. The screen shot of the login page is shown in Figure 10.4.

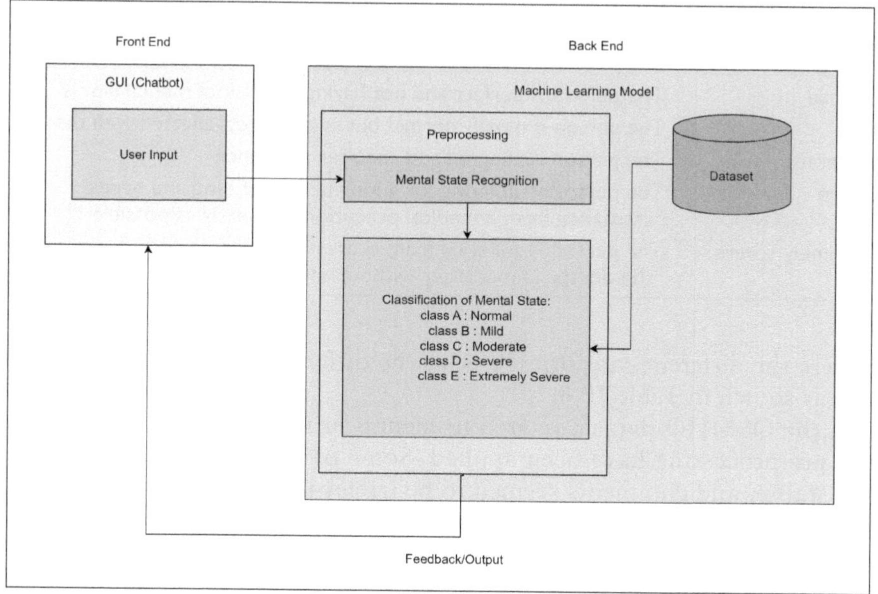

Figure 10.2 The work flow schematic diagram of the proposed system.

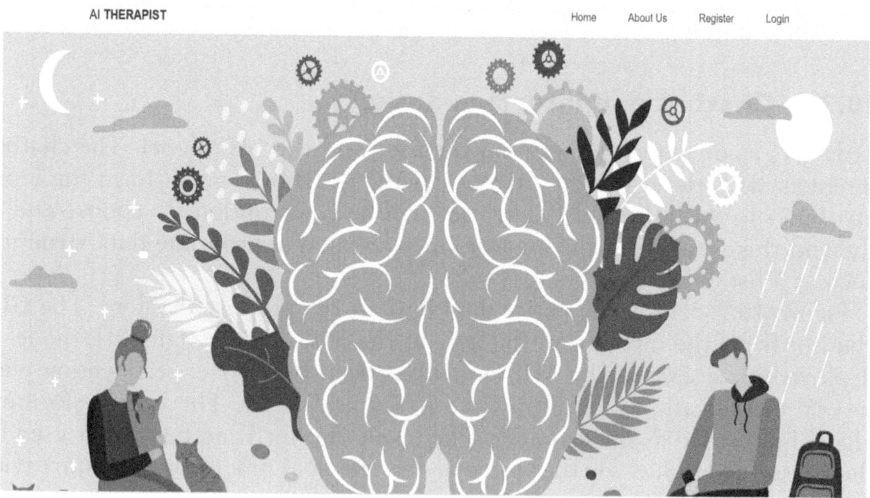

Figure 10.3 Landing page of the website.

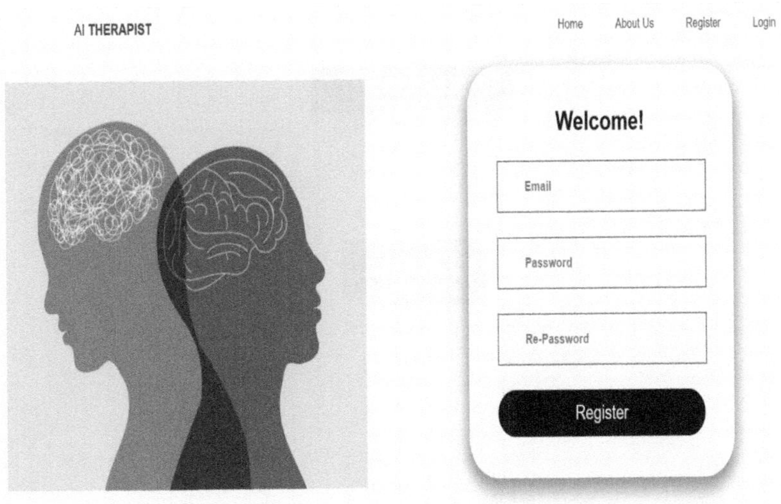

Figure 10.4 Registration page.

Figure 10.5 shows the interface design of the chatbot. The chatbot asks questions as mentioned in the DASS dataset one by one and captures the response of the user. For an undesired response from the user, the chatbot re-questions the user until it gets a valid response. One constraint that has been introduced is the user cannot pause in between the assessment. The chatbot does not store the intermediate response. After the assessment, the

Figure 10.5 Chatbot interface.

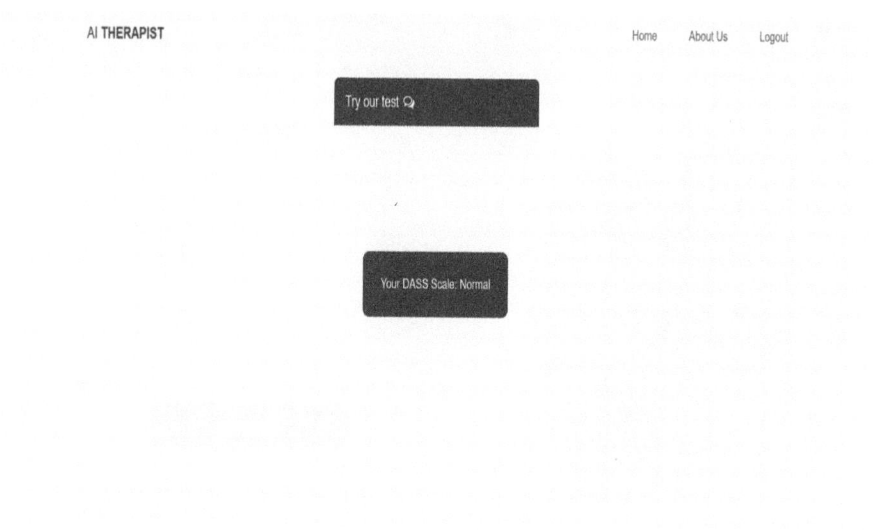

Figure 10.6 Result of DASS test.

DASS scale is shown to the user as seen in Figure 10.6. Since the response of the user contains sensitive personal information, special care should be taken to prevent data breach.

10.4 RESULTS AND DISCUSSION

After performing the pre-processing on the DASS dataset, the number of attributes of the chosen dataset reduces from 172 to 60. ML classification algorithms such as KNN, random forest, and SVM are applied and analysed.

The performance of various classifying algorithms is analysed using their classification report. Certain performance metrics are as follows:

1. *Precision:* This is a reference to the percentage of actually positive predictions out of all the positive ones.

   $$Precision\ for\ moderate\ category = True\ Moderate/(True\ Moderate + False\ Moderate)$$

2. *Recall:* This refers to what proportion of the overall positive are positive predictions.

   $$Recall\ for\ moderate\ category = True\ Moderate/(True\ Moderate + False\ Moderate)$$

Table 10.9 Classification report of random forest classifier

Class label	Precision	Recall	F1-score	Support
Extremely severe	0.92	0.86	0.86	1,085
Mild	0.76	0.62	0.68	1,233
Moderate	0.77	0.86	0.81	2,242
Normal	0.91	0.93	0.92	1,646
Severe	0.80	0.81	0.81	1,738
Accuracy	–	–	0.82	7,944
Macro avg	0.83	0.81	0.82	7,944
Weighted avg	0.82	0.82	0.82	7,944

3. *F1-score:* This is given by the following formula:

$$f\text{1-score} = 2 * precision\_moderate * recall\_moderate / \left(precision\_moderate + recall\_moderate\right)$$

The random forest algorithm, SVM, and KNN classification results are shown in Tables 10.9–10.11, respectively.

Table 10.9 presents the classification result of random forest classifier. We see the accuracy of the correct positive predictions is less for the mild and moderate categories. This implies that the model cannot distinguish between mild and moderate categories effectively. The extreme categories are distinguished with much better accuracy.

From the classification report in Table 10.10, we can conclude that the multi-class classification using RBF kernel for SVM classifiers gives significant accurate results. Here each class label has values of precision, recall, and *f*-score. Therefore, this model can be used in predicting mental illness with less chance of misclassification. In the classification report of KNN as in Table 10.11, the score for the mild category is significantly less and it is not considered for building the model.

Table 10.10 Classification report of support vector classifier

Class label	Precision	Recall	F1-score	Support
Extremely severe	0.97	0.96	0.96	1,085
Mild	0.94	0.92	0.93	1,233
Moderate	0.95	0.96	0.96	2,242
Normal	0.97	0.98	0.98	1,646
Severe	0.95	0.95	0.95	1,738
Accuracy	–	–	0.96	7,944
Macro avg	0.96	0.95	0.95	7,944
Weighted avg	0.96	0.96	0.96	944

Table 10.11 Classification report of KNN

Class label	Precision	Recall	F1-score	Support
Extremely severe	0.84	0.87	0.86	1,127
Mild	0.66	0.71	0.68	1,201
Moderate	0.80	0.78	0.79	2,212
Normal	0.90	0.90	0.90	1,710
Severe	0.79	0.75	0.77	1,694
Accuracy	–	–	0.80	7,944
Macro avg	0.80	0.80	0.80	7,944
Weighted avg	0.80	0.80	0.80	7,944

From the performance comparison of different algorithms [22] shown in Figure 10.7, it can be considered that the model performs better with SVM classifiers in comparison with other algorithms and this is used further in developing the AI therapist. On plotting the precision score for each class label for SVM classifier in Figure 10.8, we see the efficiency of correctly predicting the true positive out of all the positive predicted is very high for all the class labels. For instance, out of 100 predicted extreme severe category patients, 97 of them actually have extremely severe mental illness.

Similarly for the OSMHO dataset, the various ML models have been trained [23] and the results have been derived as shown in Tables 10.12–10.14.

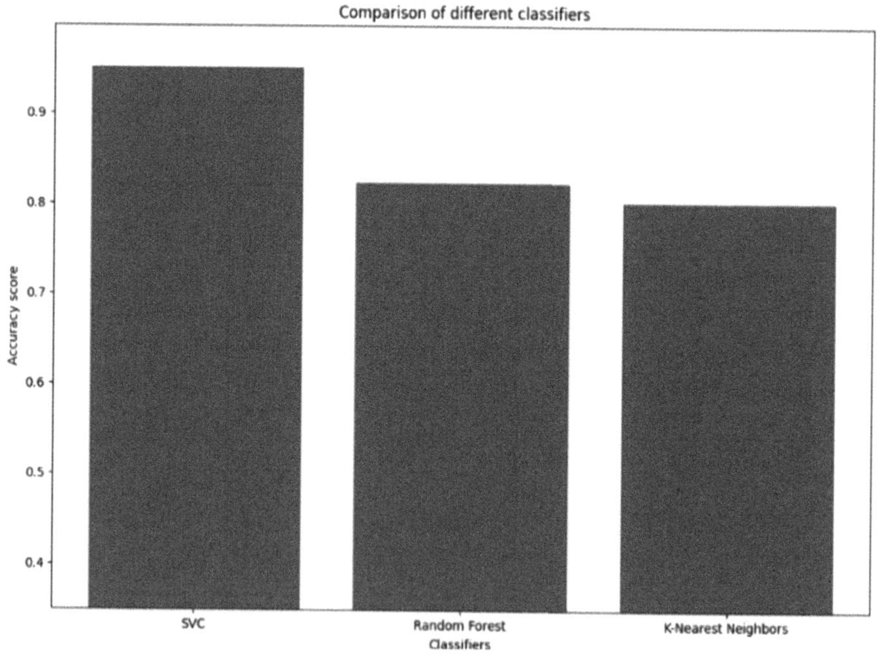

Figure 10.7 Comparison of different classifiers in terms of accuracy.

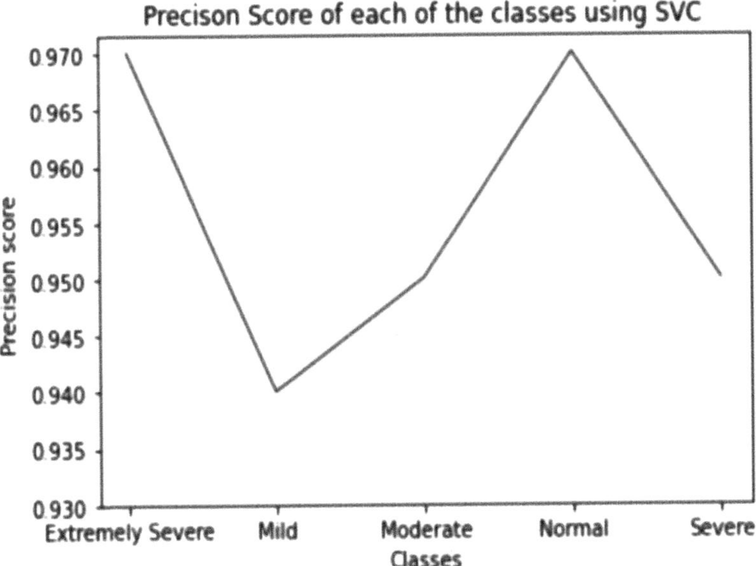

Figure 10.8 Precision score of SVM algorithm.

For the OSMHO dataset, we perform a binary classification on whether a person should take treatment for mental health or not. This can be further adopted by companies for ensuring the well-being of their employees. The classification report of random forest classifier in Table 10.12 infers that this algorithm is stable and the efficiency in which it can predict both the classes are mostly similar with F1-score close to 83%. The recall value for treatment taken class is 0.93, which means out of 100 employees who have actually taken the treatment, the model can predict 93 of them. For SVM and KNN shown in Tables 10.13 and 10.14, the recall values are comparatively less. For a small binary dataset, the random forest algorithm gives better results.

The results obtained from the experimental analysis on the OSMHO dataset suggest that the random forest classifier has outperformed compared to other classifiers with almost 83% accuracy, as shown in Figure 10.9. We tried

Table 10.12 Classification report of random forest classifier

Class label	Precision	Recall	F1-score	Support
Treatment not taken	0.93	0.74	0.82	138
Treatment taken	0.75	0.93	0.83	114
Accuracy	–	–	0.83	252
Macro avg	0.84	0.83	0.83	252
Weighted avg	0.85	0.83	0.83	252

Table 10.13 Classification report of support vector classifier

Class label	Precision	Recall	F1-score	Support
Treatment not taken	0.85	0.78	0.82	137
Treatment taken	0.76	0.83	0.79	113
Accuracy	–	–	0.81	252
Macro avg	0.80	0.81	0.80	252
Weighted avg	0.81	0.81	0.81	252

Table 10.14 Classification report of KNN

Class label	Precision	Recall	F1-score	Support
Treatment not taken	0.78	0.74	0.76	138
Treatment taken	0.70	0.75	0.72	114
Accuracy	–	–	0.74	252
Macro avg	0.74	0.74	0.74	252
Weighted avg	0.74	0.74	0.74	252

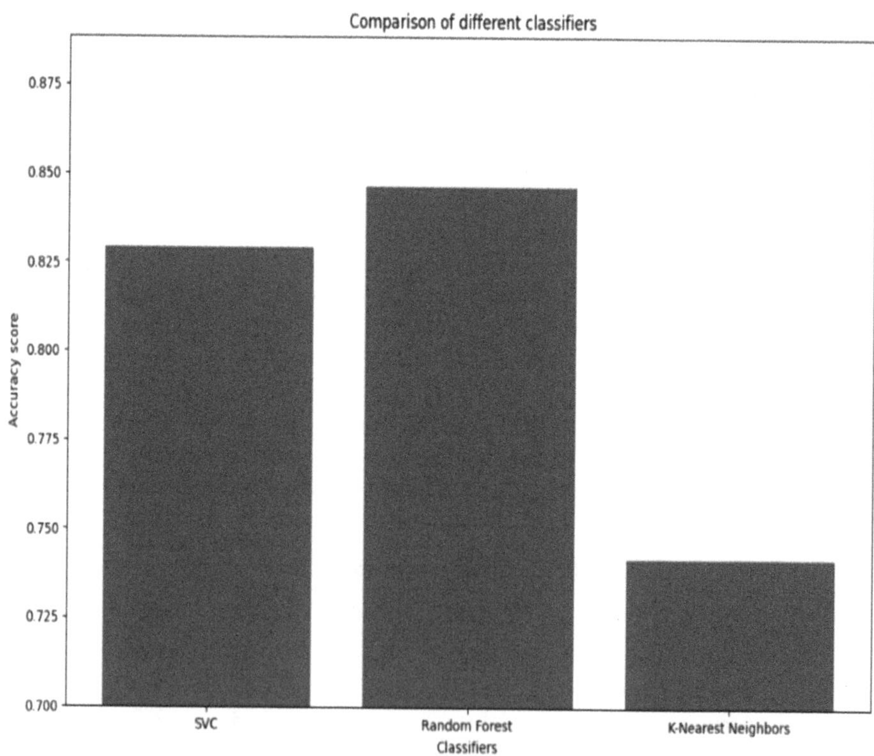

Figure 10.9 Comparison of different classifiers for the OSMHO dataset.

Table 10.15 Performance metrics of classifiers on different datasets

Classifiers	Accuracy score (in %) in DASS dataset	Accuracy score (in %) in OSMHO dataset
Random forest	82.40	84.63
SVM	95.50	82.92
KNN	80.17	74.20

to further increase the accuracy of the random forest classifier by changing the hyper-parameters. GridSearchCV is used by varying n_estimators, max_features, and max_depth to find the optimal hyper-parameter values. With these values of the hyper-parameters, the random classifier provides an accuracy close to 85%.

10.4.1 Observation on the two datasets

It is observed that SVM works as a better classifier on the DASS dataset, whereas the random forest is better for the OSMHO dataset. This is due to the varying nature of the dataset. The DASS dataset is more generic to the OSMHO dataset which is more oriented towards working professionals. The time frame while these two datasets were captured is different. Moreover, the sample size of DASS is more than the OSMHO dataset with many more attributes.

The result and performance analysis of the various ML algorithms applied to the given datasets is shown in Table 10.15.

10.5 CONCLUSION AND FUTURE WORK

In this chapter, a web-based chatbot for mental health prediction using ML techniques is introduced. This application can be used as a preliminary self-check as well as a first-level prognosis by the medical practitioners for patients at risk of mental illness. We applied various classification models such as KNN, SVM, random forest, and performed training and testing on it, which helped the user to handle depression and anxiety. The key advantage of this model lies in its ML model accuracy. The SVM classifier performs well with the DASS dataset while random forest performs well with the OSMHO dataset. The chatbot also creates an interactive interface for acquiring the user input. The chatbot has certain limitations, for example, it allows users to choose an option from the given choices, it is not able to perform semantic analysis and extract the meaning of the user's input. The AI Therapist can be extended to predict other mental health disorders such as bipolar disorder and anxiety. Many other common health-related issues such as coronary and neural diseases can be included in this system which would be available to medical practitioners only as a cross-validation tool and first level of diagnosis.

The interactive questionnaire used in accessing a person's mental state can lead to a subjective outcome. To overcome the issues of the questionnaire, this ML model can be integrated with several IOT devices and mobile-embedded sensors as highlighted in Section 10.1. These devices and sensors support real-time data acquisition and can be used to capture more dynamic mood swings and a person's current state. Furthermore, mobile applications and handheld sensors embedded in wrist bands used in conjugation to this proposed system will alert the user right at the moment. The model usage can be enhanced by using this data in a recommendation engine that suggests some remedies to the user as per the severity of their mental wellness. It is left for the readers of this chapter to extrapolate the usage of this proposed ML model to a next level.

Link to Mental Health Detector: https://github.com/arunabha212/AI-Therapist

REFERENCES

1. James, S. L. et al. *Global, Regional, and National Incidence, Prevalence, and Years Lived with Disability for 354 Diseases and Injuries for 195 Countries and Territories, 1990–2017: A Systematic Analysis for the Global Burden of Disease Study 2017.* Lancet, 2018, 392, 1789–1858.
2. Mental Health in India: Statistics and Facts, 2023. Available at: https://www.statista.com/topics/6944/mental-health-in-india/#topicOverview
3. 2022 Available at: https://www.analyticsinsight.net/can-machine-learning-be-used-to-improve-mental-health/
4. The dataset DASS, 2022. Available at: http://www2.psy.unsw.edu.au/dass/
5. The dataset on Mental Health in Workspace, 2022. Available at: https://osmhhelp.org/index.html
6. Pedrelli, P., Fedor, S., Ghandeharioun, A., Howe, E., Ionescu, D.F., Bhathena, D., Fisher, L.B., Cusin, C., Nyer, M., Yeung, A., Sangermano, L., Mischoulon, D., Alpert, J.E., Picard, R.W. *Monitoring Changes in Depression Severity Using Wearable and Mobile Sensors.* Frontiers in Psychiatry, 2020, 11, 584711. https://doi.org/10.3389/fpsyt.2020.584711
7. Mahendran, N., Vincent, D. R., Srinivasan, K., Chang, C.-Y., Garg, A., Gao, L., Reina, D. G. *Sensor-assisted Weighted Average Ensemble Model for Detecting Major Depressive Disorder.* Sensors, 2019, 19, 4822. https://doi.org/10.3390/s19224822
8. Fukuda, S., Matsuda, Y., Tani, Y., Arakawa, Y., Yasumoto, K. *Predicting Depression and Anxiety Mood by Wrist-Worn Sleep Sensor.* 2020 IEEE International Conference on Pervasive Computing and Communications Workshops (PerCom Workshops), Austin, TX, USA, 2020, pp. 1–6. https://doi.org/10.1109/PerComWorkshops48775.2020.9156176
9. Deepbots: A Webots-based Deep Reinforcement Learning Framework, 2022. Available at: https://www.ncbi.nlm.nih.gov/pmc/articles/PMC7256566/
10. 2021 Available at: https://trialsjournal.biomedcentral.com/articles/10.1186/s13063-021-05301-w
11. Balzan, E., Farrugia, P., Casha, O., Camilleri, L., *Design Considerations for Therapeutic Devices: An Investigation of Preschoolers' Preferences for an Artefact's Basic Characteristics.* International Conference On Engineering Design, ICED 19, 5–8 August 2019, Delft, The Netherlands.

12. Kotsiantis, S., Kanellopoulos, D., Pintelas, P. *Data Preprocessing for Supervised Learning*. International Journal of Computer Science, 2006, 1, 111–117.

13. Available at: https://www.v7labs.com/blog/data-preprocessing-guide

14. *(PDF) Random Forests*, 2011. Available at: https://www.researchgate.net/publication/236952762_Random_Forests

15. Lee, K. S., Ham, B. J. *Machine Learning on Early Diagnosis of Depression*. Psychiatry Investigation. 2022, 19(8), 597–605. https://doi.org/10.30773/pi.2022.0075

16. Ng, A., CS229 Lecture notes, Support Vector Machine. Available at: https://see.stanford.edu/materials/aimlcs229/cs229-notes3.pdf

17. Hu, L. Y. et al. *The distance function effect on k-nearest neighbor classification for medical datasets*. SpringerPlus, 2016, 5, 1304. https://doi.org/10.1186/s40064-016-2941-7

18. Guleria, P. *Predictions on diabetic patient datasets using big data analytics and machine learning techniques*, Editor: Pantea Keikhosrokiani, Big Data Analytics for Healthcare, Academic Press, 179–199, 2022, ISBN 9780323919074. https://doi.org/10.1016/B978-0-323-91907-4.00018-2.

19. Gosling, S. D., Rentfrow, P. J., Swann, W. B., Jr. *A Very Brief Measure of the Big Five Personality Domains*. Journal of Research in Personality, 2003, 37, 504–528.

20. Al-Wesabi, F.N., Alsolai, H., Hilal, A., Hamza, M.A., Al Duhayyim, M., Negm, N. Machine Learning Based Depression, Anxiety, and Stress Predictive Model during COVID-19 Crisis, Computers, Materials & Continua Tech Science Press, 2022.

21. Kumar, P., Garg, S., Garg, A., *Assessment of Anxiety, Depression and Stress Using Machine Learning Models*. Procedia Computer Science, 171, 2020. https://doi.org/10.1016/j.procs.2020.04.213

22. Source Code for Machine Learning Models on DASS Dataset, 2022. Available at: https://colab.research.google.com/drive/1NSO3tIyeAbGlj98w6PCKWwRq7AIobWXh?usp=sharing

23. Source Code for Machine Learning Models on Second Dataset, 2022. Available at: https://colab.research.google.com/drive/1s5hrAZZiL1pA-u1oJ0HHuzGu6AJZr0y9?usp=sharing

Medical image analysis based on deep learning approach and Internet of Medical Things (IoMT) for early diagnosis of retinal disease

S. Karkuzhali, Thendal P., and Senthilkumar S.

11.1 INTRODUCTION: BACKGROUND AND DRIVING FORCES

In recent years, the convergence of cutting-edge technologies, particularly deep learning (DL) and the Internet of Medical Things (IoMT), has revolutionized the field of healthcare, bringing forth transformative solutions for early disease diagnosis and improved patient care. One area where these advancements have had a profound impact is the early diagnosis of retinal diseases, a critical aspect of ophthalmic healthcare. Retinal diseases, such as glaucoma, age-related macular degeneration (ARMD), and diabetic retinopathy (DR), can lead to irreversible vision loss if not detected and treated in their initial stages. Medical image analysis, bolstered by the power of DL algorithms and IoMT, has emerged as a pivotal approach in enhancing the accuracy, efficiency, and accessibility of retinal disease diagnosis.

DL, a subset of artificial intelligence (AI), has exhibited remarkable capabilities in processing and interpreting complex medical images. By leveraging neural networks, particularly convolutional neural networks (CNNs), DL models can autonomously extract intricate patterns and features from medical images, including retinal scans. This ability is invaluable in identifying subtle abnormalities and early signs of retinal diseases, often imperceptible to the human eye. Furthermore, the integration of IoMT devices, such as specialized retinal imaging cameras and wearable sensors, has enabled real-time data acquisition and seamless transmission of retinal images to healthcare professionals and specialized diagnostic centers. This connectivity ensures timely analysis, allowing for swift medical interventions and personalized treatment plans tailored to individual patient needs.

This chapter explores the synergistic relationship between DL techniques and IoMT in the context of medical image analysis for the early diagnosis of retinal diseases. By delving into the advancements in neural network

DOI: 10.1201/9781003487647-11

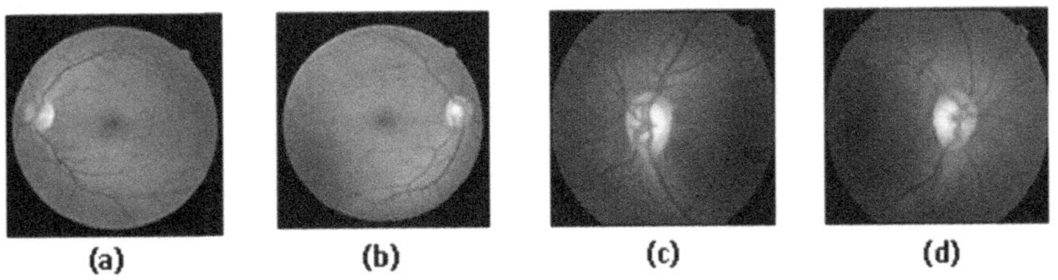

Figure 11.1 Various types of retinal images. (a) MCLE. (b) MCRE. (c) ODCLE. (d) ODCRE.

architectures, data augmentation, and transfer learning, we aim to elucidate the strides made in accurately detecting retinal abnormalities. Additionally, we investigate the role of IoMT in facilitating the seamless collection, transmission, and storage of retinal images, thereby bridging the gap between patients, healthcare providers, and specialized ophthalmologists. Through an in-depth analysis of existing research studies, technological innovations, and clinical applications, this chapter sheds light on the promising future of early retinal disease diagnosis, paving the way for proactive and targeted healthcare interventions, ultimately preserving the vision and enhancing the quality of life for millions of individuals worldwide (Figures 11.1 and 11.2).

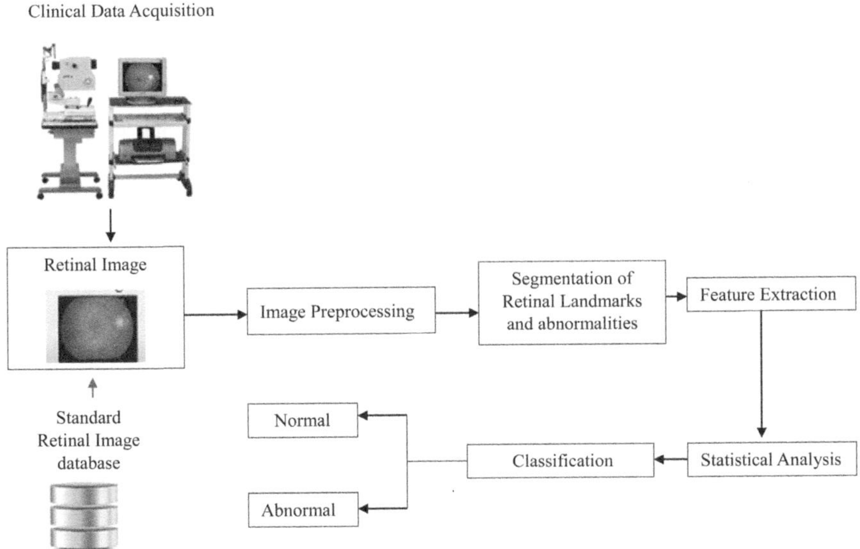

Figure 11.2 Flow diagram of RIAS.

11.2 EXITING METHODS IN DL-BASED APPROACH

Shi et al.'s (2020) description about blockchain indicates its incredible potential in changing the conventional social insurance industry. Be that as it may, there stay various exploration and operational difficulties, when endeavoring to completely coordinate blockchain innovation with existing EHR frameworks (Figure 11.3) [1].

Kermany et al. [2] established an indicative tool based on a DL system to screen patients with common treatable retinal diseases causing blindness. Schmidt-Erfurth et al. [3] incorporated three recent advancements in ophthalmology: precise diagnosis through SD-OCT imaging, the effectiveness of anti-VEGF treatment, and the potential use of AI-based tools to enhance disease management.

In the study conducted by Alsaih et al. [4], ten systems developed within a 2D framework were assessed for the segmentation of retinal diseases using OCT volumes (Table 11.1). Rayan et al. [5] presented an outline of the difficulties, pipeline, and procedures of keen well-being. An efficient pipeline of information preparing is obliged for traditional savvy well-being, covering information procurement, information handling, information scattering, information security and protection, and systems administration and processing advances. Despite various possibilities and philosophies for information examination in medical services introduced in their work, there are various orientation to be explored concerning various parts of medical services information, for example, quality, security, etc. [5].

Hsieh et al. [6] and Chaki et al. [7] conducted an analysis covering the detection of DR and diagnosis of diabetes mellitus (DM).

Schmidt-Erfurth et al. [8] explored the potential of solo ML for DR detection. In the work by Huyen et al. (2013), a disease progression model was proposed for three-dimensional visualization of treatment effects. To detect changes in abnormal areas, an automated measurement method for retinal thickness in OCT images was applied [9].

Alamelu et al. [10] employed morphological operations to identify blood vessels. To overcome existing system limitations, they introduced the exudate image identification (EII) method. The parametric analysis method was then utilized for quick evaluation of exudates in diabetic retina images, allowing for rapid exudate assessment [10].

Dash and Bhoi [11] introduced an automated method for extracting retinal veins from fundus images. The approach involved preprocessing the image for augmentation, segmentation using mean-C thresholding to isolate

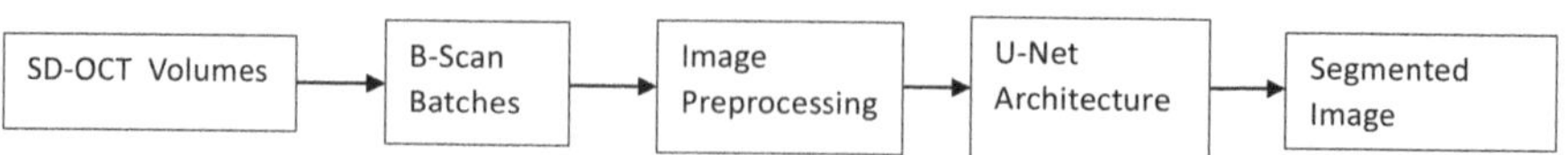

Figure 11.3 Segmentation pipeline for retinal diseases.

Table 11.1 Comparison of characteristics of the DL approach and Internet of Things (IoT)

Characteristics	DL approach	IoMT
Data source	Retinal images and scans	IoT devices, sensors, wearables
Data volume	Requires large labeled datasets	Continuous data streams
Data preprocessing	Preprocessing, augmentation	Data filtering, noise reduction
Feature extraction	Automatic feature learning	Sensor data interpretation
Model complexity	Deep neural networks	Varies (depends on sensors)
Training time	Longer training times	Real-time or periodic updates
Interpretability	Black-box models	Interpretability varies
Accuracy and performance	High accuracy in image analysis	Varies depending on sensors
Early diagnosis capability	Detects retinal anomalies	Real-time monitoring and alerts
Scalability	Scalable with GPUs/TPUs	Scalable with IoT infrastructure
Cost and infrastructure	Requires GPU/TPU, infrastructure	Sensor deployment and networks
Privacy and security	Privacy concerns with images	Data security and privacy
Clinical adoption	Common in ophthalmology	Emerging in healthcare
Challenges	Data annotation, overfitting	Data integration, standards
Applications	Various retinal diseases	General health monitoring
Examples of technologies/ models	CNNs, transfer learning	Wearable health trackers, IoT

veins, and post-processing with morphological operations to remove quarantined pixels.

11.3 EXISTING METHODS IN IoT-BASED APPROACH

Ghani [12] emphasized the importance of looking beyond traditional technological advancements for clinical technologists entering the healthcare industry. They highlighted the potential of IoT devices in providing early detection of complications, enabling immediate treatment. Their research focused on designing an optoelectronic regulator chip to control the micro-light-emitting diode (LED) grid used in retinal prostheses. The chip, developed using German foundry X-FAB 0.35-μm complementary metal-oxide-semiconductor (CMOS) technology, demonstrated applicability in various healthcare and consumer devices, incorporating both low-level driving circuits and high-level communication components. To address issues related to driving current for micro-LEDs, a specialized circuit was implemented, allowing up to 9 V output. Additionally, a custom-designed Peltier cooler was integrated to address heat dissipation concerns, significantly improving the chip's performance and surface temperature [12].

Sabanayagam et al. [13] utilized data from population-based studies in Singapore and China to develop and validate a DL algorithm for distinguishing prolonged kidney disease. Their study aimed to assess if retinal photography alone, without specific retinal signs information, could accurately identify chronic kidney disease.

Bhardwaj et al. [14] provided an overview of key principles in AI and computer vision used in the biomedical field, highlighting the shift from human expert–based interpretation to AI-based automated systems. They discussed the limitations of traditional methods, such as unreliability and human error, and emphasized the effectiveness of AI-based models in image interpretation.

Aceto et al. [15] explored the connection between ICTs and healthcare, highlighting popular ICTs-based healthcare models and their supporting technologies. Through an analysis of over 300 papers, they identified ICT-based healthcare principles and applications facilitated by technological advancements. The review provided insights into novel healthcare applications enabled by ICTs, focusing on specific research challenges. It aimed to guide readers, both from technical and clinical backgrounds, through the complex landscape created by advanced ICTs in healthcare applications [15].

Asghari et al. [16] conducted a systematic review and classification of research methods in IoT applications from 2011 to 2018. Their study analyzed IoT applications in various domains, including healthcare, environmental monitoring, smart cities, industry, and general aspects.

In 2014, Bourouis et al. [17] introduced a groundbreaking, affordable intelligent system that utilized smartphones and a small lens. This innovation allowed remote and isolated patients to undergo routine eye examinations and receive disease diagnoses. Das et al. [18] presented a similar low-cost smartphone-based intelligent system integrated with a tiny lens for remote eye examinations and disease diagnosis. Dash and Senapati [19] incorporated illumination normalization techniques like Gamma correction for contrast enhancement. The proposed method demonstrated superior performance in vessel segmentation compared to traditional methods, enhancing accuracy and detail in retinal images. The technique showcased potential for clinical evaluation and DR diagnosis, although challenges like uneven vessel walls required further exploration.

In 2018, Jebadurai and Peter [20] introduced a hybrid IoT healthcare architecture, enhancing retinal images through multikernel support vector regression (SVR). Their approach, implemented in smartphone fundoscopy, surpassed existing algorithms in quality metrics like PSNR and MSE. This innovation provides ophthalmologists with high-resolution retinal images for accurate diagnosis.

Jebaseeli et al. [21] developed a glucose level estimation system using Dexcom G4 Platinum sensors, integrating IoT technology for DR prevention. The proposed IoT-based approach utilized a custom-designed method called adaptive spatial kernel separation measure based fuzzy C-means (ASKFCM) for accurate retinal vessel segmentation. The system demonstrated high accuracy, sensitivity, and specificity in diagnosing DR, showcasing its potential for real-time analysis of large datasets and early disease detection [21].

Kapoor et al. [22] provided an overview of fundamental AI principles and their application in healthcare, specifically in ophthalmology. They emphasized the potential of AI to improve patient care through prescreening, evaluation, and treatment recommendations, particularly in specialty and rare diseases. They highlighted the need for active learning and understanding AI theory for effective implementation in patient care [22].

Pratap and Kokil [23] proposed a CNN and transfer learning for cataract classification. Their approach achieved a high accuracy of 92.91% in classifying cataracts into different stages. The system also incorporated an image quality selection module to ensure accurate diagnosis. The authors emphasized the potential of CNN-based techniques for nonintrusive cataract detection, particularly in rural areas. They highlighted the integration of IoT and automatic feature extraction methods for further enhancing clinical facilities, emphasizing the importance of AI in rural healthcare [23].

Qu et al. [24] introduced a fully automated DR diagnosis system, which could capture fundus images, analyze them, and grade DR. The system achieved an accuracy of up to 85% and enabled patients to monitor their retinopathy status. Their approach reduced the workload of clinicians and offered cost-effective solutions for mass screening, potentially preventing vision loss in diabetic patients.

Raja and Gangatharan developed a hybrid system for automated glaucoma diagnosis, incorporating preprocessing, wavelet transformation, feature extraction, and classification modules, utilizing hyper-analytical wavelet transformation (HWT)-based statistical features [25]. Grewal et al. [26] discussed the integration of DL in ophthalmic care, emphasizing its potential benefits for patients and clinicians, including various diagnostic modalities such as digital photographs, optical coherence tomography (OCT), and visual fields.

Haleem et al. [27] conducted a systematic review that highlighted the importance of accurate feature extraction in glaucoma diagnosis, aiming to provide clinicians with precise information for effective treatment. Huang et al. [28] developed an approach utilizing summary data from Stratus OCT to classify eyes as either glaucomatous or normal. The ANFIS classifier demonstrated promising results, providing a valuable tool for glaucoma diagnosis. They emphasized the need for continuous improvement and human intervention in utilizing ANFIS for accurate glaucoma diagnosis [28].

Badar et al. [29] highlighted the need for better feature extraction methods and the potential of combining DL with the IoT for improved rural healthcare.

Liu et al. [30] developed an approach that outperformed fully supervised methods, demonstrating the effectiveness of semisupervised learning in joint segmentation tasks. The authors highlighted the importance of considering spatial information and multiscale features for accurate segmentation, emphasizing the potential of their approach in clinical applications.

In their 2019 study, Liu et al. introduced an innovative spatial-aware joint segmentation technique that took into account the specific spatial regions of individual pixels and incorporated the learning of multiscale spatially dense features. To validate the effectiveness of their spatial-aware segmentation technique, the researchers conducted experiments on two widely used public datasets: ORIGA and DRISHTI. Leveraging the segmentation masks obtained, they computed the cup-to-disk ratios and applied them in the context of glaucoma screening. The study demonstrated a strong correlation between the computed cup-to-disk ratios and the risk levels of glaucoma, a relationship that was empirically validated using the ORIGA dataset. This innovative methodology holds promise for enhancing the accuracy and reliability of glaucoma screening processes [31–40].

11.4 METHODOLOGY

Using a DL approach in combination with the IoMT for the early diagnosis of retinal diseases is a promising field in healthcare. This approach can revolutionize the way we detect and treat eye conditions, providing faster and more accurate diagnoses. Let's break down the analysis and potential outcomes of this approach:

1. *Data Collection and Connectivity*
   IoMT devices, like retinal cameras and OCT machines, are capable of capturing detailed retina images. These devices can instantly transmit data to a central system or cloud for analysis. Patient information is securely stored and can be accessed by medical professionals for remote diagnosis.
2. *DL Models*
   CNNs are commonly used for image analysis in retinal disease detection. Utilizing transfer learning involves using pretrained models on extensive datasets, enhancing the training process's efficiency. Annotated retinal image datasets play a vital role in training the models effectively. These datasets should include various types of retinal diseases and conditions.
3. *Image Preprocessing*
   Methods for preprocessing images can improve image quality by eliminating noise and standardizing data, ensuring consistency. Employing data augmentation can enhance the training dataset's diversity, thereby bolstering the model's robustness.
4. *Disease Detection*
   The DL model analyzes the retinal images to detect abnormalities or signs of retinal diseases. Classifications may include DR, ARMD, glaucoma, and more. The model can provide a probability score for each diagnosis, aiding in risk assessment.

5. *Early Diagnosis*

    Early detection of retinal diseases is crucial for timely intervention and prevention of vision loss. The use of IoMT ensures that patients can undergo routine screenings without visiting a healthcare facility, increasing the likelihood of early diagnosis.

6. *Telemedicine and Remote Monitoring*

    IoMT enables telemedicine, allowing patients in remote or underserved areas to receive expert diagnosis and guidance. Continuous monitoring of high-risk patients can lead to timely interventions, preventing disease progression.

7. *Accuracy and Performance*

    The performance of the DL model should be regularly evaluated, and it should be fine-tuned to improve accuracy. The model should also provide explanations or visualizations to help clinicians understand its decisions.

8. *Challenges and Considerations*

    Data privacy and security are critical when dealing with medical images and patient data. Regulatory compliance, such as HIPAA in the United States, must be adhered to. Interpretability of DL models is essential for gaining trust among medical professionals.

9. *System Design*

    The system aims to develop an integrated solution for early diagnosis of retinal diseases leveraging the power of DL and the IoMT. By combining advanced image analysis algorithms with IoMT devices, the system will enable remote monitoring, efficient data collection, and accurate diagnosis of retinal diseases in their early stages.

10. *System Architecture*

    - *IoMT Devices:* Utilize specialized retinal imaging devices equipped with sensors for capturing high-resolution retinal images. These devices should be capable of securely transmitting data to a centralized server.
    - *Data Transmission:* Implement a secure and efficient data transmission protocol to transfer retinal images and related data from IoMT devices to the central server. Utilize encryption and authentication mechanisms to ensure data integrity and confidentiality during transmission.
    - *Centralized Server:* Set up a cloud-based server infrastructure capable of receiving, storing, and managing large volumes of retinal images and patient data. Implement robust data storage, ensuring scalability, reliability, and redundancy and built DL models.
    - *User Interface:* Create intuitive user interfaces for both healthcare professionals and patients. Healthcare professionals can access patient records, view analyzed images, and provide diagnoses. Patients can securely view their retinal images and receive notifications/alerts.

11. Workflow:
- *Data Collection:* IoMT devices capture retinal images and relevant metadata. The captured data is transmitted securely to the centralized server.
- *Data Preprocessing:* Preprocess the retinal images to enhance quality, normalize lighting conditions, and remove noise, ensuring that the input data for DL models is standardized and reliable.
- *DL Analysis:* Utilize trained DL models to analyze retinal images. Detect and classify abnormalities, lesions, or early signs of diseases.
- *Diagnostic Decision Support:* The system provides diagnostic reports to healthcare professionals, highlighting detected abnormalities and providing insights based on DL analysis.
- *Patient Engagement:* Patients can access their retinal images through a secure portal. The system can send notifications for appointments, test results, or follow-up procedures, fostering patient engagement.

12. *Security and Compliance*
- *Data Security:* Implement robust data encryption both during transmission and at rest. Ensure compliance with healthcare data protection standards such as HIPAA (in the United States) or GDPR (in Europe).

13. *Integration with Healthcare Systems:* Integrate the retinal disease diagnosis system with existing Electronic Health Record (EHR) systems, allowing seamless sharing of patient data and diagnostic reports. Ensure compatibility and interoperability with various healthcare IT infrastructures.

14. *Continuous Improvement:* Implement mechanisms for continuous model training and improvement based on new data. Regularly update DL models to enhance accuracy and incorporate the latest research findings in the field of retinal disease diagnosis.

11.5 SYSTEM ARCHITECTURE

1. *IoT Devices Layer*
- *Retinal Imaging Devices:* Specialized IoT devices equipped with high-resolution cameras and sensors capture retinal images. These devices are designed for easy handling and patient comfort.
- *Data Preprocessing Unit:* The data preprocessing unit attached to IoT devices handles initial processing tasks such as noise reduction, image enhancement, and metadata extraction. It ensures the raw data is standardized before transmission.
- *Secure Data Transmission:* Utilize secure communication protocols (e.g., TLS/SSL) for encrypted data transmission from IoT devices to the cloud server. Implement authentication mechanisms to verify the identity of devices and ensure data integrity during transmission.

2. *Cloud Computing and Storage Layer*
   - *Cloud Servers:* A cloud-based server infrastructure receives and processes data from IoT devices. Cloud servers handle data storage, DL model execution, and analysis tasks. Cloud resources can scale dynamically based on demand.
   - *Data Storage:* Store retinal images, metadata, and patient records securely in a scalable and redundant database system. Implement backup and disaster recovery mechanisms to prevent data loss.
   - *DL Model Repository:* Store pretrained DL models for retinal disease detection. Regularly update and maintain these models to ensure accurate analysis based on the latest research and medical knowledge.
3. *DL and Image Analysis Layer*
   - *DL Models:* Deploy CNNs or other advanced DL architectures for retinal image analysis. These models are trained to identify patterns, lesions, and abnormalities associated with various retinal diseases.
   - *Model Training and Update:* Implement a continuous learning system where the models are periodically retrained with new data to enhance accuracy. Integrate feedback loops to improve model performance based on diagnostic outcomes and expert annotations.
   - *Anomaly Detection:* Utilize anomaly detection algorithms to identify outliers and rare cases that might be indicative of novel or uncommon retinal conditions.
4. *Diagnostic Decision Support Layer*
   - *Diagnostic Algorithms:* Develop algorithms that interpret the output from DL models. These algorithms analyze the detected abnormalities, cross-reference patient history, and generate diagnostic reports.
   - *Clinical Decision Support System (CDSS):* Integrate the diagnostic algorithms into a CDSS that provides healthcare professionals with actionable insights, highlighting potential issues and suggesting appropriate follow-up actions or treatments.
5. *User Interface and Patient Engagement Layer*
   - *Healthcare Professional Interface:* Create a user-friendly interface for healthcare professionals, allowing them to view patient records, retinal images, diagnostic reports, and historical data. Provide tools for annotations and collaboration among medical experts.
   - *Patient Portal:* Develop a secure patient portal where individuals can access their retinal images, diagnostic reports, and educational materials related to retinal health. Implement features for appointment scheduling, teleconsultations, and medication reminders.
   - *Real-time Notifications:* Implement a notification system that alerts healthcare professionals and patients about critical findings, upcoming appointments, or changes in the patient's condition.
6. *Security and Compliance Layer*
   - *Data Encryption and Privacy:* Encrypt data both in transit and at rest to ensure confidentiality. Comply with healthcare data protection regulations such as HIPAA, GDPR, or regional equivalents.

7. *Continuous Improvement and Feedback Loop*
  - *Feedback Mechanisms:* Establish mechanisms for healthcare professionals to provide feedback on diagnoses and suggestions for model improvement. Use this feedback to enhance the DL models and diagnostic algorithms.
  - *Research Integration:* Collaborate with research institutions and medical professionals to incorporate the latest research findings into the diagnostic algorithms, ensuring the system stays up-to-date with advancements in retinal disease detection.

This integrated system architecture ensures seamless collaboration between IoT devices, cloud-based processing, DL models, healthcare professionals, and patients. It enables early diagnosis, improves patient engagement, and enhances the overall quality of care for retinal diseases.

11.6 CONCLUSION

This chapter examines the helpfulness of CAD frameworks to fairly analyze patients with retinal disease. Additionally, unique AI strategies utilized by scientists over the past decade are summarized. It has likewise been noticed that DL has points of interest over the customary machine learning procedures, whereby next to no hand-created highlights extraction and choice are required.

The potential outcomes are as follows:

- Earlier diagnosis of retinal diseases, leading to improved treatment outcomes and reduced vision loss
- Enhanced accessibility to eye care services, particularly in remote areas
- Reduced healthcare costs through preventative measures and early interventions
- Accelerated research in the field of ophthalmology through the analysis of large-scale retinal image datasets
- Improved patient engagement and empowerment through the use of IoMT devices for self-monitoring

In conclusion, the integration of DL and IoMT for early diagnosis of retinal diseases has the potential to significantly impact the field of ophthalmology and improve patient care. However, it is crucial to address technical, ethical, and regulatory challenges to ensure the safe and effective deployment of these technologies in healthcare settings.

REFERENCES

1. Shi, S., He, D., Li, L., Kumar, N., Khan, M.K. and Choo, K.K.R. (2020). Applications of blockchain in ensuring the security and privacy of electronic health record systems: A survey. Computers & Security, 97, p. 101966.

2. Kermany, D.S., Goldbaum, M., Cai, W., Valentim, C.C., Liang, H., Baxter, S.L., McKeown, A., Yang, G., Wu, X., Yan, F. and Dong, J., 2018. Identifying medical diagnoses and treatable diseases by image-based deep learning. Cell, 172(5), pp. 1122–1131.

3. Schmidt-Erfurth, U., Vogl, W.D., Jampol, L.M. and Bogunović, H. (2020). Application of automated quantification of fluid volumes to anti-VEGF therapy of neovascular age-related macular degeneration. Ophthalmology, 127(9), pp. 1211–1219.

4. Alsaih, K., Yusoff, M.Z., Tang, T.B., Faye, I. and Mŕiaudeau, F. (2020). Deep learning architectures analysis for age-related macular degeneration segmentation on optical coherence tomography scans. Computer Methods and Programs in Biomedicine, 195, p. 105566.

5. Rayan, Z., Alfonse, M. and Salem, A.B., 2019. Machine learning approaches in smart health. Procedia Computer Science, 154, pp. 361–368.

6. Hsieh, Y.T., Chuang, L.M., Jiang, Y.D., Chang, T.J., Yang, C.M., Yang, C.H., Chan, L.W., Kao, T.Y., Chen, T.C., Lin, H.C. and Tsai, C.H., 2020. Application of deep learning image assessment software VeriSee™ for diabetic retinopathy screening. Journal of the Formosan Medical Association, 120, pp. 165–171.

7. Chaki, J., Ganesh, S.T., Cidham, S.K. and Theertan, S.A., 2020. Machine learning and artificial intelligence based diabetes mellitus detection and self-management: A systematic review. Journal of King Saud University-Computer and Information Sciences, 34, pp. 3204–3225.

8. Schmidt-Erfurth, U., Sadeghipour, A., Gerendas, B.S., Waldstein, S.M. and Bogunović, H., 2018. Artificial intelligence in retina. Progress in Retinal and Eye Research, 67, pp. 1–29.

9. Huyen, N.N.A., Yamakawa, A., Kodama, D., Tsuruoka, S., Kawanaka, H., Takase, H., Uji, Y., Matsubara, H. and Okuyama, F., 2013. Disease generating model for 3D display of the effect of treatment on 3D optical coherence tomography images. Procedia Computer Science, 22, pp. 780–789.

10. Alamelu, M., Balaji, R., Mithun, J. and Hariharan, M., 2019. Diabetics retinopathy vision analysis using image identification service analysis approach. Procedia Computer Science, 165, pp. 470–477.

11. Dash, J. and Bhoi, N., 2017. A thresholding based technique to extract retinal blood vessels from fundus images. Future Computing and Informatics Journal, 2(2), pp. 103–109.

12. Ghani, A., 2019. Healthcare electronics: A step closer to future smart cities. ICT Express, 5(4), pp. 256–260.

13. Sabanayagam, C., Xu, D., Ting, D.S., Nusinovici, S., Banu, R., Hamzah, H., Lim, C., Tham, Y.C., Cheung, C.Y., Tai, E.S. and Wang, Y.X., 2020. A deep learning algorithm to detect chronic kidney disease from retinal photographs in community-based populations. The Lancet Digital Health.

14. Bhardwaj, K.K., Banyal, S. and Sharma, D.K., 2019. Artificial Intelligence Based Diagnostics, Therapeutics and Applications in Biomedical Engineering and Bioinformatics. In Internet of Things in Biomedical Engineering (pp. 161–187). Academic Press.

15. Aceto, G., Persico, V. and Pescapé, A., 2018. The role of information and communication technologies in healthcare: Taxonomies, perspectives, and challenges. Journal of Network and Computer Applications, 107, pp. 125–154.

16. Asghari, P., Rahmani, A.M. and Javadi, H.H.S., 2019. Internet of Things applications: A systematic review. Computer Networks, 148, pp. 241–261.

17. Bourouis, A., Feham, M., Hossain, M.A. and Zhang, L., 2014. An intelligent mobile based decision support system for retinal disease diagnosis. Decision Support Systems, 59, pp. 341–350.

18. Das, A., Rad, P., Choo, K.K.R., Nouhi, B., Lish, J. and Martel, J., 2019. Distributed machine learning cloud teleophthalmology IoT for predicting AMD disease progression. Future Generation Computer Systems, 93, pp. 486–498.
19. Dash, S. and Senapati, M.R., 2020. Enhancing detection of retinal blood vessels by combined approach of DWT, Tyler Coye and Gamma correction. Biomedical Signal Processing and Control, 57, p. 101740.
20. Jebadurai, J. and Peter, J.D., 2018. Super-resolution of retinal images using multi-kernel SVR for IoT healthcare applications. Future Generation Computer Systems, 83, pp. 338–346.
21. Jebaseeli, T.J., Durai, C.A.D. and Peter, J.D., 2018. IoT Based Sustainable Diabetic Retinopathy Diagnosis System. In Sustainable Computing. Informatics and Systems.
22. Kapoor, R., Walters, S.P. and Al-Aswad, L.A., 2019. The current state of artificial intelligence in ophthalmology. Survey of Ophthalmology, 64(2), pp. 233–240.
23. Pratap, T. and Kokil, P., 2019. Computer-aided diagnosis of cataract using deep transfer learning. Biomedical Signal Processing and Control, 53, p. 101533.
24. Qu, M., Ni, C., Chen, M., Zheng, L., Dai, L., Sheng, B., Li, P. and Wu, Q., 2017. Automatic diabetic retinopathy diagnosis using adjustable ophthalmoscope and multi-scale line operator. Pervasive and Mobile Computing, 41, pp. 490–503.
25. Raja, C. and Gangatharan, N., 2015. A hybrid swarm algorithm for optimizing glaucoma diagnosis. Computers in Biology and Medicine, 63, pp. 196–207.
26. Grewal, P.S., Oloumi, F., Rubin, U. and Tennant, M.T., 2018. Deep learning in ophthalmology: A review. Canadian Journal of Ophthalmology, 53(4), pp. 309–313.
27. Haleem, M.S., Han, L., Van Hemert, J. and Li, B., 2013. Automatic extraction of retinal features from colour retinal images for glaucoma diagnosis: A review. Computerized Medical Imaging and Graphics, 37(7–8), pp. 581–596.
28. Huang, M.L., Chen, H.Y. and Huang, J.J., 2007. Glaucoma detection using adaptive neuro-fuzzy inference system. Expert Systems with Applications, 32(2), pp. 458–468.
29. Badar, M., Haris, M. and Fatima, A., 2020. Application of deep learning for retinal image analysis: A review. Computer Science Review, 35, p. 100203.
30. Liu, S., Hong, J., Lu, X., Jia, X., Lin, Z., Zhou, Y., Liu, Y. and Zhang, H., 2019. Joint optic disc and cup segmentation using semi-supervised conditional GANs. Computers in Biology and Medicine, 115, p. 103485.
31. Liu, Q., Hong, X., Li, S., Chen, Z., Zhao, G. and Zou, B., 2019. A spatial-aware joint optic disc and cup segmentation method. Neurocomputing, 359, pp. 285–297.
32. Santhi, D., Manimegalai, D., Parvathi, S. and Karkuzhali, S., 2016. Segmentation and classification of bright lesions to diagnose diabetic retinopathy in retinal images. Biomedical Engineering/Biomedizinische Technik, 61(4), pp. 443–453.
33. Karkuzhali, S. and Manimegalai, D. (2017). Computational intelligence-based decision support system for glaucoma detection. Biomedical Research, 28(11), pp. 4737–4748.
34. Santhi, D., Manimegalai, D. and Karkuzhali, S., 2014. Diagnosis of diabetic retinopathy by exudates detection using clustering techniques. Biomedical Engineering: Applications, Basis and Communications, 26(06), p. 1450077.
35. Karkuzhali, S. and Manimegalai, D. (2018). Retinal haemorrhages segmentation using improved toboggan segmentation algorithm in diabetic retinopathy images. Biomedical Research, 2018(Special Issue), pp. S105–S107.
36. Karkuzhali, S. and Manimegalai, D., 2018. Detection of hemorrhages in retinal images using hybrid approach for diagnosis of diabetic retinopathy. International Journal of Pure and Applied Mathematics, 118(18), pp. 2841–2846.

37. Karkuzhali, S. and Manimegalai, D., 2019. Robust intensity variation and inverse surface adaptive thresholding techniques for detection of optic disc and exudates in retinal fundus images. Biocybernetics and Biomedical Engineering, 39(3), pp. 753–764.
38. Suriyasekeran, K., Santhanamahalingam, S. and Duraisamy, M. (2020). Algorithms for diagnosis of diabetic retinopathy and diabetic macula edema: A review. Advances in Experimental Medicine and Biology, 1307, pp. 357–373.
39. Karkuzhali, S. and Manimegalai, D., 2019. Distinguishing proof of diabetic retinopathy detection by hybrid approaches in two dimensional retinal fundus images. Journal of Medical Systems, 43(6), p. 173.
40. Karkuzhali, S. and Manimegalai, D., 2018. Microanaurysms identification using computational intelligence approach in two dimensional fundus images for detection of diabetic retinopathy. International Journal of Pure and Applied Mathematics, 118(8), pp. 485–491.

Chapter 12

Intelligent e-learning platform consolidating Web of Things and ChatGPT

Neha Katiyar, Mayank Deep Khare, Jatin Kumar, Ayush Sharma, Sachin Rawat, and Jyoti Srivastav

12.1 INTRODUCTION

Internet of Things (IoT) connects hardware devices to the internet and the web. The connectivity procedure is increasing day by day. All kinds of IoT applications work through sensing in various ways. IoT is designed for intelligent traffic systems, inventory management, farming, low-cost power consumption, etc. The use of IoT, the Web of Things (WoT), and enabling technologies has increased after COVID-19. This COVID-19 era changed personal, professional, and educational human life. Things turned out from offline to online. To develop online skills, people have started to learn many computational skills. The demand for online course content on e-learning websites is increasing daily. The whole education system shifted from offline to online. While staying home during the pandemic, gaining knowledge of IoT was more accessible for students. The higher education system took this opportunity as an advantage and now several courses on IoT are offered online. Its implementation designed different web applications for IoT learning platforms. However, it is a traditional form to create any website and upload the content so that people can gain knowledge of the site. These websites are mainly designed for those who need help in understanding the concept of unambiguous computing.

IoT is an emerging technology that is changing the way we interact with our world. As the number of IoT devices continues to increase, it has become increasingly important for individuals to understand the implications and potential applications of this emerging technology. However, learners seeking to acquire knowledge about IoT are often faced with the challenge of navigating multiple sources of information, leading to a need for more centralized and comprehensive resources for learning. To address this issue, we have developed a website for learning about IoT that provides a centralized and accessible platform for acquiring knowledge about this emerging technology, as shown in Figure 12.1. Our website aims to provide comprehensive and accessible information about IoT, including its history, current trends, and future user directions. It includes interactive components such as simulations and quizzes to facilitate accessible information about IoT, including its engagement and learning. The e-learning platform is designed and developed

DOI: 10.1201/9781003487647-12

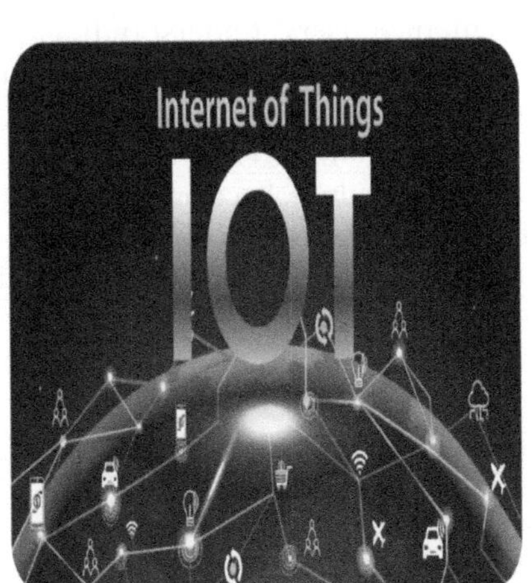

Figure 12.1 IoT e-learning website homepage.

using open-source web development technologies, such as HTML, CSS, and JavaScript, to ensure that it is user-friendly and accessible to a broad range of learners. In addition to providing [1] comprehensive information about IoT, our website also features a user-friendly interface and a search function, which enable users to find the information they require quickly. WoT provides Quantitative and qualtitative methods for the better understanding of IoT. By providing a website that offers complete information, interactive components, and a user-friendly interface, we hope to enhance users' understanding [2] of IoT and increase their interest in the topic. We represent a valuable resource for learners seeking to acquire knowledge about IoT and serve as a foundation for future research and development in this area. The problem that this research aims to address is the need for a centralized platform for learning about IoT. Currently, learners interested in acquiring knowledge about IoT must rely on multiple websites and search engines to gather information. This can be time-consuming and overwhelming, as the data must be complete and more consistent. Moreover, learners may need help finding reliable sources and more expertise to evaluate the quality of the information they find. This fragmented approach to learning can hinder the acquisition of a comprehensive understanding of IoT and limit the potential for its application. Thus, a centralized platform for learning about IoT is essential, providing learners with complete, reliable, and accessible information on this emerging technology [3]. This research seeks to fill the gap by providing an educational website offering comprehensive and accessible information about IoT and its applications. It includes interactive components to facilitate user engagement and learning and a user-friendly interface enabling learners to find the information they require quickly. Overall, this research aims to enhance users' understanding of IoT and increase their interest in the topic by addressing the need for a centralized platform for learning about this technology.

This chapter is organized in seven sections. Section 12.1 is an Introduction to the IoT e-learning platform and its designing procedure. Section 12.2 Web technology and ChatGPT. Section 12.3 discusses the methodology of Designing procedure of IoT website. Section 12.4 focuses on the ChatGPT integration searching procedure in IoT e-learning platform. Section 12.5 provides the results. Section 12.6 gives an insight into website's future use and implementation, including artificial intelligence (AI) technology. Finally, Section 12.7 concludes the chapter.

12.2 LITERATURE SURVEY

In this section, we briefly show the main principle of IoT e-learning platform. We have analyzed web technology, IoT, WoT, and ChatGPT to enhance our research work.

a. *Web Technology:* The web has many web pages interconnected with networks and the internet. Tim Berners Lee first created this. The website development project established is named "Information Management System: A Proposal." Reference [4] focuses on the year 2022; the website was the base of Hypertext Markup Language (HTML), Uniform Resource Finder (URF), and Hypertext Transfer Protocol (HTTP). At that time, the web became an essential tool for connecting to the internet. It has been enhancing various features to improve web users' usability. In 1990, the first phase of Web [1.0] was developed. At that time, it had only static websites and static web pages. It could only show the content to the user. The website management was done manually by the web developer. There were no web standards for static websites or protocols. Web hosting procedure was very simple to host the website on the internet. Website developments have so many generations to pass on the WoT. In 2022, Subedi et al. [5] worked on website connectivity with Software Development lifecycle (SDLC). They used the common approach of building an SDLC in web development. The old methods used in web development are spiral and waterfall models. In their research, they also focused on the security of web development. They provided a security methodology for web development that consists of inception, construction, and transition. The first stage, inception, works on stages of traditional development life cycle process analysis and transition refers to the stage of security assurance before deployment. In contrast, the construction phase is an iterative process of developing secure applications. It also focuses on the factors of common risk variations in web development. In 2022, Ferreira and Mamede [6] performed research on web development security threats. Web security prevention from cyber threats and attacks has become a major concern for web developers. Cybersecurity is essential for website maintenance and protecting digital assets, including sensitive content, from unauthorized access, misuse, or damage. It secures various organizations from financial losses, reputational damage, and legal liability. Proper data protection and security can avoid legal consequences and maintain customer trust. Secure web applications have become more important regarding web development due to the growing cybersecurity attacks in today's digital landscape. In 2023, Kästner et al. [7] focused on the web development platform using autonomous navigation approaches. They provide a concept of Arena-Web, a web-based development and evaluation suite for training, testing, and development. The platform is created to be intuitive and engaging to appeal to non-experts and make the technology accessible to several people. With the development of Arena-Web and its interface, training and developing deep reinforcement learning trainers is simplified, making coding easy. Their user interface comprises a file system, trained agents, plots, evaluation data, and log files. In 2023, Dela Rosa [8] focused on the e-learning platform. They developed an e-learning website to study the Mandarin language and studied the pros and cons of the website. This website was developed well, with more functionalities, features, and content. Its implementation consists of this Mandarin Chinese language web application. The technical experts worked so much so that end users can easily understand it. In 2023, Lo Chung Kwan [9] have done a systemetic review. The objective of this rapid literature review is to enhance our understanding of the capabilities of the AI-based chatbot, ChatGPT, across various subject domains, particularly in the context of its use in education, within the first three months following its launch. The review aims to explore how ChatGPT can function as both an assistant for instructors and a virtual tutor for students, assessing its potential and identifying the challenges highlighted by researchers. Additionally, it seeks to provide insights into necessary actions such as updating assessment methods and institutional policies, as well as the importance of instructor training and student education to effectively integrate ChatGPT into the educational environment. In 2024, Elbanna and Armstrong [10] preformed research on personalized learning. The main objective of this article is to explore the benefits and potential of integrating the generative AI technology, specifically ChatGPT, into educational settings. It aims to investigate how ChatGPT can be utilized for personalized learning, assessment, and content creation, while also addressing the management of its limitations and ethical considerations. The goal is to foster a discussion on how ChatGPT can effectively serve as a tool for enhancing learning and skill development, ensuring that its application is ethically sound and mindful of associated challenges. In 2016, Gyrard et al. [11] concentrated on constructing a knowledge web for IoT applications. Their research on IoT applications was conducted in three stages. The first stage involved accessing things, the second stage focused on deducing new knowledge (virtualization), and the third stage dealt with composing services (cyber). To establish such an architecture with semantic interoperability, their research presents an effective approach to integrating metadata information and modeling ontology for the application domain.

In 2014, Han et al. [3] performed research on web services. They researched on the device profile of web services. This paper created a DPWSim to support the use of technology. This sim has all the features like secure messaging, dynamic discovery, service description, etc. The DPWSim has a GUI interface on the web consisting of three scenarios: (a) Product integrating, (b) product prototyping, and (c) resource sharing. DPWSim is a Java-based application that uses the techniques of Apache Tomcat application. In 2021, Lánczky and Győrffy [12] focused on survival analysis as the cornerstone of healthcare, permitting the computation of clinical outcomes for disease breakthrough and treatment proficiency. They designed a web-based device capable of fulfilling univariate and multivariate Cox proportional risks survival tests using data generated by genomic, transcriptomic, proteomic, or metabolomic research. The web tool is built on an Apache 2.4 web server and hosted by a Linux-based server. The user interface is written in JavaScript, J Query, and PHP7. They used the Postgre SQL 12 database.

b. *WoT:* In 2016, Paganelli et al. [13] focused on the research of WoT. In this paper, they proposed a framework for intelligent things and web services. The web resources develop API for them. The interface provides a restful application programming interface. These APIs are used in web resource information model middleware and tools for developing and publishing intelligent things. WoT is access to promote value-added services to non-value-added web resources. This is used as resource-type definition and for designing web portals. This is also used as a web publishing tool. In 2022, Tzavaras et al. [14] focused on the research of WoT. They implemented an OpenAI that achieves uniformity of WoT functionality. It consists of every factor of the WoT entities. It is an open API that consists of the World Wide Web Consortium (W3C) architecture standards. The WoT model consists of behavior, interaction affordances, data schemas, security configuration like API key, and protocol binding such as Hypertext Transfer Protocol (HTTP), Hypertext Transfer Protocol Secure (HTTPS), Message Queuing Telemetry Transport (MQTT). In 2021, Zyrianoff et al. [15] focused on a WoT ecosystem. They implemented a two-way integration web service ecosystem. The W3 and WoT platforms are easily integrated through the application domain. It is a descriptive approach. WoT is also an essential asset of Industry 4.0. The

WoT has OpenAPI Specifications and is a fully functional platform. The two-way model design description is given as follows. At the lower layer, three or more web technologies are combined. In 2021, Mezenner et al. [16] focused on the WoT used in healthcare. The use of WoT in the healthcare sector is a positive approach. This technology is also used to save the life of patients. In this paper, they designed a model for the healthcare sector. It is a part of intelligent medical things. The difference between WoT and web technology is clearly shown in the web tech approach. It has four parts – measuring body temperature, providing drug injections, informing the doctor, and recording treatment in a database. In contrast, the WoT consists of a launch process and a return message. In 2023, Bashir and Warraich [17] focused on the e-learning method through the semantic web. The semantic web is an extended version of the classical web. Semantic web is one of the hottest topics of this year. It is a powerful tool that makes information more meaningful and easily understandable by people and computers. Semantic web applications set a new trend in educational opportunities for educators and students. Virtual education platforms are designed using the semantic web. These platforms break out the geographical boundaries and the educational limit for studies.

c. *IoT:* In 2019, Lin et al. [18] focused on developing NB-IoT (narrowband–Internet of Things). It is communication technology that supports the outdoor environment. NB-IoT technology is used to visualize a map to the user. In this paper, they created an NB-IoT talk platform for the fast development of NB-IoT talk applications. It has so many advanced features that an IoT platform doesn't have. It also provides many proposals for future techniques like original modeling of event-triggered NB-IoT message delivery. In 2021, Emu and Choudhury [19] focused on the IoT virtual network functionality. In this paper, they investigate deep learning functionality on virtual network function (VNF). VNF orchestration is based on the deep neural network and ensemble convolution neural network. The deep learning functionality with VNF also allocates cloud resources efficiently. The VNF deployment strategies based on two methods are optimization and AI. AI is categorized into meta-heuristics and deep learning. In 2022, Baccour et al. [20] researched on the systematic study of IoT applications. They study the communication-efficient techniques from both algorithmic and system architectures. Distributive functionality is on IoT devices, servers, and cloud servers. In this study, the most essential features of IoT devices were that they worked with deep neural networks and pervasive AI. The five features in the study are cloud computing, edge computing, data source layer, data management layer, and application layer. In 2023, Katiyar et al. [21] focused on the various trending platforms of IoT. Different companies use these platforms to get security. These platforms are used in IoT to provide an intelligent environment that can perform all the tasks quickly. These platforms support the various industry tasks so that industries can utilize them easily. In 2022, Katiyar et al. [22] also focused on the 6G connecting technology with IoT devices. They showed

6G technology connectivity with various advancements in IoT devices and focused on this technology working with space and terrestrial equipment. In 2019, Bellochet et al. [23] focused on developing IoT-based environments with an emphasis on energy-efficient techniques. They concentrated on healthcare applications within these environments. They designed an IoT-based platform that operates on a modern system-on-chip, consuming low power through a multimode preprocessor. This platform is designed to leverage both CPU and GPU capabilities in parallel, optimizing energy consumption. This platform is designed to perform parallel CPU and GPU capabilities regarding energy consumption. In 2023, Al-Taai et al. [24] focused on IoT and its education. They researched why IoT education is important in its aspects and structural components. This research deals with IoT technology in the educational fields and solves the educational problem of IoT. This study consists of an IoT teaching staff of 152 people using smart board and smart devices to deliver lectures smoothly to students during the coronavirus crisis. In year 2023, Shevchuk, Strebkov, and colleagues [25] focused on designing digital e-learning platforms. Their research highlighted trends such as spatial decentralization, feminization, occupational diversification, maturing, educational mismatch, strengthening freelance careers, planarization, and the legalization of websites for studying online work. These platforms are highly appealing, but users are often reluctant to share their property and information. The rise of these educational platform workers may make another process that develops the economies and opens new opportunities. The rise of these educational platform workers may make another process that develops the economies and opens new opportunities.

In 2023, Desai and Kim [26] focused on IoT applications in education, observing a general increase in the IoT education landscape. The IoT education system comprises smart device controllers, actuators, communication technology, and cloud-based computing, connecting humans to the internet. IoT implementations include intelligent classrooms, smart energy solutions, and cloud-based systems, effectively replacing traditional education methods. IoT implementations are based on intelligent classrooms, intelligent energy, and cloud- based solutions. IoT education system replaces the traditional education system. In 2023, Özgül and Ocak [27] focused on the distance education of IoT. It is an interdisciplinary field, and various studies have been carried out on this. They conducted analysis on 35 students and made them study through the online platform Edpuzzle, where they presented interactive videos. They also compared this platform with the Zoom application. Those students studying from the Edpuzzle platform achieved good academic scores compared to those studying from Zoom platform.

d. *ChatGPT:* In 2023, Wu et al. [28] focused on the study of ChatGPT. They focused on developing ChatGPT's future and the challenges this platform faces. They also focused on the context of learning procedure. ChatGPT includes large-scale learning models. It is an AI-based platform consisting of machine learning techniques called reinforcement learning. ChatGPT is used in various fields. It also acknowledges various studies for humankind in various fields. ChatGPT is an intelligent robot that responds according to an instruction prompt. It has shown its powerful features and performs various tasks – multilingual machine translation, story writing, project writing, content writing, etc. It is a platform designed to perform multimodal tasks and solve various challenges quickly. In 2023, Castillo et al. [29] studied the impact of Chat-GPT on university students, focusing on 216 participants. Their research examined how Chat-GPT influences the learning process, finding that the tool provides fast and accurate answers, making it practical, motivating, and engaging for students. The data collected from the 216 students was used in a descriptive analysis or qualitative analysis. This paper details the data analysis performed on the dataset.

In 2023, Božić and Poola [30] focused on the ChatGPT and its uses in education. ChatGPT is a multilanguage model that can transform education. It uses deep learning techniques to create human-based responses on a text-based model. A basic example is chatbots, which can simulate real-time conversations with students and reply to them accordingly. Chatbots also improve the policy of the feedback system. ChatGPT helps students with their writing skills. It provides them with feedback on their writing procedure. Students must know where to put punctuation and exclamation marks in writing. It also helps students to improve their grammar. In 2023, Tajik [31] focused on ChatGPT and its three phases– student-facing, system-facing, and teacher-facing tools. The student-facing tool focused on intelligent tutoring systems that help students learn new concepts. With this tool, students can improve deep learning, critical thinking, programming, etc. Teacher-facing tools help students to deliver the concept quickly and much more easily. It helps design lesson plans, syllabus outliners, create quizzes, and context. System facing refers to educational platforms that are designed to interact closely with and leverage the underlying system infrastructure, such as hardware, software, and network capabilities, to deliver educational content and services. These platforms are typically integrated with various technologies and system components to enhance the learning experience and improve the efficiency of educational processes. In 2023, Biswas [32] also focused on the concept of ChatGPT in the field of education. It is an impressive language system from OpenAI that crossed one million users in just five days. Attractive platforms like Instagram, YouTube, Netflix, and Twitter took a long time to reach this number, with 300, 1,200, 75, and 720 days, respectively. ChatGPT generate writing, closely mimics human language, and has capacity for multiple ongoing conversations in online chat mode. ChatGPT is a versatile tool that can be added to new advancements in open education by providing personalized support, direction, and feedback to autodidactic learners, thus increasing students' motivation and engagement. In 2023, Firat [33] focused on ChatGPT, its origin, and its popularity. ChatGPT is a chatbot that generates replies in response to user input. Generative Pretrained Transformer 3, or GPT 3, is a large-scale language model that can produce text with 175 billion parameters. It used natural language processing (NLP) techniques to produce pertinent answers.

In 2023, Mhlanga [34] focused on the concept of ChatGPT personalized learning. ChatGPT is a smart e-learning platform that responds to the requirements of each student. For instance, ChatGPT can suggest educational materials to students depending on their interests and learning preferences. It also helps student progress and proposes additional reading or study materials. ChatGPT evaluates a learner's vocabulary proficiency and produces a unique strategy for vocabulary development. In 2023, Rathore [35] focused on the ChatGPT research, which has created advancements in AI. The steps involved in ChatGPT processing include having the end user and getting some information from the end user. Then, the data from the end user is scrutinized. It recognizes the content from the end user. It then processes the AI-related tools and obtains the response according to the information.

12.3 METHODOLOGY

To begin with, the first step involved is conducting research on IoT and analyzing its existing resources to identify the gaps in the currently available information and resources. Our study found that, although there are numerous online resources for learning about IoT, there isn't a single centralized platform that offers comprehensive information in one place. Learners often have to rely on multiple websites and search engines to gather information on different aspects of IoT, which can be time-consuming and challenging. To address this issue, we decided to create a website that would serve as a one-stop shop for learners to access all the information related to IoT. For building the website, we opted to use open-source web development technologies such as HTML, CSS, and JavaScript, which provided us with flexibility and control over the design and functionality of the website [8].

We utilized Visual Studio Code (VSCode) as the primary integrated development environment (IDE) for creating the website. VSCode offered a wide range of features, such as code highlighting, debugging tools, and extensions, which made the development process more efficient and streamlined. To test and debug the website, we used Google Chrome and Mozilla Firefox browsers, which allowed us to identify and resolve any compatibility issues that caused chaos during the development process. One of the website's key features was incorporating interactive components such as simulations and quizzes using JavaScript. These interactive elements helped to enhance user engagement and facilitate learning by providing a more hands-on experience. Additionally, we utilized Node.js to develop the website's back-and-forth and interactive learning end functionalities, including search functionality and user authentication. Node.js allowed us to create a scalable web application with minimal overhead and easy integration with other web services.

Proposed Methodology

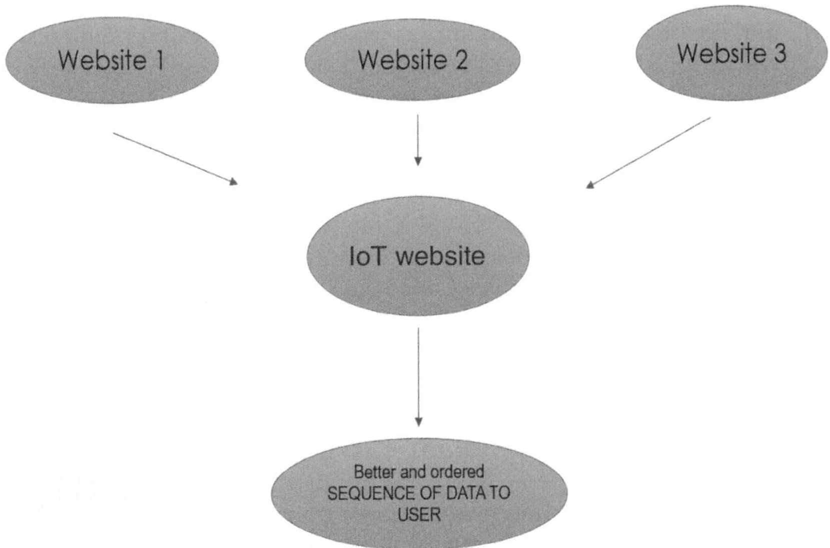

Figure 12.2 IoT learning platform for e-learning website.

We also employed quantitative and qualitative methods to evaluate the website's effectiveness in improving users' knowledge and understanding of IoT. This included collecting and analyzing data on user engagement, learning outcomes, and user satisfaction through user surveys and website usage analytics. In conclusion, the methodology for creating the website for learning IoT involved thorough analysis of the existing resources, use of open-source web development technologies, incorporation of interactive components, and evaluation of the website's effectiveness using quantitative and qualitative methods. The result is an effective and user-friendly website, which provides comprehensive information on IoT and addresses the need for a centralized platform for accessing data (Figure 12.2).

This e-learning platform enables different technologies:

a. *Technology Stack:* The project was developed using various web development technologies like HTML, CSS, and JavaScript for creating the front end of the website. For the backend, we used Node.js which is a server-side JavaScript runtime environment. We also used Chrome and Firefox browsers for testing the website and Visual Studio Code as the code editor.

b. *Website Design:* We focused on creating a user-friendly design for the website that would make it easy for learners to navigate and find the information they need. We used HTML and CSS to create the layout and styling of the website, and JavaScript to add interactivity and functionality.

c. *Content Creation:* We researched and compiled information related to IoT from various sources to ensure that our website provides comprehensive and accurate information on the topic. We used our knowledge of the subject matter to organize the information into different sections and create engaging content that would keep the learners interested.

d. *Interactive Components:* To make the learning experience more engaging, we incorporated interactive components like quizzes, simulations, and exercises into the website. We used JavaScript to create these interactive components to enhance the user experience.

e. *Backend Implementation:* To ensure that the website functions smoothly and efficiently, we used Node.js for the backend implementation. We created a server using Node.js that would handle user requests, retrieve data from the database, and send the response back to the user.

In Figure 12.3, the sitemap of IoT website is shown having all the main menu items of a webpage. It is having total six items.

Figure 12.3 shows IoT projects and ideas for designing an IoT project and its linkup to IoT simulator with IoT websites like Tinkercad, Proteus, etc. In this e-learning platform, many IoT examples and their designing processes are available, so students can design their projects efficiently. Overall, our research work involved extensive research, design, and implementation using various web development technologies and tools; as shown in

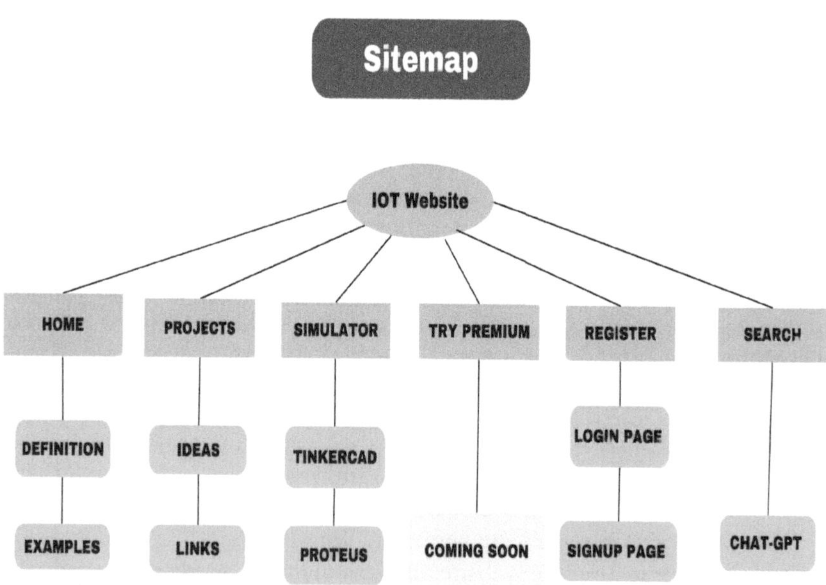

Figure 12.3 Site map consists of all the titles on the IoT website.

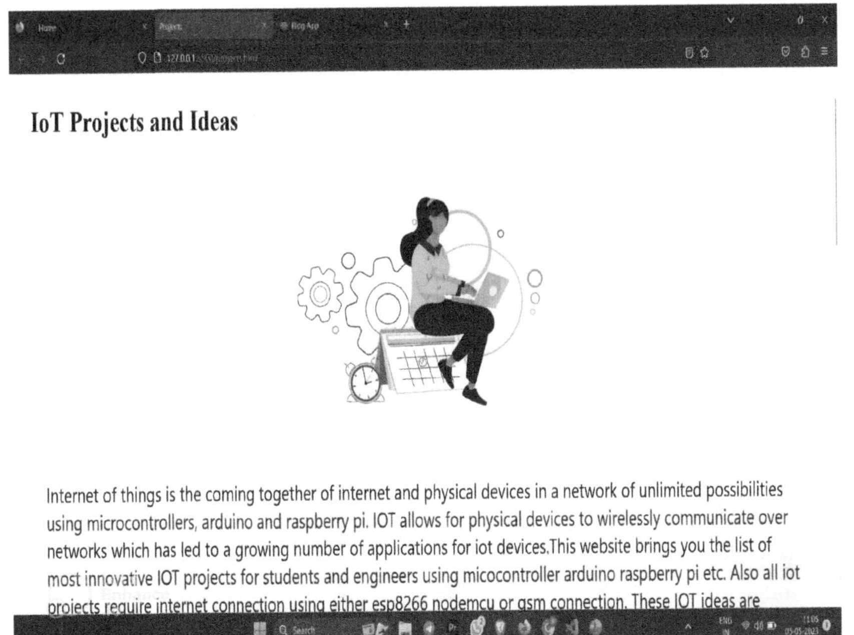

Figure 12.4 Information of IoT projects and ideas.

Figure 12.4, the platform has all the details of currently running IoT projects – the popular projects that students rapidly use for learning IoT platforms and their applications. By creating a comprehensive website for learning about IoT, we aimed to provide an accessible and user-friendly platform for learners to access all the information they need without relying on multiple websites and search engines. This e-learning platform enables the latest topic that covers IoT-related information. As shown in Figure 12.5, the e-learning platform consists of all trending issues of IoT. It consists of the basics of IoT, IoT learning and designing concepts, and IoT tools architecture like Arduino and Raspberry Pi. It also consists of IoT security as well as information about IoT devices connectivity to a different layer.

12.4 CHATGPT INTEGRATION SEARCHING PROCEDURE IN THE IOT E-LEARNING PLATFORM

Creating a website that utilizes ChatGPT for enhanced interactivity and user experience involves integrating a sophisticated language model developed by OpenAI, as shown in Figure 12.6. By incorporating this advanced language model into a website, users can enjoy seamless and more engaging conversational interactions with the website. The integration process entails utilizing the ChatGPT API provided by OpenAI. This API allows developers to send

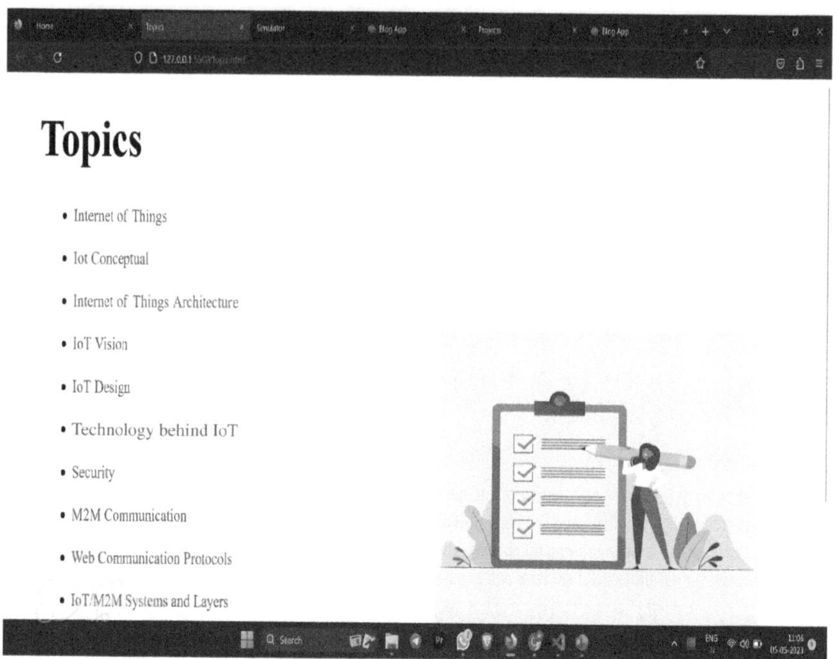

Figure 12.5 Information of IoT latest topics.

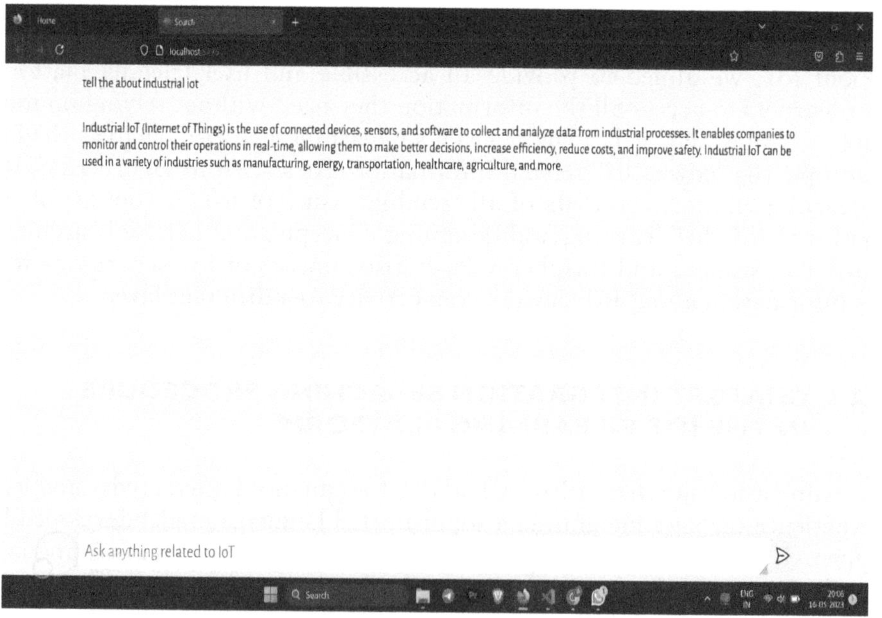

Figure 12.6 ChatGPT working procedure in the IoT learning platform.

user prompts or queries to the ChatGPT model and receive a generated text as a response. We have incorporated ChatGPT API in our search bar; so, whenever any user searches anything about IoT, that searched word or sentence is treated as a prompt for our ChatGPT API and sent to the ChatGPT server to fetch its answer. Leveraging this API empowers website owners to enhance various aspects of their website, including search functionality, customer support, recommendation systems, and interactive conversational experiences. A primary application for a ChatGPT-enabled website involves improving the search feature. Integrating ChatGPT into the search bar enables users to input their queries conversationally, resulting in more accurate and relevant search results. The ChatGPT model's natural language understanding capabilities help refine and clarify user queries, improving search accuracy and user satisfaction in finding their desired answer.

Furthermore, a ChatGPT-enabled website can offer dynamic conversational experiences, allowing users to engage in meaningful conversations with the website itself. Users can ask questions, seek clarifications, or request assistance, while the ChatGPT model generates responses that closely resemble human-like interactions. This creates an engaging and immersive user experience. Customer support is another area where ChatGPT integration proves valuable. By leveraging ChatGPT, websites can incorporate chatbots or virtual assistants to provide automated and personalized support to users. The model can effectively address frequently asked questions, offer guidance (such as user can request a roadmap to plan their study routine on IoT), and even escalate complex inquiries to human agents when necessary. Additionally, ChatGPT integration enables personalized recommendations and content filtering. The model delivers tailored suggestions and content by understanding user preferences and context. This capability enhances user engagement, ensuring that users receive relevant and captivating content aligned with their interests and needs and making them satisfied with the answers. To create a ChatGPT-enabled website, developers must obtain an API key from OpenAI and configure the necessary backend infrastructure. They install the provided libraries or Software Development Kit and handle API requests and responses in the server-side code. The integration typically involves capturing user input, submitting it to the ChatGPT API, and presenting the generated responses in a user-friendly format. ChatGPT-enabled website capitalizes on the remarkable capabilities of the ChatGPT model to provide enhanced interactivity, natural language processing, and immersive conversational experiences. Through integrating ChatGPT into a website, website owners can improve search functionality, offer interactive customer support, deliver personalized recommendations, create engaging conversational interfaces for their users, clarify their doubts, and prevent waste of time by giving everything they need on a single platform.

AIGPT-based platforms for users to complete different application aspects are shown in Table 12.1. This survey finds websites capable of generating mind maps, coding suggestions, voiceovers, and images from text.

Table 12.1   Findings of literature survey based on different AI tools available

Sr. No.	AI tools	Launch date	Features	Advantages	Disadvantages
1	Xmind.io	2007	AI platform to generate mind maps for learning topics.	Advanced mind mapping. Improves brainstorming and idea generation.	Properly not organized.
2	Scikit Learn	2007	AI tool simplifies the complexity of machine learning for the Python programming language.	Easy implementation in machine learning models.	Provides fewer preprocessing tools.
3	OpenAI	2015	Set of various AI tools like Chat GPT or Azure AI.	Personalized recommendation natural language search capabilities.	Increased cost, lack of transparency.
4	Synthesis	2017	AI platform to generate media content.	Support multilevel language, user-friendly.	Expensive and limited video credits.
5	Pictory.AI	2022	AI platform to generate photos/ videos using the prompt.	User-friendly, cloud-based convenience.	Limited video credits and transcribing hours.
6	Writesonic	2020	AI writing tool to create content.	Produce, publish, and post bulk content.	More integration, especially for blog content.
7	DALL-E	2021	AI tool that generates images from text/ prompt.	Digital art generation, editing, and manipulation.	Difficulty in understanding complex language.
8	Lovo.ai	2021	AI-based voice generator.	Voice assistant, unique voice for avatars and chatbots.	Less use of freelancer voice actors.
9	GitHub Copilot	2021	Cloud-based AI tools to generate coding suggestions.	Save time and provide suggestions.	Distraction and loss of concentration.
10	Mi- journey	2022	AI platform to generate photos using the prompt.	Refine images according to text, user-friendly.	Public generated images.

12.5 RESULTS

This section is not essential for Web Tool papers. The field of IoT is growing rapidly, and professionals with expertise in this area are in high demand. To address this demand, educational websites have emerged as a popular platform for students to learn about IoT and its practical applications. The primary outcome of an educational website for IoT is an increased understanding of the subject matter. By providing access to a variety of resources, such as e-books, video tutorials, and blog posts, students can gain a deeper understanding of IoT and its components. This can enhance their academic performance and help them apply IoT concepts to real-world scenarios.

Furthermore, educational websites can help students develop practical skills that are highly valued in the industry. By providing interactive tools such as simulators, virtual labs, and quizzes, students can gain hands-on experience in designing and implementing IoT solutions. This can help them develop critical skills for success in the IoT field, including programming, data analysis, and project management. Another significant outcome of educational websites for IoT is the opportunity for students to earn certifications. Certifications recognize students' proficiency in IoT and demonstrate their knowledge and practical skills to potential employers. Additionally, educational websites can offer customized learning paths tailored to student's interests and skill levels, helping them learn at their own pace and achieve optimal learning outcomes. Educational websites for IoT can also facilitate the development of a sense of community among IoT enthusiasts. By connecting students with experts and peers from around the world, these websites can foster collaboration and knowledge-sharing. This can help students build professional networks, gain exposure to different perspectives and ideas, and stay connected with the latest trends and developments in the advanced IoT sector.

12.6 FUTURE USE OF WEBSITE

This section consists of this website's future use and implementation, which may include AI technology. It is also used to run real-time projects at different locations. Students can add more of the latest topics and tasks that enable IoT, Industrial IoT, IoT security, etc. Students can quickly get many ideas from this website for their project development and understanding. This website may create a boom in personalized learning for students.

12.7 CONCLUSION

In conclusion, an educational website for learning IoT can offer a range of benefits to students interested in pursuing a career in this field. By providing access to various resources, interactive tools, and certification programs, the e-learning platforms using a WoT can help students gain a deeper understanding of IoT and develop practical skills that employers highly value. Furthermore, the website can facilitate collaboration and knowledge-sharing among students, experts, and peers worldwide, which can help them build professional networks and prepare for the global nature of the IoT industry. Due to the growing demand for IoT professionals, educational websites have become a valuable platform for students to learn about this technology and its practical applications by offering customized learning, customized learning paths, and virtual labs. These websites can give students the flexibility and convenience to learn at their own pace and schedule.

Adding More Advanced Topics: As IoT is an ever-evolving field, it is essential to keep updating the website's content with the latest technologies and advancements. Collaborating with IoT companies can provide students with opportunities to work on real-world projects and get some practical experience. Including case studies of successful IoT projects can give the students insight into the practical applications of IoT.

Expansion of Community Forums: Building an online community of IoT enthusiasts can help students share their knowledge and experience with others and seek expert guidance and support. Providing customized learning paths based on student's interests and skill levels can help them learn at their own pace and maximize their learning outcomes.

Integration with AI and Machine Learning: Integrating the website with AI and machine learning technologies can provide personalized learning experiences to students based on their learning styles and preferences. An e-learning platform for IoT is crucial for students interested in pursuing a career in this exciting and rapidly evolving field. Such a platform provides students with the knowledge, skills, and professional networks necessary for success. These websites enable students to take full advantage of the numerous opportunities available in the IoT industry. Therefore, it is vital for educational institutions and industry organizations to continue investing in IoT technology and support the next generation of IoT professionals. As such, educational institutions and industry organizations must continue investing in this WoT technology and supporting the next generation of IoT professionals.

12.8 GRANT INFORMATION

In this research work, no grants have been used to support this work.

NOMENCLATURE

API:	Application Program Interface
IoT:	Internet of Things
CPU:	Central Processing Unit
CSS:	Cascading Style Sheet
GPT:	Generative Pretrained Transformer
GPU:	Graphics Processing Unit
HTTP:	Hyper Text Transfer Protocol
NB-IoT:	Narrowband–Internet of Things
WoT:	Web of Things

REFERENCES

1. Reddy, H. B. S., R. S. Reddy, R. Jonnalagadda, P. Singh, and A. Gogineni. 2022. "Usability evaluation of an unpopular restaurant recommender web application Zomato." *Asian Journal of Research in Computer Science* 13, no. 4: 12–33. https://doi.org/10.9734/ajrcos/2022/v13i430319.
2. Acosta, T., P. Acosta-Vargas, J. Zambrano-Miranda, and S. Luján-Mora. 2020. "Web accessibility evaluation of videos published on YouTube by worldwide top-ranking universities." *IEEE Access* 8: 110994–111011. https://doi.org/10.1109/ACCESS.2020.3002175.
3. Han, S. N., et al. 2014. "DPWSim: A simulation toolkit for IoT applications using devices profile for web services." Paper presented at the 2014 IEEE World Forum on Internet of Things (WF-IoT), Seoul, South Korea, 544–547. https://doi.org/10.1109/WF-IoT.2014.6803226.
4. Mbunge, S. E., B. S. Jiyane, and B. Muchemwa. 2022. "Towards emotive sensory Web in virtual health care: Trends, technologies, challenges, and ethical issues." *Sensors International* 3, August 2021: 100134. https://doi.org/10.1016/j.sintl.2021.100134.
5. Subedi, B., A. Alsadoon, P. W. C. Prasad, and A. Elchouemi. 2016. "Secure paradigm for web application development." Paper presented at the 15th RoEduNet Conference: Networking in Education and Research, Bucharest, Romania, 1–6. https://doi.org/10.1109/RoEduNet.2016.7753243.
6. Ferreira, D., and H. São Mamede. "Advanced research on information systems security: Predicting cybersecurity risk—a methodology for assessments." Advanced Research on Information Systems Security 2: 7350–8263.
7. Kästner, L., et al. 2023. "Arena-Web: A Web-based Development and Benchmarking Platform for Autonomous Navigation Approaches." Accessed April 23, 2024. http://arxiv.org/abs/2302.02898.
8. Dela Rosa, A. P. 2023. "Development of a web application for learning basic Mandarin Chinese." *International Journal of Emerging Technologies in Learning* 18, no. 4: 235–247. https://doi.org/10.3991/ijet.v18i04.37121.
9. Lo, C. K. 2023. "What is the impact of ChatGPT on education? A rapid review of the literature." *Education Sciences* 13, no. 4: 410. https://doi.org/10.3390/educsci13040410.
10. Elbanna, S., and L. Armstrong. 2024. "Exploring the integration of ChatGPT in education: Adapting for the future." *Management & Sustainability: An Arab Review* 3, no. 1: 16–29.
11. Gyrard, A., P. Patel, A. Sheth, and M. Serrano. 2016. "Building the web of knowledge with smart IoT applications." *IEEE Intelligent Systems* 31, no. 5: 83–88. https://doi.org/10.1109/MIS.2016.81.
12. Lánczky, A., and B. Győrffy. 2021. "Web-based survival analysis tool tailored for medical research (KMplot): Development and implementation." *Journal of Medical Internet Research* 23, no. 7: 1–7. https://doi.org/10.2196/27633.
13. Paganelli, F., S. Turchi, and D. Giuli. 2016. "A web of things framework for RESTful applications and its experimentation in a smart city." *IEEE Systems Journal* 10, no. 4: 1412–1423. https://doi.org/10.1109/JSYST.2014.2354835.
14. Tzavaras, A., N. Mainas, and E. G. Petrakis. 2023. "OpenAPI framework for the web of things." *Internet of Things* 21: 100675.
15. Zyrianoff, I., L. Gigli, F. Montori, C. Kamienski, and M. Di Felice. 2021. "Two-way integration of service-oriented systems-of-systems with the web of things." In Proceedings of the 47th Annual Conference of the IEEE Industrial Electronics Society (IECON), 1–6. IEEE.

16. Mezenner, I., S. Bouyakoub, and F. M. H. Bouyakoub. 2021. "Towards a Web of Things-based system for a smart hospital." In Proceedings of the 2nd International Workshop on Human-centric Smart Environments for Health and Well-being (IHSH), 22–27. IEEE.

17. Bashir, F., and N. F. Warraich. 2023. "Systematic literature review of semantic web for distance learning." *Interactive Learning Environments* 31, no. 1: 527–543. https://doi.org/10.1080/10494820.2020.1799023.

18. Lin, Y. -B., H. -C. Tseng, Y. -W. Lin, and L. -J. Chen. 2019. "NB-IoTtalk: A service platform for fast development of NB-IoT applications." *IEEE Internet of Things Journal* 6, no. 1: 928–939. https://doi.org/10.1109/JIOT.2018.2865583.

19. Emu, M., and S. Choudhury. 2021. "Ensemble deep learning assisted VNF deployment strategy for next-generation IoT services." *IEEE Open Journal of the Computer Society*: Volume 2. https://doi.org/10.1109/OJCS.2021.3098462.

20. Baccour, E., et al. 2022. "Pervasive AI for IoT applications: A survey on resource-efficient distributed artificial intelligence." *IEEE Communications Surveys & Tutorials* 24, no. 4: 2366–2418. https://doi.org/10.1109/COMST.2022.3200740.

21. Katiyar, N., P. Kumari, S. Sakhshi, and J. Srivastava. 2023. "Trending IoT platforms on middleware layer." In *Intelligent Analytics for Industry 4.0 Applications*, 131–147. CRC Edited by-Avinash Chandra Pandey, Abhishek Verma, Vijaypal Singh Rathor, Press.

22. Katiyar, N., J. Srivastava, and K. P. Singh. 2022. "A perspective toward 6G connecting technology." In Micro-Electronics and Telecommunication Engineering: ICMETE 2021, Lecture Notes in Networks and Systems, vol. 373, edited by D. K. Sharma, S. L. Peng, R. Sharma, and D. A. Zaitsev. Springer, Singapore. https://doi.org/10.1007/978-981-16-8721-1_70.

23. Belloch, J. A., J. M. Badía, F. D. Igual, and M. Cobos. 2019. "Practical considerations for acoustic source localization in the IoT era: Platforms, energy efficiency, and performance." *IEEE Internet.*

24. Al-Taai, S. H. H., H. A. Kanber, and W. A. M. al-Dulaimi. 2023. "The importance of using the Internet of Things in education." *International Journal of Emerging Technologies in Learning* (Online) 18, no. 1: 19.

25. Shevchuk, A., and D. Strebkov. 2023. "Digital platforms and the changing freelance workforce in the Russian Federation: A ten-year perspective." *International Labour Review* 162, no. 1: 1–22.

26. Desai, R. R., and J. Kim. 2023. "Bibliographic and text analysis of research on implementation of the Internet of Things to support education." *Journal of Information Systems Education* 34, no. 2: 179–195.

27. Özgül, E., and M. A. Ocak. 2023. "The effect of education through distance education on student success and motivation." *Journal of Educational Technology and Online Learning* 6, no. 2: 403–420.

28. Wu, T., et al. 2023. "A brief overview of Chat-GPT: The history, status quo, and potential future development." *IEEE/CAA Journal of Automatica Sinica* 10, no. 5: 1122–1136. https://doi.org/10.1109/JAS.2023.123618.

29. Castillo, A. G. R., et al. 2023. "Effect of Chat-GPT on the digitized learning process of university students." *Journal of Namibian Studies: History Politics Culture* 33: 1–15.

30. Božić, Velibor, and Indrasen Poola. 2023. "Chat GPT and education." Preprint.

31. Tajik, E., and F. Tajik. 2023. "A comprehensive examination of the potential application of Chat-GPT in higher education institutions." *TechRxiv* Volume 2 Year 2021: 1–10.

32. Biswas, S. 2023. "Role of Chat-GPT in Education." SSRN. Accessed year. http://ssrn.com/abstract=4369981.
33. Firat, M. 2023. "How Chat GPT Can Transform Autodidactic Experiences and Open Education." Department of Distance Education, Open Education Faculty, Anadolu University.
34. Mhlanga, D. 2023. "The Value of Open AI and Chat GPT for the Current Learning Environments and the Potential Future Uses." SSRN. Accessed year 5 May 2023. http://ssrn.com/abstract=4439267.
35. Rathore, B. 2023. "Future of AI & Generation Alpha: Chat-GPT Beyond Boundaries." *Eduzone: International Peer Reviewed/Refereed Multidisciplinary Journal* 12, no. 1: 63–68.

Chapter 13

Issues and challenges in security and privacy with e-Healthcare

A thorough literature analysis

Manikandan A., Sanjay T., Gautham Menon, Aswin R., Parthiv Bijumon Bhaskar, Mahadev Govind R., and Ramprasad OG

13.1 INTRODUCTION

In the age of digitalization, the healthcare landscape is undergoing a profound transformation. The digitalization of the healthcare system encompasses a significant shift from manual procedures to robotic surgery and a transition from traditional paper-based methods to smart, digitized healthcare systems. This paradigm shift entails the utilization of smart devices to record healthcare data, thereby leveraging the power of the Internet. Consequently, healthcare professionals and hospitals can seamlessly track individuals' health records, facilitating timely assistance and intervention. Nevertheless, amidst these advancements, inherent concerns exist about the security and privacy of electronic healthcare systems. These concerns include access control, data breaches, and data sharing. This chapter highlights the security issues in healthcare systems that need to be addressed by the electronic healthcare manufacturers in the system design architectures that prioritize user security and privacy. By doing so, individuals can confidently engage with digital healthcare systems, knowing their sensitive information remains safeguarded. The use of electronic devices to assist and improve healthcare services is known as e-Health (Zaman et al., 2017). It takes a thorough approach to providing electronic healthcare. It provides unlimited access to medical treatment by instantly sharing patient information over the Internet. The partial transition from paper-based to electronic medical prescriptions, particularly in most developed nations worldwide, is a stark example of this transformation (Hopkins, 2004). E-health care, also known as electronic healthcare, has recently emerged due to the revolutionary changes brought about by integrating technology into the healthcare industry (Naseer Qureshi et al., 2020). Electronic health records (EHRs), telemedicine, mobile health (mHealth) applications, wearable technology, and remote monitoring systems are just a few of the numerous digital applications that fall under the umbrella of e-healthcare (Akhila et al., 2021). While there are many advantages to these technical developments, they have also given rise to some security concerns that present serious difficulties for the healthcare sector. Due to the abundance of sensitive information, they contain medical histories, social security

DOI: 10.1201/9781003487647-13

numbers, and payment information; healthcare records are extremely valuable on the black market (Ching et al., 2018). Cybercriminals commonly use malware, ransomware, and phishing attacks to target healthcare businesses and obtain illegal access to these records. Data breaches jeopardize patient privacy, disrupt medical procedures, and cost money (Tao et al., 2019).

Additionally, many healthcare institutions must have suitable security procedures to safeguard patient information (Brach et al., 2012). Malicious actors can take advantage of vulnerabilities in old software, weak passwords, and unencrypted data transmission, to name just a few. Furthermore, healthcare organizations cannot have strong access restrictions, making patient data available to unauthorized personnel. However, not all security risks originate from outside entities insider threats to e-healthcare security, whether purposeful or accidental, present serious risks (Al-Mhiqani et al., 2020). Employees with access to patient data risk accidentally disclosing sensitive data or falling for social engineering tricks.

Patient data can be stolen or used maliciously by disgruntled workers or others looking to profit (Roy Sarkar, 2010). Security holes may result from the interoperability of various e-healthcare systems and devices. Attackers can take advantage of weaknesses at the points of connection when diverse systems are not properly integrated or upgraded to address new threats (Tarouco et al., 2012). The growth of wearable technology and connected medical devices opens up new points of vulnerability for prospective attacks (Yaqoob et al., 2019). Devices with poor security can be exploited, allowing third parties to access patient data and, in some cases, posing a risk to life if vital medical equipment is tampered; e-healthcare companies are required to abide by stringent data privacy laws, such as the Health Insurance Portability and Accountability Act (HIPAA) in the United States (Shah & Khan, 2020). In addition to facing harsh penalties, noncompliance with these rules undermines patients' confidence in the healthcare system's ability to protect their privacy. The security and privacy of patient data have become a primary priority as the healthcare industry continues to use and rely on digital technologies. Healthcare organizations may proactively protect sensitive information and uphold the confidence of patients and stakeholders in the digital era by being aware of these difficulties (Lupton, 2017). The security issues that healthcare businesses must address change along with the e-healthcare market. Building and maintaining confidence among stakeholders, including patients, healthcare professionals, and payers, depends on addressing these security concerns (Appari & Johnson, 2010). The e-healthcare sector can safely navigate the digital world and continue to unlock the full potential of technology to enhance patient care and outcomes by putting in place strong security measures, keeping up to date on new threats, and cultivating a culture of cybersecurity awareness. The most important security challenges affecting e-healthcare today will be discussed in this chapter, along with potential solutions. The potential risks and their effects on patients, healthcare providers, and the entire healthcare system will be highlighted.

13.2 REMOTE PATIENT MONITORINGSYSTEM

The remote patient monitoring (RPM) system is a modern healthcare system that grips the concept of the Internet of Things (IoT), which connects healthcare experts with the patients for the continuous recording and monitoring of their health information; this includes pulse rate stress level, ECG, and EEG blood oxygen levels. All this vital information are gathered through wearable trackers like smartwatches (Pramanik et al., 2019). Despite easy mobility and cost-effectiveness advantages, these smart devices may have accuracy issues. Nevertheless, they have proven especially valuable for elderly individuals, allowing healthcare providers to closely monitor their health and promptly respond to subtle changes in their readings. RPM's real-time monitoring and intervention capabilities can lead to more efficient and effective healthcare delivery, improving patient outcomes and reducing hospital readmissions. As RPM technology continues to evolve, it holds great promise in transforming patient care, enhancing healthcare accessibility, and revolutionizing the healthcare industry.

13.2.1 Existing remote patient monitoring system

Several existing remote patient monitoring systems are available in the healthcare industry already. These include a range of IoT embedded systems and software such as mobile applications and cloud-based platforms that allow healthcare professionals to monitor the patient's health continually and remotely; some eminent devices are trackers, smartwatches, and mobile health apps. These systems collect and transmit data on vital signs, chronic condition management, medication adherence, and more, providing real-time insights to healthcare professionals for proactive care and timely interventions. With technological advancements, new and improved remote patient monitoring systems continue to emerge, transforming healthcare delivery.

13.2.2 Data theft and unauthorized access

Data theft and unauthorized access have become significant cybercrimes that pose serious risks to the healthcare system. With the vast reach of the Internet, attackers can retrieve or breach healthcare information from any part of the world, potentially leading to harmful consequences. For instance, attackers may send false health data to medical facilities, resulting in incorrect treatment decisions and delayed patient medication. Healthcare data breach statistics reveal the scale of the problem. The reported data breaches include incidents with 500 or more records and are disclosed to the U.S. Department of Health and Human Services Office for Civil Rights (OCR). Smaller breaches are not publicly disclosed. Between October 21, 2009, and December 31, 2022, OCR received reports of 5,150 data breaches, out of which 882 were still under investigation at the end of 2022 (HIPAAJournal, 2017). The impact of these breaches can be severe, compromising patients' privacy, trust, and the overall integrity of the healthcare system. Healthcare organizations and entities must take robust measures to safeguard sensitive patient information, adhere to HIPAA (Health Insurance Portability and Accountability Act) regulations (Shuaib et al., 2021), and implement strong cybersecurity practices. Preventing data breaches and unauthorized access requires a multilayered approach, including data encryption, access controls, regular security assessments, employee training on cybersecurity best practices, and proactive monitoring for suspicious activities. Strengthening partnerships between the healthcare sector and cybersecurity experts is crucial to combat evolving cyber threats effectively. As healthcare embraces digital transformation and telemedicine, securing patient data becomes even more critical. Continuous efforts to raise awareness about cybersecurity risks and enforce compliance with data protection regulations are essential to ensure patient safety and maintain the trust of individuals in the healthcare system. By proactively addressing these challenges, the healthcare industry can safeguard sensitive information and protect patient well-being in an increasingly connected world.

13.2.3 Challenges in RPMS in terms of attacks

Remote patient monitoring systems face significant challenges regarding cyberattacks, primarily due to the sensitive nature of the healthcare data they handle. The major challenge is the data breach, as the RPMS collects and transmits the patient's sensitive health information through the channel of IoT (Paul et al., 2023) Cybercriminals are mostly engaged in retrieving such sensitive data. These kind of data breaches can lead to the exposure of patient's health condition Ransomware attacks also pose a serious threat to the RPMS, where the attackers encrypt the transmitted data. These types of attacks can lead to temporary and permanent loss of access and connection to the patient's device, disrupting the patients care. Weak access controls or compromised credentials can lead to unauthorized access to RPMS data, enabling data manipulation, theft, or misuse, compromising patient safety and privacy. Also, vulnerabilities in IoT devices, such as wearable fitness trackers and smartwatches used in RPMS, can be exploited by attackers to enter the RPMS infrastructure. Insider threats pose an unavoidable challenge to RPMS security. Individuals with legitimate access to RPM data may inadvertently cause harm, leading to the leaking of sensitive information. Thus, ensuring cybersecurity in RPMS is essential. The healthcare organization can minimize security issues by implementing robust security measures, conducting regular updates, and providing employee training (Nifakos et al., 2021). Through these measures, patient data can be safeguarded, ensuring the integrity of the remote patient monitoring system.

13.2.4 Workable solutions for addressing attacks

Due to the sensitive nature of healthcare data, RPMS is an appealing target for hackers; therefore, addressing assaults on RPMS necessitates a thorough and proactive approach to cybersecurity. Implementing robust authentication procedures, such as multifactor authentication, is crucial to enhancing RPMS security since it guarantees that only authorized users have access to patient data. Additionally, end-to-end encryption protects data against interception and illegal use while being sent and stored. While ongoing employee training on cybersecurity best practices aids healthcare staff in recognizing and responding to potential threats like phishing and social engineering attacks, regular security audits and vulnerability assessments are crucial in identifying and addressing potential weaknesses in the RPMS infrastructure. Developing a well-defined incident response plan enables healthcare organizations to respond swiftly and efficiently to cybersecurity incidents, minimizing their impact and mitigating potential damages. Secure software development practices, regular software updates, and network segmentation help protect RPMS from known vulnerabilities and limit the impact of breaches. Implementing time monitoring and anomaly detection mechanisms allows for early identification of suspicious activities, facilitating timely intervention. Secure handling of IoT devices used in RPMS and regular firmware updates ensure their resilience against potential exploits. Having robust data backup and disaster recovery plans ensures data availability and recovery in case of data loss or ransomware attacks. Assessing the security practices of third-party vendors and business associates who have access to RPMS data is essential to maintain compliance. Adherence to compliance protection regulations, such as HIPAA, is imperative to safeguard patient privacy and comply with cybersecurity standards. By adopting these comprehensive solutions, healthcare organizations can bolster the security of their RPMS, safeguard sensitive patient data, and mitigate the risks posed by cyberattacks, ensuring the confidentiality and trustworthiness of their remote patient monitoring systems.

13.3 DATA MANAGEMENT AND ANALYSIS

Data management in healthcare is a crucial process that involves organizing and maintaining a comprehensive database of health-related information for individuals (Abbas et al., 2021). It encompasses the effective management of the entire life cycle of health data. Within healthcare organizations, a wealth of data is gathered, ranging from medical reports and lab results to insurance information and more. Consequently, safeguarding this data becomes paramount, as it is pivotal in protecting patient privacy. In healthcare, data management adopts a well-structured and systematic approach. Its primary focus lies in the seamless collection, storage, updating, and accessibility of vital patient information (Altohami et al., 2021).

The integration of sophisticated database management systems assumes paramount importance to effectively handle the vast volume of data arising from diverse healthcare interactions. Initially, the pivotal phase revolves around the meticulous collection of data from diverse sources, encompassing vital information from EHRs, medical tests, and specialized medical devices (Koushik Reddy et al., 2023). Subsequently, utmost attention is devoted to securely storing the acquired data, ensuring its steadfast reliability and seamless accessibility when needed. This imperative task demands the adept utilization of advanced big data storage systems, with cloud-based solutions being a great choice to manage the ever-increasing volume of healthcare data efficiently.

Data management in healthcare systems encompasses more than data storage; it also involves meticulously maintaining and regularly updating this data to ensure its safety, relevance, and currency (model depicted in Figure 13.1). This aspect holds paramount importance as it enables precise clinical decision-making, facilitates effective patient care, and supports advancements in medical research. Despite offering numerous benefits, healthcare data management also has drawbacks. The sensitivity of this data necessitates stringent security measures to ensure its protection. Healthcare organizations must prioritize safeguarding patient data and implementing robust measures to thwart unauthorized access, breaches, and potential misuse of the information (Firouzi et al., 2022).

In summary, data management is pivotal in the modern era of healthcare systems. By adeptly handling the vast array of health data, healthcare

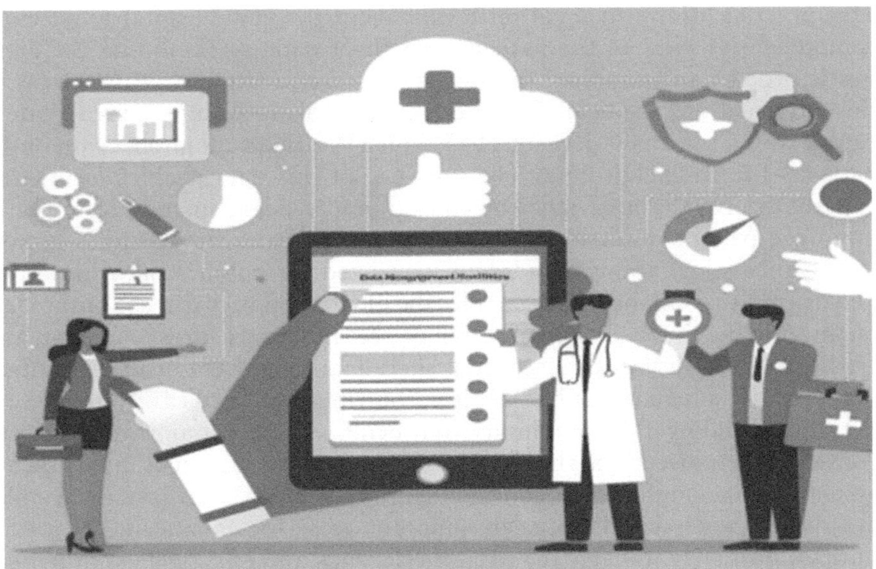

Figure 13.1 Data management in healthcare.

professionals can make well-informed decisions with greater ease and precision, thanks to the valuable insights it offers. Consequently, this significantly contributes to enhanced patient outcomes and the continuous improvement of healthcare services.

13.3.1 Importance of data management in healthcare

The primary rationale for prioritizing data management in healthcare lies in its ability to significantly enhance the diagnostic process. With improved data quality, healthcare professionals can obtain more accurate and timely information, enabling quicker and more effective diagnosis and treatment for individuals. Consequently, data management assumes the utmost significance within the healthcare sector. Moreover, in critical scenarios, such as medical emergencies, time becomes crucial, and rapid access to relevant data becomes indispensable for effectively managing a patient's health. Healthcare research represents another significant factor that underscores the importance of data management in the healthcare domain (Upadhyay & Hu, 2022). With the ability to analyze extensive volumes of data, researchers can discern intricate patterns and correlations, thus making substantial contributions to the progress of the medical field. This potential for in-depth data analysis empowers researchers to unveil novel insights, propel medical advancements, and consequently improve healthcare outcomes.

A critical factor underscoring the significance of data management is the ease of healthcare data accessibility. Patients who require a transfer between hospitals can request their medical information from the previous facility. This practice allows medical professionals at the new hospital to access a comprehensive view of the patient's pertinent data, streamlining the diagnostic process and enabling prompt and precise treatment. With access to this information, medical practitioners can ensure uninterrupted patient care, making informed decisions based on a thorough comprehension of the patient's health background. The presence of this data enables healthcare experts to provide more efficient and tailored care, ultimately resulting in improved patient results. Data management in healthcare assumes utmost importance when anonymized data is utilized for public health initiatives and disease surveillance. This enables the identification of disease outbreaks, facilitating the timely implementation of preventive measures to combat and eradicate these diseases. Leveraging such data empowers healthcare organizations to safeguard public health, contributing significantly to disease prevention and overall community well-being. Another important aspect to consider when discussing the significance of data management in healthcare systems is the emphasis on continuous improvement. This process enables healthcare professionals to easily pinpoint areas for enhancement, which, in turn, positively impacts the overall efficiency and effectiveness of patient outcomes.

13.3.2 Issues with storage

Healthcare organizations handle large amounts of data for patient care, but security remains a significant concern (Iijima et al., 2021). Healthcare systems are prime targets for data breaches, as attackers use advanced methods to gain unauthorized access and expose sensitive information. Implementing effective security measures in healthcare is complex and challenging due to the evolving sophistication of attack techniques. Healthcare data storage is a critical aspect that requires careful consideration due to the continuously increasing volume of information generated within the medical industry (Aceto et al., 2020). With the advent of the new age, data collection has surged significantly, necessitating the development of a novel storage solution that offers high scalability and cost-efficiency. This system should handle substantial quantities of data while maintaining cost-effectiveness seamlessly. Data breaches and thefts are unfortunately common in data management within healthcare applications.

Consequently, storage systems should incorporate robust mechanisms for data backup, ensuring data distribution across various nodes to enhance both its availability and safety. Storage systems must not only ensure data backup, distribution across nodes, and enhanced security, but should also strictly adhere to the regulations set forth by the regulatory authorities. Compliance with these regulations is crucial to safeguard patient privacy and maintain the ethical handling of sensitive healthcare data. Likewise, there exist many issues with the storage of healthcare data management. Measures should be taken to avoid the recurrence of such issues.

13.3.3 Issues with data protection

Cybersecurity threats pose one of the most significant risks to healthcare organizations, making them vulnerable to constant attacks. These threats can result in data breaches, amplifying concerns over patient privacy and security. Furthermore, many healthcare organizations still rely on outdated systems lacking robust security features. It is imperative to prioritize promptly updating these systems to ensure the delivery of even more effective and secure healthcare services. Inadequate employee training in various organizations can lead to data protection concerns as they might unintentionally cause data breaches. Hence, ensuring that employees undergo comprehensive training to minimize the risk of such breaches and uphold the security of sensitive data is crucial.

Additionally, data sharing among healthcare systems can create potential security challenges. Therefore, it is vital to establish a secure and well-structured framework for data sharing to avoid significant data breaches. By implementing a strong system, the data-sharing process becomes more efficient, ensuring enhanced protection of sensitive healthcare information (Vilela et al., 2019). Similarly, numerous challenges emerge concerning data protection, necessitating thorough evaluations. Proactive measures should be implemented to fortify security, thereby preventing the recurrence of such issues.

The number of data breaches in the healthcare sector compares poorly with other sectors. An analysis of data breaches recorded on the Privacy Rights database between 2015 and 2022 showed that 32% of all recorded data breaches were in the healthcare sector – almost double the number recorded in the financial and manufacturing sectors (HIPAAJournal, 2017). Surprisingly, only a small fraction, ranging from 4% to 7%, of the health system's information technology (IT) budget is allocated to cybersecurity.

Negligent employees contribute significantly to the risk, with around 61% of healthcare data breaches originating from this group. During the first half of 2022, the healthcare sector suffered close to 337 breaches, according to Fortified Health Security's mid-year report. In that same period, these 337 healthcare incidents impacted a staggering 19,992,810 individuals, as the U.S. Department of Health and Human Services reported. Between 2009 and 2022, 5,150 healthcare data breaches of 500 or more records have been reported to the HHS' Office for Civil Rights. Those breaches have resulted in the exposure or impermissible disclosure of 382,262,109 healthcare records. That equates to more than 1.2× the population of the United States. In 2018, healthcare data breaches of 500 or more records were being reported at a rate of around 1 per day. Fast forward 5 years and the rate has more than doubled. In 2022, an average of 1.94 healthcare data breaches of 500 or more records were reported each day (HIPAAJournal, 2017), as depicted in Figure 13.2.

Most of these incidents have been attributed to IT/ hacking-related events and some to loss or theft. The graph clearly indicates a steady rise in data breaches over the years, with a dip observed in 2023. It mainly increased during 2019–2021 due to the COVID-19 outbreak, where cyberattacks mostly targeted healthcare organizations. It is crucial to implement robust security

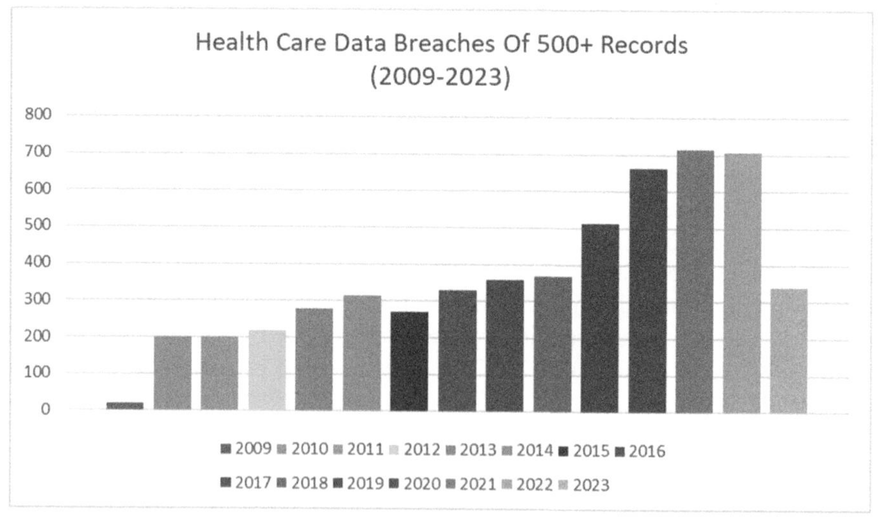

Figure 13.2 Healthcare data breaches from 2009 to 2023.

measures to prevent such occurrences and safeguard patients from harm. By doing so, healthcare organizations can effectively protect sensitive data and uphold patient privacy, mitigating potential breaches. Constant vigilance and continuous improvement in cybersecurity protocols are essential to stay ahead of evolving threats and maintain the trust and safety of patients and their information. These statistics underscore the crucial necessity for meticulous data management to protect patients and prevent data thefts or breaches. Implementing robust data security measures safeguards sensitive healthcare information and ensures uninterrupted quality care.

Negligent data management can have far-reaching implications, necessitating fortifying data systems, enhancing cybersecurity, and promoting responsibility among healthcare professionals. By upholding stringent data management practices, the healthcare industry can enhance its resilience against potential threats, ensuring patient data's confidentiality, integrity, and availability and creating a safer healthcare landscape.

13.3.4 Workable solutions for data management issues

13.3.4.1 EHRs

EHRs are pivotal in healthcare organizations as they provide a digital repository for storing comprehensive patient details. This secure and accessible platform facilitates seamless data access, significantly mitigating the likelihood of errors and ensuring optimized patient care.

13.3.4.2 Cloud-based data storage

In cloud-based data storage solutions, the vast capacity allows us to store massive volumes of data, catering to a wide array of information types. This cost-effective approach not only provides us with the ability to scale our storage needs seamlessly but also grants easy accessibility to the data.

13.3.4.3 Blockchain technology

Leveraging blockchain technology for data management in healthcare systems offers significant benefits, including improved data traceability, enhanced security, and streamlined sharing capabilities. Nevertheless, it demands thorough attention and careful consideration during the implementation process to ensure its successful integration and optimal functioning within the healthcare ecosystem.

13.4 TELEMEDICINE

Telemedicine refers to the remote medical consultations and treatments using technology, such as video calls and mobile apps, for patient care. Telemedicine proved highly valuable during the COVID-19 pandemic when physical visits to doctors were restricted. Telemedicine, despite not fully replicating in-person visits, emerged as a vital option during the pandemic when direct consultations were unavailable (Prasad et al., 2020). Over time, advancements have bridged the gap, almost matching the experience of face-to-face visits. As a result, telemedicine's progress continues, solidifying its position as an invaluable asset for people's healthcare needs.

13.4.1 Telemedicine applications

Telemedicine's crucial role lies in facilitating patients to discuss medical conditions, receive diagnoses, and obtain prescriptions through secure video conferencing or data transmission, leading to considerable time and resource savings (Haleem et al., 2021). Telemedicine revolutionizes healthcare accessibility by eliminating the need for arduous travel to receive medical care. This innovative approach enhances convenience, making healthcare more reachable and efficient for patients worldwide. Telemedicine encompasses diverse applications, including virtual medical consultations for diagnosis and treatment, remote monitoring and assistance for chronic conditions, psychological support through virtual therapy, medication advice via tele pharmacy, physical therapy conducted via video calls, remote radiology image transmission and interpretation, critical care support in distant locations through tele-ICU, and initial assessments and medical guidance provided through tele triage. With numerous additional applications, telemedicine firmly establishes itself as a fundamental pillar within the healthcare industry of the new era.

13.4.2 Existing telemedicine systems

There is a wide range of telemedicine systems, such as Teladoc, Amwell, Doctor on Demand, MDLIVE, PlushCare, and Doxy.me, Zoom for Healthcare, etc. Some of the famous applications are depicted in Table 13.1 (Elliott & Yopes, 2019).

The number of telemedicine systems continues to grow over time. Telemedicine services are expanding and evolving, providing diverse healthcare solutions. Additional services include remote patient monitoring (RPM), telepsychiatry, tele stroke services, teleophthalmology, telecardiology, teledermatology, telerehabilitation, and more.

Though the applications are readily accessible to the public, the significant risk of data theft in telemedicine emerges due to information being shared via media platforms. Consequently, data privacy becomes a crucial aspect to consider in telemedicine services. Telemedicine services must implement a confidential protocol safeguarding patients' rights to access information and ensuring transparency. Additionally, they should prioritize non-leachable data and regularly delete unnecessary information. Security in data processing becomes paramount due to data transfer, necessitating meticulous measures to preserve content privacy and safety. During the COVID-19

Table 13.1 Famous telemedicine applications

Application	Description
Teladoc	Teladoc is considered one of the largest and main telemedicine companies, offering doctor visits through the virtual platform, mental health services, and skin care centers
Amwell	Amwell is one of the telemedicine systems that provide telehealth solutions for various medical needs, including primary care, specialty care, and mental health services
Doctor on demand	This telemedicine platform interconnects patients with licensed healthcare providers for video consultations, allowing users to seek medical advice and treatment from their homes comfortably
MDlive	This system offers telehealth services for non-emergency medical conditions like mental health counseling and psychiatric care
PlushCare	PlushCare allows patients to schedule video appointments with doctors for various health conditions, and the patient will get personalized treatment plans
Doxy. me	It is a simple, free, and secure telemedicine platform that healthcare providers can use for virtual consultations with their patients through the Doxy app
Zoom for healthcare	As we know, Zoom, a widely used video conferencing tool, also offers Telemedicine services for healthcare providers for secure telemedicine sessions
Telepathology	Telepathology includes transmitting digital pathology images like tissue samples, X-rays, etc. to pathologists for remote examination and diagnosis
Telerehabilitation services	Services are related to mental health conditions, providing remote consultation, counseling, and support to deal with mental health problems
Cerner's Virtual Health solution	Designed to enable healthcare providers to deliver telemedicine services, engage with patients, and manage remote care

pandemic, several data theft incidents were recorded worldwide, including India. For instance, a hacker sold telemedicine data from the Philippines to the dark web, while a UK-based provider faced a cyberattack that exposed patient video consultations. Teladoc Health, a major company, also suffered a cyberattack leading to a data breach of over 25,000 patient records, attributed to weak authentication (Dash, 2020). Such incidents highlight the need for robust security measures in telemedicine to safeguard sensitive medical information.

13.4.3 Device authentication issues and challenges

Device authentication in telemedicine involves using multiple methods to confirm access to an account. Its purpose is to address data theft and hacking concerns by safeguarding patient's private and classified medical information.

However, various challenges and issues must be addressed to ensure a secure data authentication process in telemedicine

Data Security: As Telemedicine includes transferring sensitive information about patients and storing it on servers, it is a main target for cyber-attacks. Therefore, weak authentication leads to data breaches, which severely affect patients and doctors.

Securing Endpoints: Telemedicine relies on various endpoints, such as smartphones, tablets, computers, and medical devices. Each endpoint must be properly authenticated to prevent unauthorized devices from accessing the telemedicine platform.

User Authentication: Properly authenticating healthcare providers, patients, and authorized personnel is crucial. Traditional username/password authentication might need to be revised, and stronger authentication methods like two-factor authentication (2FA) or multifactor authentication (MFA) should be implemented.

Device Diversity: Healthcare providers and patients may use various devices and operating systems. Ensuring compatibility and security across different devices can be challenging.

Mobile Device Security: Many telemedicine interactions occur on mobile devices, which may be more susceptible to loss, theft, or malware. Ensuring the security of these devices and protecting patient data is crucial.

Compliance with Regulations: Telemedicine platforms must adhere to various healthcare regulations and data protection laws. Compliance with these regulations adds complexity to device authentication processes.

User Experience and Efficiency: While security is essential, the device authentication process should not be difficult and must balance security and user experience. Lengthy authentication procedures could disrupt the workflow and hinder the adoption of telemedicine solutions.

Integration with Existing Systems: Integrating secure device authentication with existing EHR systems and other healthcare applications can be challenging, requiring seamless interoperability and data exchange.

Authentication in Emergency Situations: Rapid and reliable device authentication is crucial to ensuring timely access to patient data and appropriate medical care in critical or emergency telemedicine scenarios.

Emerging Technologies and Standards: As telemedicine technology evolves, so do authentication methods. Staying up to date with the latest authentication technologies and industry standards is essential to address emerging security challenges effectively.

13.4.4 Workable solutions for the issues with telemedicine

- *Multifactor Authentication:* Implementing multifactor authentication will increase data security by requiring patients to give multiple identification forms, like a face ID or password before they can access the telemedicine platform.

- *Biometric Authentication:* Fingerprint scanning, face scanning, or passwords will provide the best security to users, especially if they use mobile phones or laptops.
- *Endpoint Security:* Requiring regular updates, strong passwords, and security software on devices can mitigate vulnerabilities and protect against malware and cyberattacks.
- *Two-Way Authentication:* For critical interactions, adopting two-way authentication ensures mutual verification between healthcare providers and patients.
- *Public Key Infrastructure Technology:* Use this technology enhances authentication through digital certificates and encryption to certify the identity of the users.
- *Device Certificates:* Issuing device certificates for authorized devices will ensure that only trusted devices can access the telemedicine virtual platform.
- *Role-based Access Control:* Implementing role-based access control reduces the risk of data breaches by giving users access to the resources and information necessary for their roles.
- *Regulatory Compliance:* Maintaining relevant healthcare regulations and security standards, such as HIPAA or GDPR, helps ensure proper device authentication practices are followed.
- *Identity Verification Services:* Utilizing third-party identity verification services can help authenticate patients remotely, verifying their identity and reducing the risk of fraud.
- *User Education and Training:* Educating users about device security, strong passwords, and the risks of sharing credentials can foster a security-conscious culture.
- *Remote Wipe and Lock:* The ability to remotely wipe or lock devices in case of loss or theft can prevent unauthorized access to sensitive data.
- *Session Timeouts:* Automatically logging users out of the telemedicine platform after an inactivity reduces the risk of unauthorized access if a device is left unattended.
- *Regular Security Audits:* Conducting periodic security audits and vulnerability assessments can identify weaknesses in device authentication and enable continuous improvement.
- *Secure Development Practices:* Implementing secure coding practices during the development of telemedicine platforms can help prevent security vulnerabilities.
- *Data Encryption at Rest:* Encrypting data stored on devices and servers adds a layer of protection against unauthorized access to sensitive information.
- *Logging and Monitoring:* Monitoring user activity, access attempts, and login failures can help detect suspicious behavior and potential security breaches.

- *Continuous Authentication:* This adds an extra layer of security to monitor user behavior throughout the telemedicine session.
- *Secure Network Protocols:* Using secure network protocols such as Transport Layer Security for data transmission helps protect against data interception.

Telemedicine services proved immensely helpful during the pandemic, emerging as a cornerstone in the medical industry. The attachment people developed to it during the crisis led to its continued prominence. Ensuring robust implementation of solutions against data thefts and other issues will foster telemedicine's sustained growth and enhance its value as an asset for future healthcare needs.

13.5 e-HEALTH CLOUDS

The sporadic availability of professional medical and the exorbitant cost of healthcare services has posed a challenge to the conventional healthcare system and emphasized the importance of creating an affordable and worldwide approach to medical administration. The preeminent method is that of cloud computing. This methodology puts forth many advantages and gives room for further upgradation. Despite having numerous advantages, this subject has yet to be adequately examined and explored. Health encompasses much more than simply the integration of medicine and the Internet.

13.5.1 Importance of cloud in e-Health

Hospitals and healthcare institutions must extensively use electronic medical records (EMRs) to save information about patient interactions in the e-health cloud (Zandesh et al., 2019). The goals of cloud computing in the medical field are to improve the quality, dependability, and efficacy of medical services, involve patients and their families, improve care coordination, and more effectively maintain patient confidentiality and protection. Doctors, nurses, and other healthcare professionals can digitally edit and save EHRs on the cloud. The healthcare industry has undergone an impressive transformation in an era of rapid technological advancement. This transition is spearheaded by eHealth Technologies, a groundbreaking company that has revolutionized how healthcare is delivered.

Integrating cloud storage for EHRs can streamline the process of collaborative patient care (Zandesh et al., 2019). Cloud storage simplifies the ability for doctors to access or exchange a patient's medical records collectively (model depicted in Figure 13.3). Traditionally, a patient would have separate sets of medical records at each doctor's office, specialist, or hospital they visited. This created significant challenges for physicians to collaborate on the patient's care. Cloud computing has significantly changed and improved the current

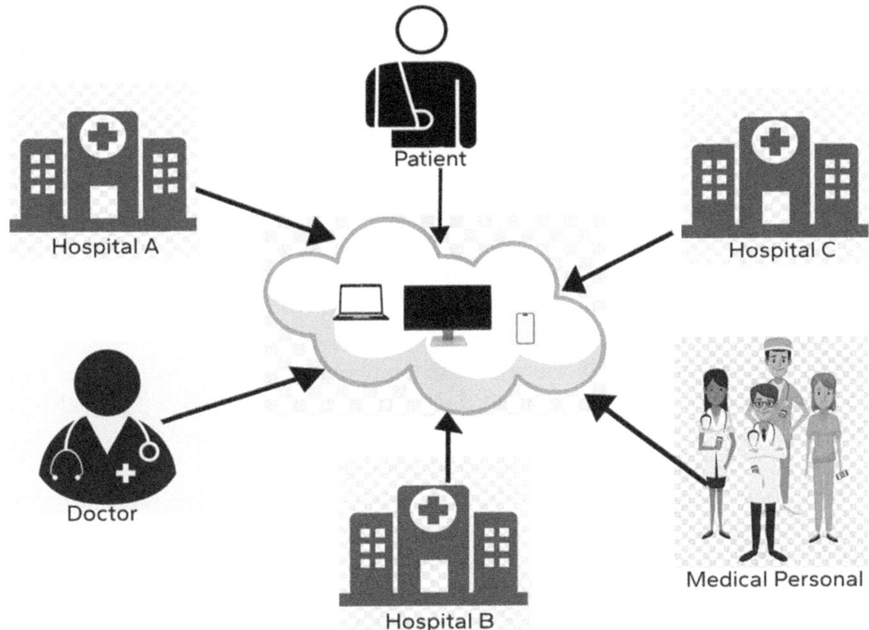

Figure 13.3 Cloud integration with healthcare.

healthcare system, making it an essential component of e-health. Large volumes of EHRs and medical data may be effectively stored and managed using cloud-based solutions, which offer a scalable and secure architecture. The real-time access to patient information made possible by this accessibility enables healthcare practitioners to make decisions that are more efficient and well-informed. It is also feasible to conduct telemedicine and offer treatment to patients in inaccessible or remote places, thanks to the capacity to access patient data remotely via cloud technology. By removing the need for costly on-premises hardware purchases and maintenance, cloud-based technologies allow healthcare companies to save operating expenses and concentrate on enhancing patient care. Additionally, cloud platforms enable seamless data exchange and interoperability between various healthcare systems and institutions, ensuring that pertinent patient information is easily accessible to authorized healthcare providers, improving patient outcomes and care coordination. As healthcare organizations' demands change, cloud-based solutions can simply scale up or scale down to meet those needs. This enables them to keep up with changing technology requirements and handle changes in data volume. This adaptability improves the capacity to utilize potent data analytics tools and machine learning algorithms, enabling healthcare providers and researchers to gain data-driven insights, conduct medical research, and discover patterns or trends that lead to better treatments and healthcare practices. Additionally, cloud computing provides reliable disaster recovery and data backup solutions, assuring the protection and prompt restoration of crucial patient data in the case of hardware failure or natural catastrophes. To secure patient data, reputable cloud service providers go above and beyond what individual healthcare companies can accomplish on their own by implementing stringent security measures and adhering to industry norms and laws, like HIPAA. Overall, modern healthcare systems must include cloud technology into e-health due to its effective data management, accessibility, cost-effectiveness, interoperability, scalability, and affordability. By utilizing cloud-based technologies, healthcare providers may enhance patient care, streamline operations, and promote innovation in the industry's always changing environment.

Suppliers of cloud-based healthcare solutions manage the management, development, and upkeep of cloud data storage services, allowing healthcare providers to decrease their initial expenses and concentrate their efforts on their core competency of delivering patient care.

In the past, doctors who used filing cabinets to save a lot of patient records were in danger of identity theft or other harm. Physical documents are easily lost or stolen; a flood, fire, or other unforeseen disaster may destroy them. The patients' safety was seriously jeopardized by the lack of adequate security measures surrounding these data. Healthcare providers can construct their on-site data storage system when the EMR mandate is implemented (Lee et al., 2020). To ensure the protection of patient information, this would call for hiring software professionals who are knowledgeable in data security. Healthcare providers now have an option in the form of HIPAA-compliant cloud storage services for data storage and protection. These providers offer patient EMR data storage that conforms to statutory mandates for data security and privacy. Every healthcare practitioner now has access to a data storage option that can appropriately safeguard sensitive patient data, thanks to "the cloud." Healthcare providers also have the choice to assign data storage and security to cloud storage services that abide by HIPAA rules (Al-Issa et al., 2019). These services provide patient EMR data storage compliant with regulatory data security and privacy requirements. Every healthcare practitioner now has access to a data storage option that will adequately protect patient privacy, thanks in part to "the cloud."

13.5.2 Available cloud models

13.5.2.1 Public cloud

A public cloud is a type of cloud computing architecture in which cloud resources and services are offered and controlled by outside cloud service providers and made available to the general public online (Tabrizchi & Kuchaki Rafsanjani, 2020). This paradigm allows numerous organizations or people to use the same underlying hardware, software, and infrastructure. Still, it also ensures data privacy and security by conceptually separating their data and applications. Anyone with an Internet connection and the proper login credentials can use the services and resources the public cloud provides. These services are accessible to users 24/7, on any device, from anywhere. Due to their tremendous scalability, public cloud services enable customers to change their computing resources in response to demand quickly. Thanks to this flexibility, organizations can effectively manage a range of workloads without making a big upfront infrastructure investment. Users of public clouds only pay for the resources they use, thanks to the pay-as-you-go concept. This economic strategy avoids significant hardware capital expenditures and enables businesses to optimize their spending based on real usage.

Public cloud service providers manage, maintain, and update the underlying infrastructure, hardware, and software (Rashid & Chaturvedi, 2019) (as depicted in Figure 13.4). This frees up organizations from managing their infrastructure, enabling them to concentrate on their main lines of business. Users may deploy their apps and services closer to their target audience for increased performance and decreased latency, thanks to public cloud providers' data centers that are dispersed across several different geographical areas. Reputable public cloud providers invest significantly in security measures to safeguard data and applications. They also adhere to various compliance standards, making it easier for healthcare organizations to meet regulatory requirements.

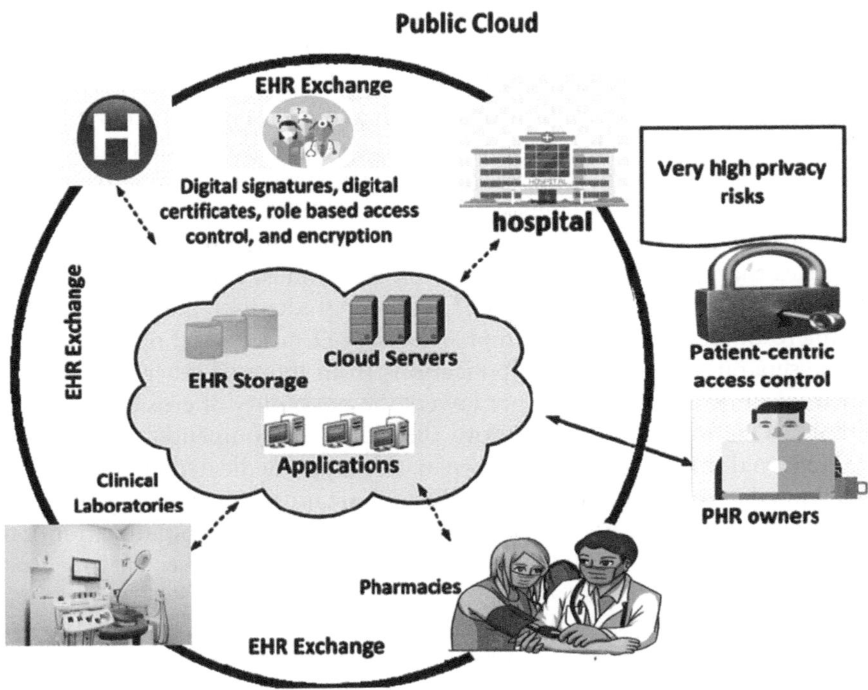

Figure 13.4 Public Cloud service with EHR.

However, regarding e-health applications and data that may involve sensitive patient information, healthcare providers must carefully evaluate the security and compliance measures provided by the public cloud provider. They should also consider data encryption, data residency requirements, and contractual agreements to ensure that the cloud services align with healthcare industry regulations and best practices.

13.5.2.2 Private cloud

A private cloud is a type of cloud computing that gives a single company or entity access to specialized infrastructure and services (Tabrizchi & Kuchaki Rafsanjani, 2020). In contrast to the public cloud, the dedicated cloud is not shared with other businesses. Therefore, all of the hardware, software, and resources are managed and run purely for the benefit of that particular business. Dedicated clouds may be housed on-site (in the company's data centers) or by a different cloud service provider.

Having complete control over their data and apps is one of the main reasons businesses select a dedicated cloud. Thanks to this degree of authority, they may put stringent security controls and alter the cloud environment to meet their unique security needs. A specialized cloud offers better data privacy and compliance for sectors like healthcare, which handle sensitive patient data subject to tight legal standards (e.g., HIPAA). Data breaches and unauthorized access are less likely because the data stays inside the organization's walls (Say & Vasudeva, 2020). Dedicated clouds may be customized to an organization's requirements, enabling them to optimize performance for the workloads and applications that make up their particular business. For firms with particular or specialized computer needs, this flexibility is valuable. Organizations with specialized infrastructure may better manage performance and reduce latency, ensuring that crucial applications and services operate at peak efficiency. Dedicated clouds often have greater upfront expenses than public clouds because businesses must invest in the appropriate infrastructure and technology. They may gradually reduce costs by fine-tuning resource allocation and improving their IT processes. Logical isolation, or the separation of data and applications from those of other businesses, is a feature of dedicated clouds that lowers the possibility of cross-tenant interference. This isolation may improve the cloud environment's dependability, and external influences can be lessened. Although dedicated clouds can provide high data privacy and security, the organization must manage and maintain compliance with industry standards. As a result, the organization must ensure all pertinent compliance requirements are met, and security measures are implemented.

A dedicated cloud is usually more appropriate for major corporations, government agencies, and organizations that need strict control, compliance, and customization over their cloud infrastructure due to the extra complexity and higher expenses involved with putting it up and operating it. An organization may use the benefits of both open and private clouds by combining aspects of both in a hybrid cloud, which enables creating of a unified, flexible, and integrated cloud environment. In a hybrid cloud setup, the open and private clouds operate independently but are linked by networking technology, facilitating data transfer and applications between them. By employing the open cloud for brief spikes in workloads and keeping their private cloud stable for routine operations, hybrid clouds allow businesses to expand their computing resources on demand. This versatility ensures effective resource management and cost reduction. Organizations may choose where to store their data using the hybrid cloud approach based on data sensitivity and regulatory needs. Less sensitive data can be retained in the open cloud for cost-effectiveness and accessibility, while more sensitive data can be housed in the private cloud for increased security. Hybrid clouds provide robust disaster recovery capabilities. In the case of a localized infrastructure breakdown, organizations may copy crucial data and apps from the private cloud to the open cloud, assuring business continuity (K.C. et al., 2019). By keeping sensitive data inside the confines of their private cloud while utilizing the benefits of open cloud services for other non-sensitive processes, a hybrid cloud enables organizations to comply with local rules for sectors with tight data residency and compliance requirements. Organizations may avoid the upfront expenditures of building their private cloud infrastructure and gain from the open cloud's pay-as-you-go approach by using it for nonsensitive applications. A hybrid cloud setup enables businesses to put certain apps and data in the private cloud, closer to the end users or devices, to improve performance. Some applications may need low-latency access to data. Organizations can "burst" into the open cloud to accommodate sudden surges in demand, guaranteeing that service-level agreements can be met without overstuffing their private cloud resources.

Careful planning and integration between the open and private cloud components are necessary to implement a hybrid cloud. To create a seamless and effective hybrid cloud environment, businesses must consider data integration, security precautions, networking, and application compatibility.

The hybrid cloud model gives businesses the flexibility to alter their cloud approach to fit particular business demands, legal regulations, and financial concerns, making it a popular option for many businesses and organizations.

13.5.3 Security issues with e-Health

Protecting patient information and maintaining data security is paramount in e-health and telemedicine. Unauthorized access can lead to identity theft, fraud, and compromised patient care, necessitating robust access controls and encryption protocols. Insider threats from healthcare employees and lost or stolen devices are significant concerns, highlighting the need for training, encryption, and password protection. External cyberattacks like ransomware pose further risks, emphasizing the importance of security updates, vulnerability assessments, and data backup. By addressing these challenges and implementing strong security measures, healthcare organizations can safeguard patient privacy and preserve the integrity of medical data, preventing financial loss and potential harm to patients.

13.5.3.1 Common security vulnerabilities

Presently, the existing Internet security protocols and approaches are inadequate in protecting the susceptibilities that e-health platforms and other related healthcare systems face. From a technical standpoint, healthcare applications are prone to all typical security susceptibilities, including inadequate authentication, cross-site scripting, SQL injection, and cross-site request forgery. Traditional safeguards such as SSL and firewalls have become feeble and essentially useless.

13.5.3.2 Authentication

User verification plays a crucial function in e-health systems to safeguard patient confidentiality and safety. Single-factor verification may be vulnerable to attacks, making it an unsuitable approach for a system that stores delicate information. Healthcare establishments should establish a more efficient multifactor verification.

13.5.3.3 SQL injection

SQL injection remains a persistent and problematic security vulnerability in electronic records databases, including EMR and EHR systems. These databases often utilize SQL as their query language, which makes them vulnerable to SQL injection if proper input data cleansing is not implemented. The user interface, represented by the GUI, interacts with the SQL database through input fields. If these fields lack appropriate data cleansing, attackers can exploit SQL injection to manipulate the database without restraint. Moreover, attackers frequently employ brute force methods on login pages to obtain unauthorized entries when SQL injection protection is inadequate. Implementing adequate security measures is crucial to mitigate the risks associated with these vulnerabilities.

13.5.3.4 Cross-site request forgery

A cross-site request forgery (CSRF) attack poses a significant threat to the security of web applications, including those used in healthcare systems. The attack tricks a logged-on user's browser into sending malicious HTTP requests to a vulnerable web application, unknowingly including the user's session cookie and authentication data. The attacker can exploit the user's browser to take actions on their behalf without their awareness because the application deems the request as valid. This can result in illegal access to patient medical records in the context of e-health systems, jeopardizing their security and privacy.

To reduce this danger and safeguard sensitive patient data, appropriate security measures are essential, such as implementing anti-CSRF tokens.

13.5.3.5 Cross-site scripting

When a web application takes untrusted data and presents it to users without sufficient validation or escaping, Cross-Site Scripting (XSS), a significant security issue, results. Because of this flaw, attackers can insert malicious scripts into the application, which are subsequently run in users' browsers. As a result, hackers can control website content, hijack user sessions, and drive people to dangerous websites. Sensitive patient information is put at risk in the context of healthcare applications because hackers may steal private information or direct users to malicious and fraudulent websites. It is essential to implement strong input validation and output encoding to stop XSS attacks and safeguard both users' data and their privacy.

13.5.4 Workable solutions

Telemedicine and e-health systems share similar prerequisites as the overall IT systems. A few of the prerequisites are delineated beneath.

13.5.4.1 Authentication

Verification is vital in telemedicine and e-health to validate the identities of individuals seeking entry to healthcare information. Insufficient verification can result in intermediary attacks. Different cryptographic algorithms assist in confirming the genuineness of endpoints, combating such assaults. Cybercriminals might focus on healthcare systems to modify or erase medical documents, creating life-threatening hazards. Medical identity theft (MIDT) is another worry where hackers pilfer records for deceptive intentions. Protecting important information, such as medical documents and visuals, necessitates strong verification measures to protect patient data and guarantee confidentiality.

13.5.4.2 Integrity

Integrity is essential in e-health to guarantee data reliability and precision, preventing unauthorized changes. Despite the objective of flawless systems, telemedicine encounters integrity problems such as record alterations. Dealing with these worries is crucial to prevent system breakdowns and potential harm to patients' well-being. HIPAA highlights the importance of implementing measures to protect medical records through verification and integrity techniques. For instance, implementing hash or checksum on data aids in identifying tampering, and if integrity checks are unsuccessful, the e-health application should notify errors and stop the procedure, ensuring data dependability and safeguarding.

13.5.4.3 Confidentiality

To avoid unauthorized access to private information, privacy is essential in e-health. Data breaches are more likely when data is stored in the cloud, which affects patient confidence and the patient–doctor relationship. Additionally, it could make patients less likely to seek medical attention. Confidentiality can be guaranteed through access control and encryption technologies. Data remanence, or the remnants of wiped data, may accidentally result in data security breaches. Inadequate methods for preserving data integrity and secrecy might emerge from failing to consider data persistence in telemedicine. It is essential to address these issues to protect patient data and keep people confident in the e-health system.

13.5.4.4 Availability

To deliver timely medical operations and address crises, especially in the face of malfeasance or security breaches, the e-health system must guarantee accessibility. High accessibility is stressed while the system must continue functioning in the face of hardware failures, DoS assaults, updates, and power outages. The system must guarantee the ongoing use of e-health data and records while keeping security and privacy requirements to comply with the HIPAA statute. In urgent circumstances, putting accessibility first and ensuring system availability improves patient care and safety.

13.5.4.5 Access control

Access control is an important method in e-health to restrict access to patient information to only authorized parties. These authorized parties include those whom third-party patients or healthcare providers have given access privileges. There are several options for solutions to access control issues. ABAC (attribute-based access control) and RBAC (role-based access control) are popular approaches in e-health cloud applications. While RBAC grants rights based on specified roles, focuses on qualities like user characteristics and environmental elements to provide safe and regulated data access in the e-health system.

13.6 CONCLUSION

One of the biggest issues preventing the healthcare sector from quickly adopting e-healthcare technology is security. e-Healthcare's advantages and strengths greatly outweigh its drawbacks and risks. Without a considerable investment in infrastructure and staff, it is getting more and more difficult to achieve security needs. The problem is that consumer convenience and security are inversely related. In other words, customers would feel less secure and so less willing to use the cloud service as security measures get more complex. In this chapter, vast issues and challenges in e-healthcare are identified and the assessed solutions are not comprehensive in nature; rather, they only partially address the security issue. The majority of those solutions only partially solve the issue and fall short of balancing all conflicting security requirements.

REFERENCES

Abbas, A., Alroobaea, R., Krichen, M., Rubaiee, S., Vimal, S., & Almansour, F. M. (2021). Blockchain-assisted secured data management framework for health information analysis based on Internet of Medical Things. *Personal and Ubiquitous Computing.* https://doi.org/10.1007/s00779-021-01583-8

Aceto, G., Persico, V., & Pescapé, A. (2020). Industry 4.0 and health: Internet of things, big data, and cloud computing for healthcare 4.0. *Journal of Industrial Information Integration, 18.* https://doi.org/10.1016/j.jii.2020.100129

Akhila, L., Megha, B. S., Santhoshlal, N. M., Sreelakshmi, B., Pradeep, V., Chalil, A., & Sreehari, K. N. (2021). IoT-enabled Geriatric Health Monitoring System. *Proceedings of the 2nd International Conference on Electronics and Sustainable Communication Systems, ICESC 2021.* IEEE. https://doi.org/10. 1109/ICESC51422.2021.9532781

Al-Issa, Y., Ottom, M. A., & Tamrawi, A. (2019). EHealth cloud security challenges: A survey. *Journal of Healthcare Engineering2019* https://doi.org/10.1155/ 2019/7516035

Al-Mhiqani, M. N., Ahmad, R., Abidin, Z. Z., Yassin, W., Hassan, A., Abdulkareem, K. H., Ali, N. S., & Yunos, Z. (2020). A review of insider threat detection: Classification, machine learning techniques, datasets, open challenges, and recommendations. *Applied Sciences (Switzerland), 10*(15). https://doi.org/10. 3390/app10155208

Altohami, A. B. A., Haron, N. A., Ales@Alias, A. H., & Law, T. H. (2021). Investigating approaches of integrating BIM, IoT, and facility management for renovating existing buildings: A review. *Sustainability (Switzerland), 13*(7). https://doi.org/10.3390/su13073930

Appari, A., & Johnson, M. E. (2010). Information security and privacy in healthcare: Current state of research. *International Journal of Internet and Enterprise Management, 6*(4). https://doi.org/10.1504/ijiem.2010.035624

Brach, C., Keller, D., Hernandez, L. M., Baur, C., Parker, R., Dreyer, B., Schyve, P., Lemerise, A. J., & Schillinger, D. (2012). Ten Attributes of Health Literate Health Care Organizations.National Academy of Sciences

Ching, T. et al. (2018). Opportunities and obstacles for deep learning in biology and medicine. *Journal of the Royal Society Interface, 15*(141). https://doi. org/10.1098/rsif.2017.0387

Dash, S. P. (2020). The impact of IoT in healthcare: Global technological change & the roadmap to a networked architecture in India. *Journal of the Indian Institute of Science, 100*(4). https://doi.org/10.1007/s41745-020-00208-y

Elliott, T., & Yopes, M. C. (2019). Direct-to-consumer telemedicine. *Journal of Allergy and Clinical Immunology: In Practice, 7*(8). https://doi.org/10.1016/j. jaip.2019.06.027

Firouzi, F., Farahani, B., Barzegari, M., & Daneshmand, M. (2022). AI-driven data monetization: The other face of data in IoT-based smart and connected health. *IEEE Internet of Things Journal, 9*(8). https://doi.org/10.1109/JIOT.2020.3027971

Haleem, A., Javaid, M., Singh, R. P., & Suman, R. (2021). Telemedicine for healthcare: Capabilities, features, barriers, and applications. *Sensors International 2* https://doi.org/10.1016/j.sintl.2021.100117

HIPAAJournal. (2017). What is considered PHI under HIPAA? *www.Hipaajournal.Com.*

Hopkins, R. (2004). Information retrieval: A health and biomedical perspective. *Health Information & Libraries Journal, 21*(4). https://doi.org/10.1111/j.1471-1842.2004.00530.x

Iijima, K., Arai, H., Akishita, M., Endo, T., Ogasawara, K., Kashihara, N., Hayashi, Y. K., Yumura, W., Yokode, M., & Ouchi, Y. (2021). Toward the development of a vibrant, super-aged society: The future of medicine and society in Japan. *Geriatrics and Gerontology International, 21*(8). https://doi.org/10.1111/ggi.14201

Koushik Reddy, P., Mohana Vamsi, P., Revanth Kumar, C., Yokesh Kumar, K. V., Jagruth Reddy, P., & Nisha, K. L. (2023). Predictive Analysis from Patient Health Records Using Machine Learning. *2023 4th International Conference for Emerging Technology, INCET 2023*. IEEE. https://doi.org/10.1109/INCET57972.2023.10170221

Lee, H. A., Kung, H. H., Udayasankaran, J. G., Kijsanayotin, B, Marcelo, M. P., Chao, A. B., & Hsu, L. R. (2020). An architecture and management platform for blockchain-based personal health record exchange: Development and usability study. *Journal of Medical Internet Research, 22*(6). https://doi.org/10.2196/16748

Lupton, D. (2017). Digital health now and in the future: Findings from a participatory design stakeholder workshop. *Digital Health, 3*. https://doi.org/10.1177/2055207617740018

Naseer Qureshi, K., Din, S., Jeon, G., & Piccialli, F. (2020). An accurate and dynamic predictive model for a smart m-Health system using machine learning. *Information Sciences, 538*. https://doi.org/10.1016/j.ins.2020.06.025

Nifakos, S., Chandramouli, K., Nikolaou, C. K., Papachristou, P., Koch, S., Panaousis, E., & Bonacina, S. (2021). Influence of human factors on cyber security within healthcare organisations: A systematic review *Sensors, 21*(15 https://doi.org/10.3390/s21155119

Paul, M., Maglaras, L., Ferrag, M. A., & Almomani, I. (2023). Digitization of healthcare sector: A study on privacy and security concerns. *ICT Express*. https://doi.org/10.1016/j.icte.2023.02.007

Pramanik, P. K. D., Upadhyaya, B. K., Pal, S., & Pal, T. (2019). Internet of things, smart sensors, and pervasive systems: Enabling connected and pervasive healthcare. *Healthcare Data Analytics and Management*. https://doi.org/10.1016/B978-0-12-815368-0.00001-4

Prasad, A., Brewster, R., Newman, J. G., & Rajasekaran, K. (2020). Optimizing your telemedicine visit during the COVID-19 pandemic: Practice guidelines for patients with head and neck cancer. *Head and Neck, 42*(6). https://doi.org/10.1002/hed.26197

Rashid, A., & Chaturvedi, A. (2019). Cloud computing characteristics and services A brief review. *International Journal of Computer Sciences and Engineering, 7*(2). https://doi.org/10.26438/ijcse/v7i2.421426

Roy Sarkar, K. (2010). Assessing insider threats to information security using technical, behavioural and organisational measures. *Information Security Technical Report, 15*(3). https://doi.org/10.1016/j.istr.2010.11.002

Say, G. D., & Vasudeva, G. (2020). Learning from digital failures? The effectiveness of firms' divestiture and management turnover responses to data breaches. *Strategy Science, 5*(2). https://doi.org/10.1287/stsc.2020.0106

Shah, S. M., & Khan, R. A. (2020). Secondary use of electronic health record: Opportunities and challenges. *IEEE Access, 8.* https://doi.org/10.1109/ACCESS.2020.3011099

Shuaib, M., Alam, S., Shabbir Alam, M., & Shahnawaz Nasir, M. (2021). WITHDRAWN: Compliance with HIPAA and GDPR in blockchain-based electronic health record. *Materials Today: Proceedings.* https://doi.org/10.1016/j.matpr.2021.03.059

Tabrizchi, H., & Kuchaki Rafsanjani, M. (2020). A survey on security challenges in cloud computing: Issues, threats, and solutions. *Journal of Supercomputing, 76*(12). https://doi.org/10.1007/s11227-020-03213-1

Tao, H., Bhuiyan, M. Z. A., Rahman, M. A., Wang, G., Wang, T., Ahmed, M. M., & Li, J. (2019). Economic perspective analysis of protecting big data security and privacy. *Future Generation Computer Systems, 98.* https://doi.org/10.1016/j.future.2019.03.042

Tarouco, L. M. R., Bertholdo, L. M., Granville, L. Z., Arbiza, L. M. R., Carbone, F., Marotta, M., & De Santanna, J. J. C. (2012). Internet of Things in healthcare: Interoperatibility and security issues. *IEEE International Conference on Communications.* https://doi.org/10.1109/ICC.2012.6364830

Ujjwal, K.C., Garg, S., Hilton, J., Aryal, J., & Forbes-Smith, N. (2019). Cloud computing in natural hazard modeling systems: Current research trends and future directions. *International Journal of Disaster Risk Reduction, 38.* https://doi.org/10.1016/j.ijdrr.2019.101188

Upadhyay, S., & Hu, H. F. (2022). A qualitative analysis of the impact of electronic health records (EHR) on healthcare quality and safety: Clinicians' lived experiences. *Health Services Insights, 15.* https://doi.org/10.1177/11786329211070722

Vilela, P. H., Rodrigues, J., Solic, P. C., Saleem, P., & Furtado, K., V. (2019). Performance evaluation of a Fog-assisted IoT solution for e-Health applications. *Future Generation Computer Systems, 97.* https://doi.org/10.1016/j.future.2019.02.055

Yaqoob, T., Abbas, H., & Atiquzzaman, M. (2019). Security vulnerabilities, attacks, countermeasures, and regulations of networked medical devicesA review. *IEEE Communications Surveys and Tutorials, 21*(4). https://doi.org/10.1109/COMST.2019.2914094

Zaman, S. B., Hossain, N., Ahammed, S., & Ahmed, Z. (2017). Contexts and opportunities of e-health technology in medical care. *Journal of Medical Research and Innovation, 1*(2). https://doi.org/10.15419/jmri.62

Zandesh, Z., Ghazisaeedi, M., Devarakonda, M. V., & Haghighi, M. S. (2019). Legal framework for health cloud: A systematic review. *International Journal of Medical Informatics132.* https://doi.org/10.1016/j.ijmedinf.2019.103953

Harnessing the power of distributed cloud and edge computing for advanced healthcare systems

Sampath Boopathi

14.1 INTRODUCTION

In recent years, the healthcare industry has been witnessing a significant transformation, driven by advancements in technology and the increasing demand for efficient and personalized patient care. One of the key technological advancements that has the potential to revolutionize healthcare systems is the integration of distributed cloud and edge computing. Distributed cloud computing refers to the decentralization of cloud services and infrastructure, allowing them to be located closer to the end users or data sources. On the other hand, edge computing involves processing and analyzing data at or near the source, rather than relying solely on centralized cloud servers. By combining the capabilities of distributed cloud and edge computing, advanced healthcare systems can overcome the limitations of traditional centralized architectures and unlock new possibilities for improved patient care, real-time analytics, and enhanced data security (Saranya & Fatima, 2022). This chapter explores the potential of harnessing the power of distributed cloud and edge computing in the context of advanced healthcare systems. We will discuss the key benefits and challenges associated with these technologies and delve into various use cases and applications within the healthcare domain. Furthermore, we will examine the implications for data privacy and security and explore strategies for effective implementation and adoption. By leveraging distributed cloud and edge computing, healthcare providers can achieve faster and more efficient data processing, enable real-time monitoring and decision-making, enhance patient engagement, and enable remote access to healthcare services. Additionally, these technologies can facilitate the integration of emerging technologies such as artificial intelligence (AI), Internet of Things (IoT), and big data analytics, further amplifying their potential to transform healthcare delivery (Hartmann et al., 2022).

Distributed cloud and edge computing are innovative technologies that have the potential to revolutionize healthcare systems by bringing computation and data processing closer to the point of care. Distributed cloud computing involves the decentralization of cloud services and infrastructure. Instead of relying on a centralized cloud server located in a remote data center, distributed cloud computing brings cloud resources closer to the end users or data sources. This proximity

DOI: 10.1201/9781003487647-14

improves the latency and response time for healthcare applications, enabling faster data processing and real-time analytics. Distributed cloud computing reduces network latency, improves scalability and reliability, and enhances data privacy and compliance by bringing cloud services closer to healthcare facilities or devices. This reduces network latency and enables real-time interactions and data processing (Muhammad et al., 2018; Thota et al., 2018).

Edge computing brings computation closer to the point of care, enabling faster data processing, reducing network bandwidth requirements, and improving privacy and security. Edge computing in healthcare enables real-time analytics and decision-making, reduced network bandwidth, and enhanced data privacy. It enables data to be processed and analyzed locally, minimizing the need for transmitting sensitive patient information. Edge computing in healthcare is used for wearable health-monitoring devices, remote patient monitoring, smart ambulances, and mobile clinics, where real-time data analysis and immediate response are essential. The combination of distributed cloud and edge computing can provide a powerful solution for advanced healthcare systems. Distributed cloud and edge computing enable efficient data processing, seamless collaboration, hybrid deployments, remote diagnostics, real-time image analysis, predictive analytics, and personalized healthcare delivery. Use cases include remote diagnostics, real-time image analysis, predictive analytics, and personalized healthcare delivery (Atieh, 2021; Hao et al., 2022).

While cloud computing advances service platforms and infrastructure, fog and edge computing solutions address data processing challenges. The primary study topics include big data, security, network latency, and energy efficiency. However, big data takes up 63% of publications, whereas energy efficiency only makes up 17%. Researchers can use this knowledge to focus on unexplored areas in their hunt for more potent treatments (Hammad et al., 2023).

Because of the rapid development of the Internet of Biomedical Things, cloud computing, and edge computing, real-time healthcare monitoring is a difficulty in the biomedical sectors. The healthcare sector needs to accurately diagnose illnesses. To solve healthcare concerns, a unique computing architecture blends cloud and edge computing. However, because of the considerable community latency, cloud computing is not recommended for real-time applications (Gautam et al., 2023).

By classifying these technologies into complementary collections and examining the many ways in which they are presented, this study explores how cloud, edge, and fog computing are used in healthcare informatics. It analyses trade-offs between these activities and healthcare requirements and illustrates how well these tasks function in terms of growth using examples from the actual world (Patra & Mohapatra, 2021).

With an emphasis on automated patient monitoring, activity tracking, heart rate measurement, and calorie intake/burn, the chapter examines the integration of fog and cloud computing in IoT-based healthcare systems. The IoT–fog–cloud continuity and research issues in this area are also covered (Kumar et al., 2021).

Due to the vastly expanding and varied nature of medical data, smart healthcare is a crucial issue. To improve productivity and convenience, technologies like IoMT, big data, and cloud computing are being deployed. These technologies do, however, come with certain drawbacks, such as high bandwidth costs, data security risks, and delays. This chapter addresses intelligent healthcare, lists current fixes, and suggests directions for further research (Moujahid et al., 2023).

In an integrated IoT–edge–cloud computing system, the study introduces Health Edge, a smart healthcare framework for type 2 diabetes prediction based on ML. It may be seen through a comparison of random forest and logistic regression that RF predicts diabetes on average more accurately (Liu & Li, 2023).

This chapter provides insights into the potential benefits and challenges of distributed cloud and edge computing in advanced healthcare systems, allowing healthcare organizations to make informed decisions and develop strategies to harness the power of these technologies.

14.1.1 Objectives

- To introduce the reader to the concept of distributed cloud- and edge-enabled networked healthcare systems and highlight their importance in modern healthcare.
- To elucidate why healthcare organizations are increasingly adopting distributed computing architectures. This includes the proliferation of connected devices, IoT, and the demand for real-time data processing.
- To establish a solid conceptual framework by covering key concepts, architectures, and technologies relevant to distributed cloud- and edge-enabled healthcare systems.
- To provide a comprehensive overview of the technologies involved in these systems, such as cloud computing, edge computing, and IoT, and explain how they are integrated into healthcare settings.
- To explore the crucial aspects of distributed data storage and processing, emphasizing the need for efficient data management in healthcare environments.
- To delve into the infrastructure required for edge computing in healthcare, including hardware and software components.
- To discuss the importance of network connectivity in ensuring seamless data transfer and communication within distributed healthcare systems.

14.2 DISTRIBUTED CLOUD COMPUTING

Multi-cloud Architecture: In this architecture, cloud services are distributed across multiple cloud providers. It allows organizations to leverage the strengths and offerings of different cloud providers, ensuring redundancy, scalability, and flexibility (Sen et al., 2015).

Fog Computing: Fog computing refers to a distributed computing infrastructure that extends cloud capabilities to the edge of the network. It brings computing resources and services closer to the edge devices, enabling real-time data processing, low latency, and bandwidth savings.

Mobile Edge Computing (MEC): MEC focuses on bringing cloud computing capabilities to the edge of the mobile network, enabling efficient data processing and content delivery for mobile devices. It reduces network congestion and latency by processing data closer to the end users (Rahamathunnisa et al., 2023).

14.2.1 Characteristics

- *Proximity:* Distributed cloud computing emphasizes the idea of bringing cloud resources closer to the point of use, reducing the distance between the data source and the computing infrastructure. This proximity minimizes network latency and enables real-time data processing and analysis (S. M. & Raj, 2020).
- *Scalability:* Distributed cloud architectures are designed to be highly scalable. By leveraging multiple distributed nodes, resources can be dynamically allocated and scaled up or down based on demand. This ensures efficient resource utilization and responsiveness to changing workload requirements.
- *Fault Tolerance:* Distributed cloud computing introduces redundancy and fault tolerance mechanisms to ensure high availability and reliability. If one node or data center fails, the workload can be seamlessly shifted to other available nodes, minimizing disruptions in service.
- *Data Privacy and Security:* Distributed cloud computing offers improved data privacy and security. Since data can be processed and analyzed closer to the source, there is less need for transmitting sensitive information over the network. This reduces the exposure to potential security threats and ensures compliance with data privacy regulations.
- *Interoperability:* Distributed cloud computing requires interoperability among distributed nodes and services to enable seamless communication and collaboration. Standardized protocols and interfaces are necessary to ensure compatibility and smooth integration of different components within the distributed cloud infrastructure.

14.2.2 Edge computing infrastructure and its role in healthcare

Edge computing infrastructure plays a crucial role in healthcare by bringing computational capabilities and data processing closer to the point of care. It involves deploying edge devices, gateways, and edge servers at or near healthcare facilities, devices, or IoT endpoints (Dave et al., 2021; Muthukumari & Raj, 2020).

Edge Devices: These are the endpoints where data is generated, such as wearable health monitoring devices, medical sensors, or IoT-enabled medical equipment. These devices capture and collect patient health data, vital signs, and other relevant information. Edge devices are equipped with processing power and storage capabilities to perform initial data preprocessing and filtering, reducing the amount of data that needs to be sent to centralized cloud servers.

Edge Gateways: Edge gateways serve as intermediaries between edge devices and cloud services. They provide connectivity, protocol translation, and data aggregation functions. Gateways can collect and preprocess data from multiple edge devices, performing local analytics and filtering before forwarding selected data to the cloud or edge servers. They enhance data security by controlling access to edge devices and enabling encryption and authentication mechanisms.

Edge Servers: Edge servers are deployed at the edge of the network or within healthcare facilities, enabling local data processing and analytics. These servers have higher computational power and storage capacity compared to edge devices, allowing for more complex analysis and decision-making. Edge servers can run applications, algorithms, and ML models for real-time data analysis, anomaly detection, and immediate response.

14.2.3 The role of edge computing infrastructure in healthcare

Role of edge computing infrastructure in healthcare is illustrated in Figure 14.1.

- *Real-time Data Processing:* Edge computing enables real-time data processing at or near the point of care. It allows for immediate analysis of patient data, vital signs, and sensor readings, facilitating timely interventions and decision-making. Real-time data processing is critical for applications like remote patient monitoring, emergency response systems, and telemedicine (Dave et al., 2021).

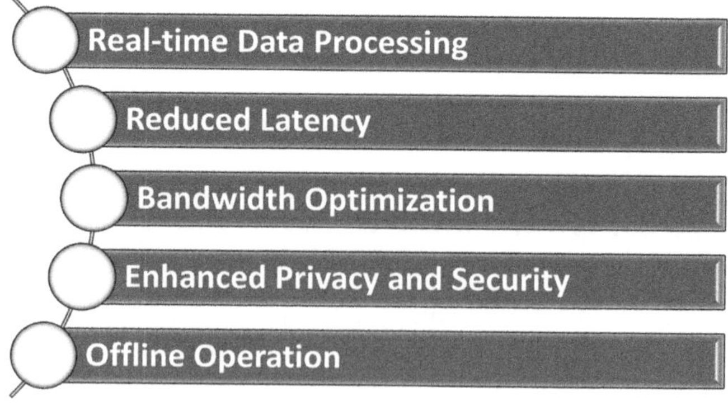

Figure 14.1 Role of edge computing infrastructure in healthcare.

- *Reduced Latency:* By processing data locally, edge computing significantly reduces the latency associated with transmitting data to centralized cloud servers. This is particularly important for applications requiring real-time interactions, such as remote diagnostics, teleconsultations, and surgical assistance. Low latency ensures timely and accurate delivery of information, leading to improved patient outcomes.
- *Bandwidth Optimization:* Edge computing minimizes the need for transmitting large volumes of data over the network. Data preprocessing and filtering at the edge devices or gateways help reduce bandwidth requirements, especially in scenarios where network connectivity is limited or unreliable. This is particularly valuable in remote or resource-constrained areas where internet connectivity may be intermittent (Domakonda et al., 2022).
- *Enhanced Privacy and Security:* Edge computing enhances data privacy and security by processing sensitive patient information locally. Only aggregated or anonymized data may be transmitted to the cloud for further analysis or storage. This approach reduces the risk of data breaches during data transfer, ensuring compliance with privacy regulations like HIPAA (Karthik et al., 2023).
- *Offline Operation:* Edge computing allows certain healthcare applications to continue functioning even when there is limited or no internet connectivity. Edge devices and servers can store and process data locally, ensuring uninterrupted operation and enabling healthcare services in remote or disconnected environments.

14.2.4 Integration of cloud and edge resources in networked healthcare systems

Integrating cloud and edge resources in networked healthcare systems involves a systematic procedure to ensure seamless collaboration and efficient utilization of resources (Andriopoulou et al., 2017; Oueida et al., 2018). The cloud and edge resources in networked healthcare systems are illustrated in Figure 14.2.

Needs Assessment: Begin by identifying the specific requirements and needs of the healthcare system. Consider factors such as data processing speed, latency requirements, scalability, data privacy, and security. Determine the use cases and applications that can benefit from the integration of cloud and edge resources.

Infrastructure Planning: Assess the existing infrastructure and identify the necessary upgrades or additions to support cloud and edge computing. Determine the optimal locations for edge devices, gateways, and edge servers based on the network topology and proximity to healthcare facilities and devices. Consider factors such as power supply, network connectivity, and environmental conditions.

Edge Device Selection: Evaluate different edge devices and select the ones that are best suited for the healthcare system's requirements. Consider factors

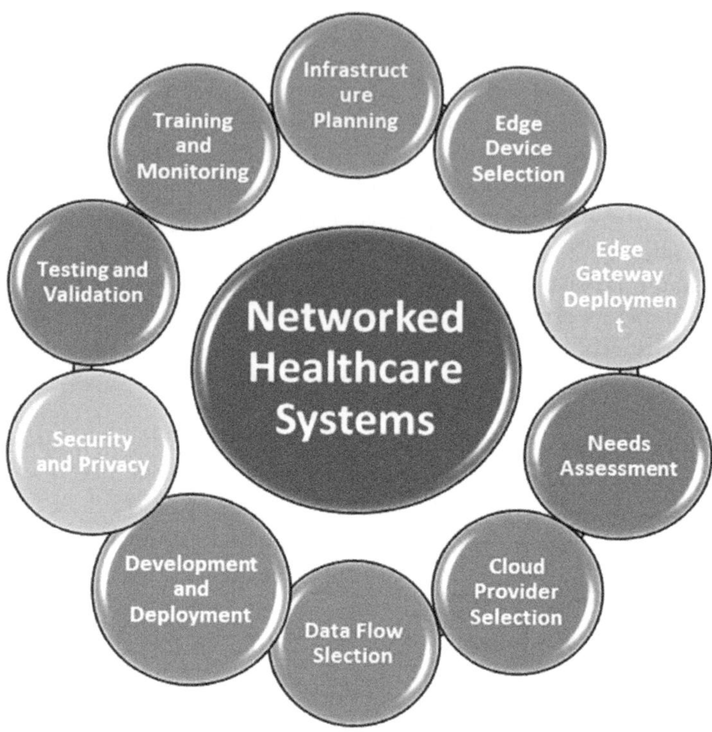

Figure 14.2 The cloud and edge resources in networked healthcare systems.

such as computational capabilities, storage capacity, connectivity options, compatibility with existing systems, and security features. Ensure that the selected edge devices can effectively collect and preprocess the required data.

Edge Gateway Deployment: Deploy edge gateways at suitable locations within the network. These gateways should have the capability to aggregate data from edge devices, perform local analytics, and establish secure connections with cloud resources. Select gateways that support the necessary communication protocols and ensure compatibility with edge devices and cloud services.

Cloud Provider Selection: Choose the cloud provider(s) that align with the healthcare system's requirements. Consider factors such as scalability, reliability, security measures, compliance with data privacy regulations, and integration capabilities with edge resources. Evaluate the available cloud services and features that are needed for the healthcare applications, such as storage, computing power, and analytics tools (Agrawal et al., 2024; Syamala et al., 2023).

Data Flow Design: Design the data flow architecture that integrates cloud and edge resources. Determine which data needs to be processed locally at the edge and which data should be sent to the cloud for further analysis and storage. Define the communication protocols and interfaces between edge devices, gateways, edge servers, and cloud resources to ensure seamless data transmission and interoperability.

Application Development and Deployment: Develop or adapt healthcare applications that leverage both cloud and edge resources. Implement edge algorithms, real-time analytics, and decision-making capabilities at the edge devices and servers. Develop cloud-based components for centralized analytics, long-term storage, and collaboration. Ensure compatibility and smooth integration between edge and cloud components.

Security and Privacy Considerations: Implement robust security measures to protect sensitive healthcare data. Apply encryption techniques, access controls, authentication mechanisms, and data anonymization where necessary. Comply with relevant regulations, such as HIPAA, to ensure data privacy and security. Regularly monitor and update security protocols to mitigate emerging threats.

Testing and Validation: Conduct thorough testing and validation of the integrated system. Verify the performance, scalability, reliability, and interoperability of the cloud and edge components. Test data transmission, latency, response times, and system resilience under different conditions. Perform user acceptance testing to ensure that the integrated system meets the healthcare providers' and patients' needs.

Training and Adoption: Provide training and education to healthcare professionals and staff members on how to effectively use the integrated cloud and edge resources. Ensure they understand the benefits, functionalities, and limitations of the system. Foster a culture of innovation and continuous improvement by encouraging feedback and suggestions for optimizing the use of cloud and edge resources in healthcare operations.

Monitoring and Maintenance: Establish a monitoring and maintenance plan to ensure the ongoing performance and reliability of the integrated system. Monitor edge devices, gateways, edge servers, and cloud resources for issues such as performance degradation, security vulnerabilities, and software updates. Regularly evaluate the system's efficiency and make necessary adjustments to optimize resource utilization.

14.3 DISTRIBUTED DATA STORAGE AND PROCESSING

14.3.1 Scalable and fault-tolerant distributed storage solutions

Scalable and fault-tolerant distributed storage solutions are essential for managing and storing large volumes of healthcare data in distributed cloud and edge environments. The medical data storage and processes are illustrated in Figure 14.3.

- *Replication and Data Distribution:* Distributed storage systems replicate data across multiple nodes or data centers to ensure redundancy and fault tolerance. Replication allows for high availability, as data can

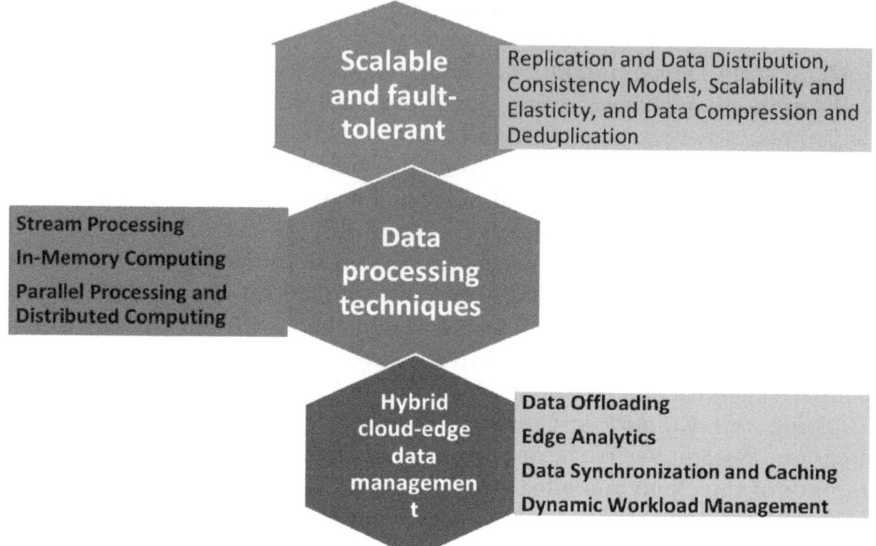

Figure 14.3 Data storage and processing.

be accessed from alternative locations if a node or data center fails. Data distribution techniques, such as sharding or partitioning, enable efficient storage and retrieval of data across distributed nodes (Dhanya et al., 2023).

- *Consistency Models:* Distributed storage systems employ consistency models to ensure data consistency and integrity. Consistency models, such as eventual consistency or strong consistency, define how data updates are propagated and synchronized across distributed nodes. The choice of the consistency model depends on the application require-ments and trade-offs between data consistency and system performance (Ramudu et al., 2023).
- *Scalability and Elasticity:* Distributed storage solutions should be scal-able to handle growing volumes of healthcare data. Horizontal scaling, achieved by adding more nodes to the storage infrastructure, allows for increased storage capacity and improved performance. Elasticity enables automatic scaling based on demand, ensuring efficient resource utilization and cost-effectiveness.
- *Data Compression and Deduplication:* To optimize storage capacity and reduce bandwidth requirements, distributed storage systems often employ data compression and deduplication techniques. Compression algorithms reduce the size of data before storage, minimizing storage space and improving data transfer efficiency. Deduplication eliminates redundant data by storing only unique data segments, further reducing storage requirements.

14.3.2 Data processing techniques for real-time analytics and decision-making

Real-time analytics and decision-making in healthcare require efficient data processing techniques (Jabbar et al., 2020).

- *Stream Processing:* Stream processing techniques enable real-time analysis of continuous data streams generated by healthcare devices and systems. Stream processing platforms, such as Apache Kafka or Apache Flink, can handle high data ingestion rates and perform real-time analytics, pattern detection, and complex event processing. Stream processing allows for immediate insights and timely decision-making.
- *In-memory Computing:* In-memory computing techniques store and process data in the main memory, enabling faster data access and processing compared to traditional disk-based storage systems. In-memory databases and caching mechanisms facilitate real-time analytics by minimizing data retrieval latency. They are particularly suitable for applications requiring low-latency responses, such as real-time patient monitoring or alert systems.
- *Parallel Processing and Distributed Computing:* Distributed data processing frameworks, such as Apache Spark or Apache Hadoop, leverage parallel processing across distributed nodes for large-scale data analytics. These frameworks enable distributed computations, data transformations, and ML algorithms, improving the speed and efficiency of data processing. Distributed computing frameworks are capable of handling big data analytics and can be deployed in both cloud and edge environments.

14.3.3 Hybrid cloud–edge data management strategies

Hybrid cloud–edge data management strategies aim to optimize the utilization of cloud and edge resources for efficient data storage, processing, and management (Dinh et al., 2020).

- *Data Offloading:* Offloading involves transferring data from edge devices or gateways to the cloud for long-term storage and analysis. Data can be offloaded selectively, based on predefined criteria or data policies, to reduce storage requirements at the edge and enable centralized analytics.
- *Edge Analytics:* Edge analytics focuses on processing data locally at the edge devices or gateways, reducing the need for transmitting large volumes of data to the cloud. Edge analytics allows for immediate insights, real-time decision-making, and faster response times. Only relevant aggregated or summarized data may be transmitted to the cloud for further analysis.

- *Data Synchronization and Caching:* Data synchronization mechanisms ensure consistency and coherence between edge and cloud data repositories. Changes made at the edge are synchronized with the cloud, allowing for seamless data access and availability. Caching strategies can be employed to store frequently accessed data locally at the edge, reducing latency and enhancing data retrieval speed.
- *Dynamic Workload Management:* Hybrid cloud–edge environments require dynamic workload management strategies. These strategies involve monitoring the resource utilization, network conditions, and data processing requirements to determine the optimal allocation of tasks between cloud and edge resources. Workload management techniques, such as load balancing and task scheduling, ensure efficient utilization of available resources.

14.4 NETWORK CONNECTIVITY FOR HEALTHCARE SYSTEMS

IoT Technologies and Standards for Healthcare Connectivity: IoT technologies play a crucial role in healthcare connectivity, enabling seamless communication and data exchange between various devices and systems (Egan & Liu, 1995; Management Association, 2016; Zeadally & Bello, 2021).

- *IoT Protocols:* IoT devices in healthcare often utilize communication protocols such as MQTT (Message Queuing Telemetry Transport), CoAP (Constrained Application Protocol), and HTTP (Hypertext Transfer Protocol) for data transmission. These protocols ensure efficient and reliable connectivity between devices and facilitate interoperability in healthcare systems (Reddy et al., 2023).
- *Wireless Connectivity:* IoT devices in healthcare commonly utilize wireless connectivity technologies such as Wi-Fi, Bluetooth, Zigbee, or cellular networks (e.g., 4G/5G). Each technology has its own advantages and trade-offs in terms of range, data rate, power consumption, and deployment flexibility. The selection of wireless connectivity depends on specific use cases and requirements.
- *IoT Standards:* Various standards and frameworks have been developed to ensure interoperability and compatibility among IoT devices and systems in healthcare. Examples include HL7 (Health Level Seven), FHIR (Fast Healthcare Interoperability Resources), and IEEE 11073 (Health Informatics – Personal Health Device Communication). These standards define common data formats, communication protocols, and data exchange models for seamless integration and collaboration.

Wireless Sensor Networks and Their Role in Monitoring Patient Health: Wireless sensor networks (WSNs) are instrumental in monitoring patient health by leveraging small, battery-powered sensors that collect and transmit data wirelessly. WSNs offer the following benefits in healthcare (Koshariya et al., 2023):

- *Remote Monitoring:* WSNs enable continuous remote monitoring of patient health parameters, such as vital signs, activity levels, glucose levels, or ECG readings. Wireless sensors attached to patients or integrated into medical devices capture and transmit data in real time, providing healthcare professionals with up-to-date information for monitoring and diagnosis (Subha et al., 2023).
- *Real-time Alerts and Notifications:* WSNs can be programmed to send real-time alerts and notifications based on predefined thresholds or abnormal readings. Healthcare providers can receive timely notifications regarding critical conditions or emergencies, enabling prompt intervention and improving patient outcomes.
- *Mobility and Flexibility:* WSNs provide mobility and flexibility in healthcare settings. Patients can move freely within a healthcare facility while wearing or carrying wireless sensors. This enables continuous monitoring without restricting their mobility, allowing for a more comfortable patient experience.
- *Data Analytics and Decision Support:* WSNs generate large volumes of data, which can be processed and analyzed using data analytics techniques. These techniques help extract valuable insights, identify patterns, and support clinical decision-making. WSNs combined with analytics enable early detection of deteriorating health conditions and proactive interventions.

Integration of Wearable Devices and Medical Equipment into Networked Systems: The integration of wearable devices and medical equipment into networked systems enhances healthcare connectivity and improves patient care (Anitha et al., 2023; Subha et al., 2023).

- *Wearable Devices:* Wearable devices, such as smartwatches, fitness trackers, or biosensors, collect various health-related data from individuals. These devices can monitor heart rate, sleep patterns, physical activity, and other vital signs. Integration of wearable devices into networked systems allows continuous monitoring of patients' health status and provides valuable data for personalized healthcare, preventive medicine, and remote patient monitoring.
- *Medical Equipment:* Medical equipment, including imaging systems, patient monitors, infusion pumps, and diagnostic devices, can be integrated into networked systems to enable seamless data sharing and collaboration. Integration allows real-time transmission of patient data, imaging results, and device status to electronic health records (EHRs) or clinical decision support systems. It enhances the efficiency of healthcare

workflows, reduces manual data entry errors, and improves communication among healthcare professionals.

- *Interoperability and Data Integration:* Integration of wearable devices and medical equipment requires interoperability standards and interfaces to ensure seamless data integration and exchange. Healthcare systems must support standard communication protocols, such as HL7 or DICOM (Digital Imaging and Communications in Medicine), to enable interoperability between wearable devices, medical equipment, and other healthcare information systems.
- *Data Security and Privacy:* Integration of wearable devices and medical equipment necessitates robust data security and privacy measures. Healthcare systems must implement encryption, access controls, authentication mechanisms, and data anonymization techniques to protect patient data and comply with privacy regulations such as HIPAA (Health Insurance Portability and Accountability Act).

By leveraging IoT technologies, wireless sensor networks, and integrating wearable devices and medical equipment into networked systems, healthcare providers can enhance connectivity, improve patient monitoring, enable personalized healthcare, and facilitate data-driven decision-making.

14.5 SECURITY, PRIVACY, AND REGULATORY CONSIDERATIONS

14.5.1 Data security and privacy challenges in distributed healthcare systems

Distributed healthcare systems pose unique challenges for data security and privacy due to the distributed nature of data storage, processing, and communication (Newaz et al., 2021).

- *Data Breaches and Unauthorized Access:* The distributed nature of healthcare systems increases the risk of data breaches and unauthorized access. Malicious actors may target vulnerable points in the system, such as edge devices, gateways, or cloud infrastructure, to gain unauthorized access to sensitive patient data.
- *Data Integrity and Trustworthiness:* Ensuring the integrity and trustworthiness of healthcare data is crucial. Data may be altered or tampered with during transmission or storage, leading to incorrect diagnoses, treatment errors, or compromised patient safety (Boopathi et al., 2021; Pramila et al., 2023; Sengeni et al., 2023).
- *Insider Threats:* Insider threats refer to security risks posed by individuals within the healthcare organization who have authorized access to

sensitive data. Employees, contractors, or third-party service providers may intentionally or inadvertently misuse or disclose patient data, leading to privacy breaches.

- *Interoperability and Standardization:* Achieving interoperability between different healthcare systems and devices while maintaining data security is a challenge. Integrating diverse systems may introduce vulnerabilities and require careful consideration of security measures.

14.5.2 Secure data transmission and access control mechanisms

To address data security and privacy challenges, distributed healthcare systems should implement secure data transmission and access control mechanisms (Ahouanmenou et al., 2023).

- *Encryption:* Use encryption techniques, such as Transport Layer Security (TLS) or Secure Sockets Layer (SSL), to protect data during transmission. Encryption ensures that data remains confidential and cannot be accessed or understood by unauthorized parties.
- *Access Control:* Implement robust access control mechanisms to regulate data access based on user roles, privileges, and authentication. Multi-factor authentication, strong passwords, and role-based access control (RBAC) can help prevent unauthorized access to sensitive data.
- *Data Segmentation and Isolation:* Segment data based on sensitivity levels and isolate critical data from noncritical data. This approach limits the exposure of sensitive information and reduces the impact of potential breaches.
- *Audit Logs and Monitoring:* Maintain comprehensive audit logs to track data access, modifications, and system activities. Regularly monitor these logs to detect and respond to any suspicious or unauthorized activities promptly.
- *Secure APIs and Interfaces:* Ensure that APIs and interfaces used for data exchange between different components of the distributed system are secure. Implement authentication and authorization mechanisms for API access, and employ secure coding practices to prevent vulnerabilities and API-based attacks.

14.5.3 Compliance with healthcare regulations and standards

Compliance with healthcare regulations and standards is essential to protect patient privacy and ensure the security of healthcare data (Ahmed & Mousa, 2016).

- *HIPAA Compliance:* Adhere to the Health Insurance Portability and Accountability Act (HIPAA) regulations, which provide guidelines for safeguarding protected health information (PHI). Implement necessary administrative, technical, and physical safeguards to protect patient privacy and ensure secure data handling.
- *Data Protection Regulations:* Comply with data protection regulations such as the General Data Protection Regulation (GDPR) or other applicable regional regulations. These regulations govern the collection, storage, processing, and transfer of personal data and impose strict requirements for data security and privacy.
- *Industry Standards:* Adhere to industry-specific standards and best practices for data security and privacy, such as those defined by organizations like HITRUST (Health Information Trust Alliance) or ISO (International Organization for Standardization).
- *Data Retention and Destruction:* Implement policies and procedures for data retention and secure data destruction. Ensure that data is retained only for the necessary duration and securely disposed of when it is no longer required, following proper data destruction protocols.

14.6 APPLICATIONS OF DISTRIBUTED CLOUD AND EDGE COMPUTING IN HEALTHCARE

14.6.1 Remote patient monitoring and telehealth solutions

Distributed cloud and edge computing enable remote patient monitoring and telehealth solutions, providing healthcare services outside of traditional healthcare facilities (Newaz et al., 2021).

- *Remote Monitoring:* Distributed edge devices and sensors allow continuous monitoring of patient vital signs, medication adherence, and activity levels. Real-time data transmission to healthcare providers enables timely intervention and proactive care management (Boopathi, 2023a; Subha et al., 2023).
- *Teleconsultations:* Distributed cloud infrastructure supports secure video conferencing and communication platforms for remote consultations between healthcare providers and patients. Telehealth solutions reduce travel time, improve access to specialized care, and enhance patient convenience.
- *Home Healthcare:* Distributed edge devices and wearable technologies enable patients to receive healthcare services at home. Remote monitoring, medication management, and virtual assistance enhance patient comfort, reduce hospital readmissions, and lower healthcare costs.

14.6.2 Real-time analytics and predictive modeling for healthcare decision support

Distributed cloud and edge computing facilitate real-time analytics and predictive modeling, empowering healthcare providers with data-driven decision support tools (Ahouanmenou et al., 2023).

- *Real-time Health Monitoring:* Distributed edge analytics process streaming patient data to detect anomalies, identify critical events, and trigger alerts for immediate intervention. Real-time analytics enable timely responses to deteriorating health conditions and emergency situations.
- *Predictive Analytics:* By leveraging distributed cloud resources, healthcare systems can perform advanced predictive analytics using ML and AI algorithms. Predictive models analyze patient data, historical records, and population health data to identify disease patterns, predict outcomes, and optimize treatment plans (Boopathi, 2023b; Reddy et al., 2023).
- *Healthcare Resource Optimization:* Distributed analytics platforms optimize resource allocation by analyzing patient demand, bed availability, and staff schedules in real time. This helps healthcare facilities manage capacity, streamline workflows, and ensure efficient resource utilization (Ramudu et al., 2023).

14.6.3 Intelligent healthcare systems and personalized medicine

Distributed cloud and edge computing enable intelligent healthcare systems that leverage AI, ML, and big data analytics to deliver personalized healthcare solutions. Applications include the following:

- *Clinical Decision Support:* Distributed systems provide healthcare professionals with real-time access to patient data, medical literature, and treatment guidelines. AI-powered decision support systems assist in diagnosis, treatment planning, and medication recommendations, enhancing clinical decision-making.
- *Precision Medicine:* Distributed cloud and edge computing support the analysis of genomic data and personalized treatment plans. By integrating patient-specific genetic information with medical records, healthcare providers can tailor treatments and therapies to individual patients, improving efficacy and reducing adverse effects (Pramila et al., 2023).
- *Health Monitoring and Behavior Modification:* Distributed edge devices and AI-powered algorithms monitor patient behavior, lifestyle patterns, and environmental factors to promote healthy habits and preventive care. Intelligent systems provide personalized recommendations for physical activity, nutrition, and lifestyle modifications (Ravisankar et al., 2023).

14.7 CASE STUDIES AND PRACTICAL EXAMPLES

The power of distributed cloud and edge computing for advanced healthcare systems (Boopathi, 2023b; Ramudu et al., 2023; Satav et al., 2024): Case studies are illustrated in Figure 14.4.

14.7.1 Case study I

Remote *Patient Monitoring for Chronic Disease Management* (Boopathi, 2023a; Subha et al., 2023):

- *Implementation:* A distributed cloud- and edge-enabled remote patient monitoring system was implemented to monitor patients with chronic diseases such as diabetes, hypertension, and heart failure.
- *Solution:* Wearable devices and home-based sensors collected patient data, which was processed at the edge for real-time analysis. Critical data was securely transmitted to the cloud for further analysis and storage.
- *Impact:* The system allowed healthcare providers to remotely monitor patient vital signs, medication adherence, and lifestyle factors. Early detection of health deteriorations led to timely interventions, reduced hospital readmissions, and improved patient outcomes (Walker et al., 2019).

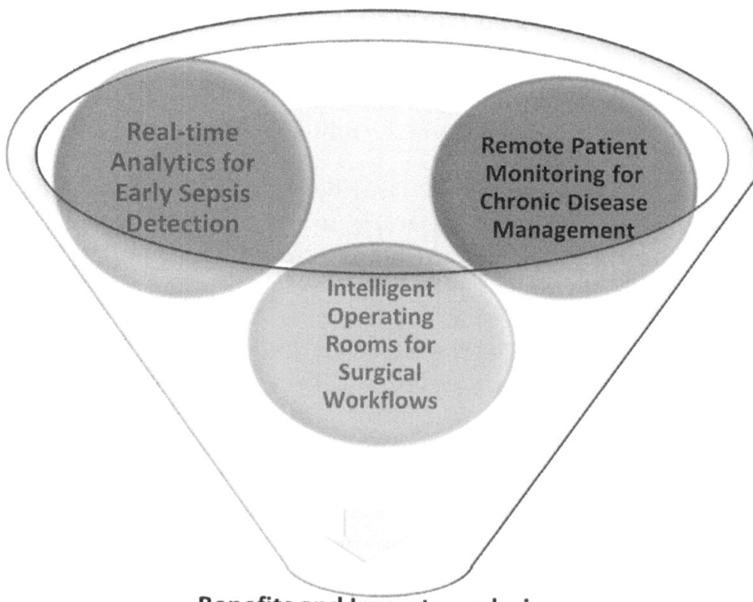

Figure 14.4 Case studies and practical examples.

14.7.2 Case study II

Real-time Analytics for Early Sepsis Detection (Ramudu et al., 2023):

- *Implementation:* A distributed cloud- and edge-enabled healthcare system was implemented in an intensive care unit (ICU) to detect early signs of sepsis, a life-threatening condition (Stanculescu et al., 2014).
- *Solution:* Edge devices collected patient data from monitoring devices and bedside sensors. Real-time analytics at the edge analyzed the data for sepsis indicators, triggering alerts for medical staff.
- *Impact:* The system enabled early detection of sepsis, allowing healthcare providers to intervene promptly. Timely treatment reduced sepsis-related mortality rates, improved patient outcomes, and reduced healthcare costs associated with prolonged ICU stays.

14.7.3 Case study III

Intelligent Operating Rooms for Surgical Workflows (Boopathi, 2023a, 2023b):

- *Implementation:* Distributed cloud and edge computing were utilized to create intelligent operating rooms, enhancing surgical workflows and patient safety.
- *Solution:* Edge devices, such as cameras and sensors, captured real-time surgical data. Edge analytics provided real-time insights, assisting surgeons with image recognition, instrument tracking, and decision support.
- *Impact:* The intelligent operating rooms improved surgical precision, reduced surgical errors, and enhanced patient safety. Surgeons had access to relevant patient data, surgical guidance, and real-time feedback, resulting in improved surgical outcomes.

14.7.4 Benefits and impacts analysis

- Successful implementations require collaboration among stakeholders, including healthcare providers, IT teams, device manufacturers, and regulatory bodies. Ensuring interoperability between different systems, devices, and data formats is crucial (Dave et al., 2021).
- Adequate planning for scalable infrastructure and resource management is essential. Considering the dynamic nature of healthcare demands, distributed systems should be designed to handle increasing data volumes and accommodate future growth.
- Robust data security measures and adherence to privacy regulations are critical. Implementing encryption, access controls, and data anonymization techniques help protect sensitive patient information (Boopathi, 2023b).
- Reliable network connectivity is vital for seamless data transmission between edge devices, cloud infrastructure, and healthcare systems. Redundancy measures should be in place to ensure uninterrupted operations.

- Training healthcare professionals and staff on using distributed cloud- and edge-enabled systems is essential. Change management strategies should be implemented to ensure smooth adoption and integration into existing healthcare workflows.

14.7.5 Impact on patient care, healthcare workflows, and cost-efficiency

- *Improved Patient Care:* Real-time monitoring, predictive analytics, and decision support systems enable early detection of health issues, personalized treatments, and proactive interventions, improving patient outcomes (Abbasi & Younis, 2007).
- *Enhanced Healthcare Workflows:* Seamless integration of data, intelligent systems, and decision support tools streamline healthcare workflows, reducing administrative burdens, minimizing errors, and improving collaboration among healthcare professionals.
- *Cost-efficiency:* Remote monitoring, telehealth solutions, and predictive analytics reduce hospital readmissions, enable early interventions, and optimize resource utilization, resulting in cost-savings for healthcare providers and patients.

14.8 FUTURE DIRECTIONS AND RESEARCH OPPORTUNITIES

- As edge computing capabilities continue to advance, there is an opportunity to explore the integration of AI and ML algorithms directly at the edge devices. This can enable real-time decision-making, predictive analytics, and personalized interventions without relying heavily on cloud resources (Hartmann et al., 2022).
- Federated learning is a distributed ML approach that allows training models across multiple edge devices while keeping data locally. Research can focus on developing privacy-preserving federated learning techniques that enable collaborative model training for healthcare applications, ensuring data security and privacy.
- Investigate novel frameworks and algorithms for efficient collaboration between edge devices and cloud resources. This can optimize resource allocation, data processing, and workload distribution to maximize system performance, scalability, and cost-efficiency.
- Explore techniques for seamless integration and fusion of data from multiple edge devices and cloud resources. This can provide a comprehensive view of patient health data, facilitating more accurate and holistic analysis for healthcare decision-making.
- Develop context-aware and adaptive systems that dynamically adjust to changing healthcare environments, patient conditions, and network

conditions. This can enable personalized and adaptive interventions, treatment plans, and resource allocations based on real-time data and patient-specific needs (Ravisankar et al., 2023; Reddy, Gaurav, et al., 2023; Reddy, Reddy, et al., 2023; Satav et al., 2024).

- Address interoperability challenges and develop standards for seamless integration of distributed healthcare technologies. This includes defining data formats, communication protocols, and security frameworks that allow different systems, devices, and platforms to communicate and exchange data effectively.
- Investigate the ethical, legal, and social implications of distributed healthcare technologies. This includes issues related to data privacy, informed consent, algorithmic bias, and equitable access to healthcare services. Research can focus on developing frameworks and guidelines that ensure responsible and ethical deployment of these technologies (Dave et al., 2021).
- The integration of edge computing and telemedicine technologies to enable real-time, high-quality remote consultations, diagnostics, and treatments. This can enhance access to healthcare services, particularly in remote areas or during emergencies.
- Investigate the role of edge computing in enabling scalable and secure connectivity for healthcare IoT devices. This includes exploring edge-based device management, data aggregation, and intelligent routing to optimize IoT-based healthcare systems.
- Emphasize human-centric design principles to ensure that distributed healthcare systems are user-friendly, intuitive, and accessible to healthcare providers and patients of diverse backgrounds and technological literacy.

14.9 CONCLUSIONS

In conclusion, the adoption of distributed cloud and edge computing in healthcare systems has the potential to revolutionize the way healthcare is delivered, monitored, and managed. Key findings and insights include the following:

- Distributed cloud and edge computing offer scalable and fault-tolerant solutions for healthcare systems, enabling real-time data processing, analysis, and decision-making at the edge of the network.
- Integration of edge computing infrastructure allows for efficient and timely data processing, reducing latency and enabling immediate interventions in healthcare workflows.
- Network connectivity technologies, such as IoT and wireless sensor networks, play a vital role in healthcare connectivity, enabling seamless integration of wearable devices and medical equipment into networked systems.
- Data security, privacy, and regulatory considerations are critical in distributed healthcare systems. Robust security measures, secure data

transmission, and compliance with healthcare regulations and standards are necessary for safeguarding patient data.

- Applications of distributed cloud and edge computing in healthcare include remote patient monitoring, real-time analytics for decision support, and intelligent healthcare systems for personalized medicine, resulting in improved patient outcomes, enhanced care management, and cost-savings.

Implications and potential benefits of distributed cloud- and edge-enabled healthcare systems are significant:

- Real-time monitoring, timely interventions, and personalized healthcare enable better management of chronic diseases, early detection of health deteriorations, and improved patient outcomes.
- Remote patient monitoring, real-time analytics, and decision support systems streamline healthcare workflows, reduce hospital readmissions, and optimize resource allocation.
- Remote patient monitoring and proactive interventions reduce healthcare costs associated with hospital stays, emergency room visits, and complications. Distributed cloud and edge computing enable cost-effective and scalable solutions.

Recommendations for future implementation and research endeavors:

- Implementers should continuously evaluate the performance and impact of distributed cloud- and edge-enabled healthcare systems to identify areas for improvement and implement best practices.
- Foster collaboration between healthcare providers, IT experts, researchers, and policymakers to address the challenges and ethical implications of distributed healthcare technologies effectively.
- Develop standards and protocols that facilitate interoperability among different systems, devices, and platforms, ensuring seamless integration and exchange of healthcare data.
- Address ethical concerns related to data privacy, informed consent, and algorithmic bias. Develop ethical frameworks and guidelines to ensure responsible and equitable deployment of distributed healthcare systems.
- Explore the integration of emerging technologies such as AI, ML, and federated learning to enhance distributed healthcare systems' capabilities, including personalized interventions and real-time decision support.

In conclusion, the integration of distributed cloud and edge computing in healthcare systems offers transformative opportunities to enhance patient care, optimize healthcare workflows, and improve cost-efficiency. By leveraging these technologies and addressing the associated challenges, healthcare systems can evolve toward more patient-centric, proactive, and data-driven models of care delivery.

REFERENCES

Abbasi, A. A., & Younis, M. (2007). A survey on clustering algorithms for wireless sensor networks. *Computer Communications, 30*(14–15), 2826–2841.

Agrawal, A. V., Shashibhushan, G., Pradeep, S., Padhi, S. N., Sugumar, D., & Boopathi, S. (2024). Synergizing Artificial Intelligence, 5G, and Cloud Computing for Efficient Energy Conversion Using Agricultural Waste. In *Practice, Progress, and Proficiency in Sustainability* (pp. 475–497). IGI Global. https://doi.org/10.4018/979-8-3693-1186-8.ch026

Ahmed, I., & Mousa, A. (2016). Security and privacy issues in e-healthcare systems: Towards trusted services. *International Journal of Advanced Computer Science and Applications, 7*(9). https://doi.org/10.14569/IJACSA.2016.070933

Ahouanmenou, S., Van Looy, A., & Poels, G. (2023). Information security and privacy in hospitals: A literature mapping and review of research gaps. *Informatics for Health and Social Care, 48*(1), 30–46. https://doi.org/10.1080/17538157.2022.2049274

Andriopoulou, F., Dagiuklas, T., & Orphanoudakis, T. (2017). Integrating IoT and Fog Computing for Healthcare Service Delivery. In G. Keramidas, N. Voros, & M. Hübner (Eds.), *Components and Services for IoT Platforms* (pp. 213–232). Springer International Publishing. https://doi.org/10.1007/978-3-319-42304-3_11

Anitha, C., Komala, C., Vivekanand, C. V., Lalitha, S., & Boopathi, S. (2023). Artificial intelligence driven security model for Internet of Medical Things (IoMT). 2023 3rd International Conference on Innovative Practices in Technology and Management (ICIPTM) (pp. 1–7). IEEE.

Atieh, A. T. (2021). The next generation cloud technologies: A review on distributed cloud, fog and edge computing and their opportunities and challenges. *ResearchBerg Review of Science and Technology, 1*(1), 1–15.

Boopathi, S. (2023a). Internet of Things–Integrated Remote Patient Monitoring System: Healthcare Application. In *Dynamics of Swarm Intelligence Health Analysis for the Next Generation* (pp. 137–161). IGI Global.

Boopathi, S. (2023b). Securing Healthcare Systems Integrated with IoT: Fundamentals, Applications, and Future Trends. In *Dynamics of Swarm Intelligence Health Analysis for the Next Generation* (pp. 186–209). IGI Global.

Boopathi, S., Gavaskar, T., Dogga, A. D., Mahendran, R. K., Kumar, A., Kathiresan, G., N., V., Ganesan, M., Ishwarya, K. R., Ramana, G. V., & others. (2021). Emergency medicine delivery transportation using unmanned aerial vehicle (Patent Grant).

Dave, R., Seliya, N., & Siddiqui, N. (2021). The benefits of edge computing in healthcare, smart cities, and IoT. *Journal of Computer Sciences and Applications, 9*(1), 23–34. https://doi.org/10.12691/jcsa-9-1-3

Dhanya, D., Kumar, S. S., Thilagavathy, A., Prasad, D., & Boopathi, S. (2023). Data Analytics and Artificial Intelligence in the Circular Economy: Case Studies. In *Intelligent Engineering Applications and Applied Sciences for Sustainability* (pp. 40–58). IGI Global.

Dinh, T. Q., Liang, B., Quek, T. Q. S., & Shin, H. (2020). Online resource procurement and allocation in a hybrid edge-cloud computing system. *IEEE Transactions on Wireless Communications, 19*(3), 2137–2149. https://doi.org/10.1109/TWC.2019.2962795

Domakonda, V. K., Farooq, S., Chinthamreddy, S., Puviarasi, R., Sudhakar, M., & Boopathi, S. (2022). Sustainable Developments of Hybrid Floating Solar Power Plants: Photovoltaic System. In *Human Agro-Energy Optimization for Business and Industry* (pp. 148–167). IGI Global.

Egan, G. F., & Liu, Z.-Q. (1995). Computers and networks in medical and health-care systems. *Computers in Biology and Medicine, 25*(3), 355–365. https://doi.org/10.1016/0010-4825(95)00016-W

Gautam, S., Bhatt, M., & Singh, K. (2023). Advancement In Healthcare By Cloud And Edge Computing. In *Handbook of Research on Artificial Intelligence and Soft Computing Techniques in Personalized Healthcare*. Academic Press.

Hammad, M. M., Banat, S., Baker, Q. B., Al-Refai, M., & Abudhais, B. (2023). A comprehensive study of cloud, fog, and edge computing technologies for health-care IoT systems.

Hao, T., Hwang, K., Zhan, J., Li, Y., & Cao, Y. (2022). Scenario-based AI benchmark evaluation of distributed cloud/edge computing systems. *IEEE Transactions on Computers, 72*, 719–731.

Hartmann, M., Hashmi, U. S., & Imran, A. (2022). Edge computing in smart health care systems: Review, challenges, and research directions. *Transactions on Emerging Telecommunications Technologies, 33*(3), e3710.

Information Resources Management Association. (2016). *Big Data: Concepts, Methodologies, Tools, and Applications*. IGI Global. https://doi.org/10.4018/978-1-4666-9840-6

Jabbar, A., Akhtar, P., & Dani, S. (2020). Real-time big data processing for instanta-neous marketing decisions: A problematization approach. *Industrial Marketing Management, 90*, 558–569. https://doi.org/10.1016/j.indmarman.2019.09.001

Karthik, S., Hemalatha, R., Aruna, R., Deivakani, M., Reddy, R. V. K., & Boopathi, S. (2023). Study on Healthcare Security System-Integrated Internet of Things (IoT). In *Perspectives and Considerations on the Evolution of Smart Systems* (pp. 342–362). IGI Global.

Koshariya, A. K., Kalaiyarasi, D., Jovith, A. A., Sivakami, T., Hasan, D. S., & Boopathi, S. (2023). AI-enabled IoT and WSN-integrated Smart Agriculture System. In *Artificial Intelligence Tools and Technologies for Smart Farming and Agriculture Practices* (pp. 200–218). IGI Global.

Kumar, D., Maurya, A. K., & Baranwal, G. (2021). IoT Services in healthcare indus-try with fog/edge and cloud computing. In *IoT-based Data Analytics for the Healthcare Industry* (pp. 81–103). Elsevier.

Liu, Z., & Li, J. (2023). A trusted computing resources optimal scheduling algo-rithm in industrial internet and healthcare integrating DRL, blockchain and end–edge–cloud. *Journal of Mechanics in Medicine and Biology, 23*(04), 2340056.

Moujahid, F. E., Aouad, S., & Zbakh, M. (2023). Smart healthcare development based on IoMT and edge-cloud computing: A systematic survey. The 3rd International Conference on Artificial Intelligence and Computer Vision (pp. 575–593). Springer.

Muhammad, G., Alhamid, M. F., Alsulaiman, M., & Gupta, B. (2018). Edge computing with cloud for voice disorder assessment and treatment. *IEEE Communications Magazine, 56*(4), 60–65.

Muthukumari, S. M., & Raj, G. D. P. E. (2020). The Pivotal Role of Edge Computing with Machine Learning and Its Impact on Healthcare. In A. Suresh, R. Udendhran, & S. Vimal (Eds.), *Deep Neural Networks for Multimodal Imaging and Biomedical Applications* (pp. 219–236). IGI Global. https://doi.org/10.4018/978-1-7998-3591-2.ch014

Newaz, A. I., Sikder, A. K., Rahman, M. A., & Uluagac, A. S. (2021). A survey on security and privacy issues in modern healthcare systems: Attacks and defenses. *ACM Transactions on Computing for Healthcare, 2*(3), 1–44. https://doi.org/10.1145/3453176

Oueida, S., Kotb, Y., Aloqaily, M., Jararweh, Y., & Baker, T. (2018). An edge com-puting based smart healthcare framework for resource management. *Sensors, 18*(12), 4307. https://doi.org/10.3390/s18124307

Patra, B., & Mohapatra, K. (2021). Cloud, edge and fog computing in healthcare. *Intelligent and Cloud Computing: Proceedings of ICICC 2019*, vol. 2, pp. 553–564.

Pramila, P., Amudha, S., Saravanan, T., Sankar, S. R., Poongothai, E., & Boopathi, S. (2023). Design and Development of Robots for Medical Assistance: An Architectural Approach. In *Contemporary Applications of Data Fusion for Advanced Healthcare Informatics* (pp. 260–282). IGI Global.

Rahamathunnisa, U., Sudhakar, K., Murugan, T. K., Thivaharan, S., Rajkumar, M., & Boopathi, S. (2023). Cloud Computing Principles for Optimizing Robot Task Offloading Processes. In *AI-enabled Social Robotics in Human Care Services* (pp. 188–211). IGI Global.

Ramudu, K., Mohan, V. M., Jyothirmai, D., Prasad, D., Agrawal, R., & Boopathi, S. (2023). Machine Learning and Artificial Intelligence in Disease Prediction: Applications, Challenges, Limitations, Case Studies, and Future Directions. In *Contemporary Applications of Data Fusion for Advanced Healthcare Informatics* (pp. 297–318). IGI Global.

Ravisankar, A., Sampath, B., & Asif, M. M. (2023). Economic Studies on Automobile Management: Working Capital and Investment Analysis. In *Multidisciplinary Approaches to Organizational Governance during Health Crises* (pp. 169–198). IGI Global.

Reddy, M. A., Gaurav, A., Ushasukhanya, S., Rao, V. C. S., Bhattacharya, S., & Boopathi, S. (2023). Bio-medical Wastes Handling Strategies during the COVID-19 Pandemic. In *Multidisciplinary Approaches to Organizational Governance during Health Crises* (pp. 90–111). IGI Global.

Reddy, M. A., Reddy, B. M., Mukund, C., Venneti, K., Preethi, D., & Boopathi, S. (2023). Social Health Protection during the COVID-Pandemic Using IoT. In *The COVID-19 Pandemic and the Digitalization of Diplomacy* (pp. 204–235). IGI Global.

Saranya, S. S., & Fatima, N. S. (2022). Exploration on IoT based Edge Cloud Computing Techniques for Improving the Patient Information Management System. *2022 International Conference on Edge Computing and Applications (ICECAA)* (pp. 1–5). https://doi.org/10.1109/ICECAA55415.2022.9936532

Satav, S. D., Hasan, D. S., Pitchai, R., Mohanaprakash, T. A., Sultanuddin, S. J., & Boopathi, S. (2024). Next Generation of Internet of Things (NGIoT) in Healthcare Systems. In *Practice, Progress, and Proficiency in Sustainability* (pp. 307–330). IGI Global. https://doi.org/10.4018/979-8-3693-1186-8.ch017

Sen, P., Saha, P., & Khatua, S. (2015). A distributed approach towards trusted cloud computing platform. *2015 Applications and Innovations in Mobile Computing (AIMoC)* (pp. 146–151). https://doi.org/10.1109/AIMOC.2015.7083844

Sengeni, D., Padmapriya, G., Imambi, S. S., Suganthi, D., Suri, A., & Boopathi, S. (2023). Biomedical Waste Handling Method Using Artificial Intelligence Techniques. In *Handbook of Research on Safe Disposal Methods of Municipal Solid Wastes for a Sustainable Environment* (pp. 306–323). IGI Global.

Stanculescu, I., Williams, C. K. I., & Freer, Y. (2014). Autoregressive hidden Markov models for the early detection of neonatal sepsis. *IEEE Journal of Biomedical and Health Informatics*, 18(5), 1560–1570. https://doi.org/10.1109/JBHI.2013.2294692

Subha, S., Inbamalar, T., Komala, C., Suresh, L. R., Boopathi, S., & Alaskar, K. (2023). A remote health care monitoring system using Internet of Medical Things (IoMT). In 2023 3rd International Conference on Innovative Practices in Technology and Management (ICIPTM) (pp. 1–6). IEEE.

Syamala, M., Komala, C., Pramila, P., Dash, S., Meenakshi, S., & Boopathi, S. (2023). Machine Learning–integrated IoT-based Smart Home Energy Management System. In *Handbook of Research on Deep Learning Techniques for Cloud-based Industrial IoT* (pp. 219–235). IGI Global.

Thota, C., Sundarasekar, R., Manogaran, G., Varatharajan, R., & Priyan, M. K. (2018). Centralized Fog Computing Security Platform for IoT and Cloud in Healthcare System. In *Fog Computing: Breakthroughs in Research and Practice* (pp. 365–378). IGI Global.

Walker, R. C., Tong, A., Howard, K., & Palmer, S. C. (2019). Patient expectations and experiences of remote monitoring for chronic diseases: Systematic review and thematic synthesis of qualitative studies. *International Journal of Medical Informatics, 124*, 78–85. https://doi.org/10.1016/j.ijmedinf.2019.01.013

Zeadally, S., & Bello, O. (2021). Harnessing the power of Internet of Things based connectivity to improve healthcare. *Internet of Things, 14*, 100074. https://doi.org/10.1016/j.iot.2019.100074

Chapter 15

Securing cloud-based IoT

Exploring the significance of lightweight cryptography for enhanced security

Gaikwad Vidya S., Nilesh P. Sable, Disha S. Wankhede, Vaishali Mishra, Madhuri P. Karnik, Nitin Ambhore, and Akshay Manikjade

15.1 INTRODUCTION TO CLOUD IoT

An Internet of Things (IoT) cloud is a cloud-based platform that enables the deployment and management of IoT devices and applications. It provides a scalable and flexible infrastructure for collecting, storing, processing, and analyzing the data generated by IoT devices in real-time.

An IoT cloud typically includes a range of components such as cloud servers, databases, middleware, and networking components. These components are designed to provide a seamless, end-to-end platform for managing IoT devices and applications. In addition to providing infrastructure and services, an IoT cloud also addresses critical security and privacy concerns related to IoT devices and data. This involves implementing robust security protocols and access controls, as well as ensuring that data is encrypted and protected throughout its life cycle. Overall, an IoT cloud serves as a critical foundation for enabling the full potential of IoT applications across a wide range of industries and use cases.

15.2 NEED OF CLOUD IoT

15.2.1 Storage of data

In a cloud-based IoT architecture, the data generated by IoT sensors is sent to a cloud server, where it is stored and processed. This approach has several advantages, including the ability to handle large volumes of data and the ability to easily scale up or scale down as needed.

In contrast, in an on-premise IoT architecture, the data is stored and processed locally, typically within the same physical location as the sensors. This approach may be preferable in some cases where there are security or privacy concerns, or where low latency is required.

DOI: 10.1201/9781003487647-15

15.2.2 Scalability

The cloud infrastructure is designed to handle large amounts of data and traffic, which makes it ideal for IoT applications that involve a large number of devices generating a significant amount of data.

Cloud IoT platforms can easily handle thousands of devices by providing scalable compute, storage, and networking resources. This allows organizations to quickly add new devices to their IoT network without having to worry about the underlying infrastructure's limitations. Additionally, cloud-based IoT platforms often provide tools and services to manage and monitor large-scale deployments.

Cloud-based IoT is that it enables organizations to easily scale their IoT applications as their needs change over time. For example, if an organization needs to add more devices or increase the amount of data being processed, they can simply allocate more resources in the cloud infrastructure without having to invest in additional hardware.

15.2.3 Flexibility

Cloud IoT offers a high level of flexibility because it allows devices to be added or removed from the system as needed without requiring a complete reconfiguration of the entire system. This flexibility is due to the fact that Cloud IoT platforms typically use a centralized management system to control and monitor the connected devices.

In addition to the ease of adding or removing devices, Cloud IoT also provides the flexibility to customize and configure the system to meet specific business requirements. For example, businesses can choose which devices to connect to the cloud, define how data is collected and analyzed, and specify how alerts and notifications are triggered. This level of flexibility can help businesses to optimize their IoT systems and gain valuable insights from their data.

15.2.4 Maintenance

In Cloud IoT, the responsibility for maintaining the servers and networking equipment lies with the (CSP). The CSP is responsible for ensuring that the infrastructure is secure, up-to-date, and functioning properly. This includes tasks such as updating software, monitoring performance, and resolving any issues that arise.

On the other hand, in other types of IoT architectures, such as on-premise or edge computing, the responsibility for maintenance may fall on the end user. This means that the end user would be responsible for maintaining and updating the hardware and software used in their IoT system, as well as monitoring performance and resolving any issues that arise.

15.2.5 Cost

Cloud-based IoT solutions can be more cost-effective over the long term compared to on-premise solutions that require significant upfront investments in hardware, software, and infrastructure. This is because cloud-based IoT solutions operate on a pay-as-you-go model, where users only pay for the resources they actually consume. This allows users to scale their IoT deployments as needed without incurring unnecessary costs. The cost-benefits of cloud-based IoT solutions make them an attractive option for many organizations looking to deploy IoT at scale.

15.3 FUNCTIONALITY OF CLOUD-BASED IoT

Cloud IoT platforms allow IoT devices to securely and reliably communicate with cloud servers, where the data can be processed, analyzed, and acted upon. This enables a wide range of applications, such as remote monitoring, predictive maintenance, and real-time control. MQTT and HTTP are two commonly used communication protocols for IoT devices to communicate with cloud servers. MQTT is a lightweight messaging protocol that is ideal for low-power, low-bandwidth devices, while HTTP is a more robust protocol that is widely used in web applications. Wired and wireless networks, such as Wi-Fi, Bluetooth, and cellular, can be used to connect IoT devices to the cloud. By integrating IoT devices with other cloud services, such as data analytics, machine learning, and automation, businesses can unlock new insights and efficiencies that were previously not possible (Figure 15.1).

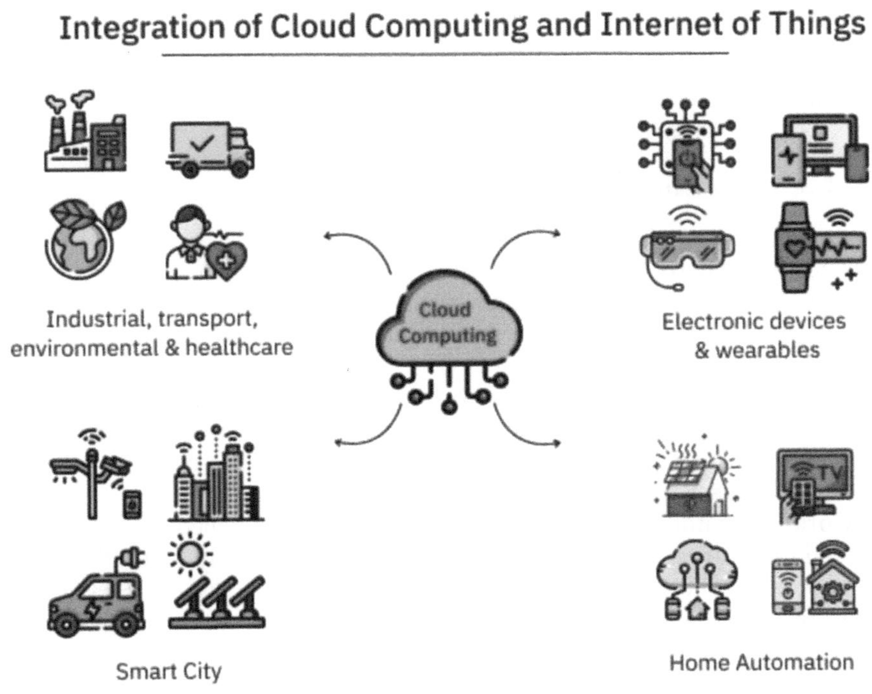

Figure 15.1 Integration of Cloud IoT.

IoT is all about connected devices and sensors that collect data and communicate with each other over the internet. This data can come from a wide range of sources, including sensors, actuators, operating systems, mobile devices, standalone applications, and analytic systems.

15.4 CHALLENGES IN IMPLEMENTING CLOUD IoT

15.4.1 Security and data breaches in Cloud IoT

Security challenges and data breaches are indeed a major concern with cloud computing. If there is a security vulnerability or bug within a cloud computing provider's network, it can potentially allow attackers to gain unauthorized access to not only an individual subscriber's data, but also all other subscribers' data.

15.4.2 Connectivity of internet

In order to access data stored in the cloud, an internet connection is typically required. Many cloud computing providers have measures in place to ensure high availability and minimize the risk of service interruptions. For example, they may have redundant systems in place, such as multiple data centers and network connections, to ensure that there are backup options available if one system goes down.

Some cloud providers offer offline access options, such as local caching or synchronization, which can allow users to continue working with their data even if they are temporarily unable to connect to the cloud.

15.4.3 Data migration

Data migration can be a complex and time-consuming process, especially when dealing with large volumes of data. However, with the help of automation solutions like robotic process automation (RPA) bots and workload automation, businesses can streamline the migration process and minimize the risk of human error.

RPA bots can be programmed to automate repetitive and manual tasks involved in the migration process, such as data extraction, transformation, and loading. They can also perform data validation and reconciliation, ensuring that data is accurately transferred from one system to another.

Workload automation, on the other hand, can help schedule and manage the data migration process, ensuring that it runs smoothly and efficiently. It can automate the movement of data between different systems and applications and provide real-time monitoring and alerts to ensure that the migration is completed on time and with minimal disruptions.

15.4.4 Cost

Setting up an IoT cloud storage infrastructure can be expensive, especially if a company requires a private domain. Private domains provide additional security and control over data, but they come with additional costs, such as purchasing and maintaining dedicated hardware and software and hiring IT personnel to manage the infrastructure.

In addition to the cost of setting up the infrastructure, there are ongoing costs associated with cloud storage, such as data storage fees, network bandwidth fees, and data transfer fees. The cost of these services can vary depending on the cloud provider and the amount of data stored and transferred.

To manage costs associated with IoT cloud storage, companies can implement strategies such as data tiering, which involves storing frequently accessed data on high-performance storage media and less frequently accessed data on lower-cost storage media. They can also optimize their network usage by scheduling data transfers during off-peak hours and compressing data to reduce bandwidth usage.

Overall, while the initial cost of setting up an IoT cloud storage infrastructure can be high, the benefits of cloud storage make it a worthwhile investment for many businesses.

15.4.5 Environment

Cloud computing can help reduce carbon footprint compared to traditional on-premise computing, it is not a completely green platform. Cloud computing still requires significant amounts of energy to power the data centers that host the cloud infrastructure, and this energy is often generated from nonrenewable sources such as coal and natural gas.

To address these environmental concerns, cloud providers are taking steps to increase the use of renewable energy sources to power their data centers. For example, some providers are building new data centers in locations where renewable energy sources such as wind and solar are abundant, while others are investing in renewable energy projects to offset their energy consumption.

In addition to increasing the use of renewable energy, cloud providers are also adopting more energy-efficient technologies and practices to reduce their energy consumption. These include server virtualization, power management, and advanced cooling systems that use less energy than traditional air-conditioning.

15.5 ATTACKS ON CLOUD IoT

15.5.1 Denial of service (DoS)

A DoS attack is a type of cyberattack that attempts to disrupt normal traffic to a targeted system, making it unavailable to users. In the context of Cloud

IoT, DoS attacks can be particularly devastating because they can impact both the cloud infrastructure and the devices connected to it.

There are several types of DoS attacks that can be carried out against Cloud IoT systems:

i. *Distributed Denial of Service (DDoS) Attacks:* In a DDoS attack, multiple devices are used to flood a system with traffic, overwhelming its resources and making it unavailable to users. IoT devices can be particularly vulnerable to DDoS attacks because they often have limited computing power and may not be able to handle large amounts of traffic.

ii. *Application Layer Attacks:* These attacks target the application layer of a system, attempting to overload it with requests or other types of traffic. In Cloud IoT, application layer attacks can target specific applications or services running on the cloud infrastructure or on IoT devices.

iii. *Protocol Attacks:* These attacks exploit weaknesses in the communication protocols used by Cloud IoT systems, causing them to become unresponsive or unavailable. For example, an attacker may flood a system with TCP SYN packets, which can cause it to become overwhelmed and unable to respond to legitimate traffic.

iv. *IoT-specific Attacks:* These attacks exploit vulnerabilities in IoT devices themselves, such as weak passwords or unsecured network connections. An attacker may compromise an IoT device and use it to launch a DoS attack against other devices or the cloud infrastructure.

15.5.2 Jamming attack in Cloud IoT

A jamming attack is a type of cyberattack that attempts to disrupt wireless communications by flooding a network or system with high levels of radio frequency (RF) signals. In the context of Cloud IoT, jamming attacks can be particularly damaging because they can prevent devices from communicating with each other and with the cloud infrastructure, making them unavailable or unresponsive.

In Cloud IoT, jamming attacks can be carried out in a number of ways:

a. *RF Jamming:* An attacker can flood the wireless spectrum used by IoT devices with RF signals, disrupting their ability to communicate with each other and with the cloud infrastructure.

b. *Protocol Jamming:* An attacker can exploit vulnerabilities in the communication protocols used by Cloud IoT systems to disrupt their ability to communicate. For example, an attacker may send invalid or malformed packets to disrupt communications.

c. *DoS Jamming:* An attacker can use jamming techniques to carry out a DoS attack, overwhelming the system with RF signals and making it unavailable to users.

15.5.3 Sybil attack in Cloud IoT

A Sybil attack is a type of cyberattack in which an attacker creates multiple fake identities, or "Sybils," in order to gain control or influence over a network or system. In the context of Cloud IoT, Sybil attacks can be particularly dangerous because they can compromise the integrity and security of the entire system.

In Cloud IoT, Sybil attacks can be carried out in a number of ways:

a. *Device Spoofing:* An attacker can create fake IoT devices that appear to be legitimate, allowing them to gain access to the cloud infrastructure or other IoT devices.
b. *Identity Spoofing:* An attacker can create fake user accounts or device identities, allowing them to gain access to the cloud infrastructure or other IoT devices.
c. *Man-in-the-Middle (MitM) Attacks:* An attacker can intercept and manipulate communication between IoT devices and the cloud infrastructure, allowing them to create fake identities or manipulate data.

To protect against Sybil attacks in Cloud IoT, it's important to implement strong security measures at every level of the system. This may include using strong access controls and authentication measures for IoT devices and cloud infrastructure, monitoring network traffic for unusual activity, and implementing encryption and secure communication protocols to protect data in transit. Additionally, it may be necessary to use techniques such as blockchain or distributed consensus algorithms to validate the identities of IoT devices and prevent Sybil attacks from occurring.

15.5.4 Black hole attack in Cloud IoT

A black hole attack in Cloud IoT refers to a security attack in which an attacker intentionally drops or discards packets or traffic that is being sent to a particular node or service in the Cloud IoT environment. This can lead to a DoS for that particular node or service, disrupting the normal functioning of the IoT network.

To prevent black hole attacks in Cloud IoT, it is important to implement security measures such as secure communication protocols, access control, and intrusion detection systems. Additionally, network administrators can monitor network traffic to detect any anomalies or suspicious activity, which can help identify and prevent black hole attacks.

15.5.5 Wormhole attack in IoT

A wormhole attack in Cloud IoT refers to a security attack in which an attacker creates a tunnel or shortcut in the network, allowing them to capture, modify, or redirect traffic between two points in the network. This can be particularly harmful in Cloud IoT environments, where a large number of devices are connected to a cloud-based infrastructure, and any disruption can lead to serious consequences.

To prevent wormhole attacks in Cloud IoT, it is important to implement security measures such as secure communication protocols, access control, and intrusion detection systems. Additionally, network administrators can deploy mechanisms such as time synchronization, distance estimation, and location verification to detect and prevent wormhole attacks. These mechanisms can help identify any discrepancies in the network, such as time differences or unexpected routing paths, which can be an indication of a wormhole attack.

15.5.6 Ransome attack on Cloud IoT

Cloud ransomware is a type of cyberattack where malicious actors exploit vulnerabilities in cloud services, applications, and infrastructure to gain unauthorized access to data stored in the cloud. Once they have gained access, they proceed to encrypt files and folders, essentially locking the victim out of their own data. To regain access, the attackers demand a ransom payment from the victim, usually in cryptocurrency, in exchange for providing the decryption key.

15.5.7 Brute force attack on Cloud IoT

A brute force attack is indeed a trial-and-error method used by malicious actors to decode sensitive data, primarily through repeated attempts until the correct value is discovered.

Brute force attacks are often automated using scripts or bots, making it possible for attackers to test thousands or even millions of combinations quickly. To defend against these attacks, organizations and individuals often implement security measures such as account lockout policies (temporary lockout after multiple failed login attempts), strong password requirements, multi-factor authentication (MFA), and intrusion detection systems (IDS) that can detect and block repeated failed login attempts.

15.6 EMPHASIS ON LIGHTWEIGHT CRYPTOGRAPHY

Lightweight cryptography refers to a class of cryptographic algorithms that are designed to operate efficiently on resource-constrained devices such as IoT devices, embedded systems, and mobile devices. These devices typically have limited processing power, memory, and energy resources.

Lightweight cryptography algorithms are designed to use less computational power, memory, and energy, while still providing a reasonable level of security.

They achieve this by simplifying the cryptographic primitives, reducing the key size, and limiting the number of rounds of encryption.

Some examples of lightweight cryptography algorithms are as follows:

- *Simon and Speck Block Ciphers:* These are family of lightweight block ciphers with small block sizes and key sizes, optimized for low-power devices.
- *PRESENT:* A lightweight block cipher designed for use in RFID tags, with a small key size and simple round structure.
- *ChaCha20:* A stream cipher designed to be highly efficient on a wide range of platforms, including mobile devices.
- *Curve25519:* A lightweight elliptic curve cryptography (ECC) algorithm that provides a high level of security with a relatively small key size.

In summary, lightweight cryptography algorithms are designed to provide cryptographic security for resource-constrained devices while minimizing the use of computational power, memory, and energy resources.

The comparison of asymmetric and symmetric encryption based on some characteristics is mentioned in Table 15.1.

Table 15.1 Comparison of symmetric and asymmetric cryptography

Characteristic	Symmetric cryptography	Asymmetric cryptography
Keys used	The same secret key is used for both encryption and decryption of the message	Two different keys are used – a public key for encryption and a private key for decryption
Size of key	Smaller than or same plaintext	Larger than or same plaintext
Efficiency in execution	The efficiency of an encryption technique can depend on several factors, such as the size of the plaintext, the encryption algorithm used, and the processing power of the system performing the encryption	It is inefficient since it works for smaller messages
Speed of execution	Faster, because it uses same single key for encryption and decryption	Slower, because it uses two different keys for encryption and decryption
Application	Symmetric encryption uses the same key for both encryption and decryption, which makes it ideal for encrypting and decrypting large volumes of data quickly	Asymmetric encryption can be used to encrypt small amounts of data
Security in Cloud IoT	Less secure, because single key is used	More secure, because two keys are used
Algorithms of security	AES, DES, RC4	Gamal and El, DSA, RSA, Diffie-Hellman, ECC

15.7 WHY LIGHTWEIGHT CRYPTOGRAPHY IS PREFERRED FOR CLOUD IoT?

15.7.1 Resource-constrained devices

Cloud IoT devices often have limited computational power, memory, and energy resources. Therefore, lightweight cryptography algorithms are preferred, as they require less processing power and memory to operate, reducing the energy consumption of the devices.

15.7.2 Communication overhead

Cloud IoT devices are typically connected to the cloud through wireless networks, which have limited bandwidth and high latency. Using lightweight cryptography algorithms reduces the size of the encrypted data, thereby reducing the communication overhead and improving the performance of the wireless network.

15.7.3 Security requirements

Cloud IoT devices need to be secure against various types of attacks, such as eavesdropping, tampering, and data manipulation. Lightweight cryptography algorithms provide a good balance between security and resource usage, making them an ideal choice for Cloud IoT devices.

15.7.4 Cost

Lightweight cryptography algorithms are often less expensive to implement than more complex algorithms, making them a cost-effective solution for Cloud IoT devices.

In summary, lightweight cryptography is preferred for Cloud IoT due to its low resource requirements, reduced communication overhead, security benefits, and cost-effectiveness.

15.8 LIGHTWEIGHT CRYPTOGRAPHIC ALGORITHMS USED IN CLOUD IoT

Table 15.2 shows the list of lightweight cryptographic algorithms used in Cloud IoT.

Table 15.3 shows the literature survey.

This chapter provides valuable insights into how well individuals and organizations understand the risks associated with cloud computing and what steps they are taking to mitigate those risks [11].

The chapter proposes a scheme designed to provide secure key exchange between devices while minimizing computational and storage requirements [12].

Table 15.2 List of lightweight cryptographic algorithms used in Cloud IoT

Sr. No.	Block cipher	Characteristics
1	AES	Key size: 128,192,256 bits Block size: 128 bits No. of rounds: 10,12,14
2	DES	Key size: 64 bits Block size: 64 bits No. of rounds: 16
3	3DES	Key size: 112,118 bits Block size: 64 bits No. of rounds: 48
4	Blowfish	Key size: 32–448 bits Block size: 64 bits No. of rounds: 16
5	Twofish	Key size: 128,192,256 bits Block size: 128 bits No. of rounds: 16
6	Curupira	Key size: 96,144,192 bits Block size: 96 bits No. of rounds: 96,144,192
7	PRESENT	Key size: 80 bits and 128 bits Block size: 128 bits No. of rounds: 32
8	KATAN	Key size: 80 bits Block size: 32,48,64 bits No. of rounds: 256
9	TEA	Key size: 128 bits Block size: 64 bits No. of rounds: 32
10	Humming bird	Key size: 256 bits Block size: 16 bits No. of rounds: 4
11	SIMON	Key size: 64–256 bits Block size: 32–128 bits No. of rounds: 32 to 2
12	TWINE	Key size: 64–256 bits Block size: 32–128 bits No. of rounds: 32 to 2

The chapter reviews the use of machine learning techniques for predicting soil nutrient levels, specifically pH, N, P, and K, in order to improve crop yield [13].

The chapter provides a survey of different approaches for word sense disambiguation (WSD) on unstructured texts and analyzes the gaps in the current literature [14].

Table 15.3 Literature survey

Reference number	IoT device application used in paper	Cryptographic algorithm
[1]	Raspberry PI	ECC: Asymmetric algorithm
[2]	Health domain sensors	ECC, identity-based encryption, and pseudonym-based cryptography techniques were used to ensure a lightweight secure IoT system
[3]	e-Health management system	Lightweight IDS based on J48 algorithm
[4]		ElGamal encryption algorithm, hash function
[5]	IoT gateway and IoT networks	A federated cloud networking security architecture so that it can secure IoT devices and networks
[6]	Baby monitoring camera	Generic cryptography
[7]		Comparative study of various lightweight cryptographic algorithms
[8]	Ehealth platform	Security solutions for IoT: i. Optimized latency for the IoT ii. Optimized energy for the IoT iii. Secure embedded computer architectures
[9]	Smart Space – smart city, light, hospital, meters, data center and gateways, toll collection	Survey of advanced cryptographic algorithms: AES, HEIGHT, TEA, PRESENT, RC5, RSA, ECC
[10]	e-Health	Identity-based cryptography (IBC)

The chapter explores the use of deep learning algorithms to predict the socio-economic status of an area based on satellite images [15].

The chapter proposes a method for storing files securely on the cloud using homomorphic encryption [16].

The chapter explores the use of deep learning algorithms for analyzing glioma brain tumors.

This is an important area of research, as gliomas are a type of brain tumor that can be difficult to diagnose and treat. By using deep learning algorithms to analyze medical images, such as MRI scans, the authors may be able to improve the accuracy of glioma diagnosis and treatment [16].

The chapter explores the use of deep learning algorithms with dynamic architecture for predicting survival outcomes in patients with glioblastoma brain tumors. This is an important area of research, as glioblastoma is a highly aggressive brain tumor with poor prognosis [17].

The chapter explores the use of image processing techniques for identifying plant diseases. This is an important area of research, as plant diseases can have significant economic and environmental impacts, and early detection and treatment is crucial for reducing their spread [18].

The chapter explores the use of tongue images for predicting the health status of internal organs.

This is an interesting area of research, as the tongue has long been used as a diagnostic tool in traditional Chinese medicine, and recent studies have shown that changes in the appearance of the tongue may be indicative of underlying health conditions [19].

The chapter explores the integration of cloud computing and wireless sensor networks. The chapter's approach of using cloud computing systems to analyze and store data collected from wireless sensor networks could provide a valuable tool for a wide range of applications, such as environmental monitoring, smart cities, and industrial control [20].

The chapter's approach of using a trust-based access control scheme that takes into account the policies and trustworthiness of the devices involved could provide a valuable tool for securing the IoT [21].

The chapter's approach of using encryption algorithms for securing data in cloud computing systems is a well-established method for ensuring data confidentiality and integrity.

The chapter provides a comprehensive overview of various encryption algorithms, including symmetric and asymmetric encryption algorithms, and discusses their strengths and weaknesses [22].

The chapter proposes a method for measuring gear parameters automatically using a combination of IoT devices and image processing techniques. This approach can overcome the limitations of traditional gear measurement methods, which are often time-consuming and require specialized equipment [23].

The chapter discusses the concept of publicly verifiable proofs for ensuring the integrity and availability of data stored in cloud storage systems. It introduces cryptographic techniques and protocols to achieve this goal while allowing public audits [24].

The chapter describes the practical implementation of P-PORR, a system designed to verify the integrity of stored and availability of data stored in the cloud storage services. P-PORR aims to provide publicly verifiable proofs, meaning anyone can verify the correctness of data replication and retrievability without relying solely on the CSP [25].

The chapter aims to provide a comprehensive analysis of cloud architecture, its relationship with security, and the state of security assessment tools and methodologies in cloud environments. It highlights the complexity and diversity of cloud security challenges and suggests that a more nuanced approach may be necessary to address security effectively in various cloud frameworks [26].

The primary objective of the proposed system is to create a secure student data portal that safeguards student and faculty information while also ensuring the integrity of examinations. This portal is designed to provide security and efficiency in managing student attendance and the examination process [27].

The chapter likely concludes by emphasizing the importance of addressing security threats in cloud computing environments and highlights the need for continuous research and development of security solutions. It may also suggest that a comprehensive and multilayered approach to security is essential for safeguarding cloud-based resources effectively [28].

The chapter likely explores cryptographic techniques and algorithms that are designed to be lightweight. Lightweight cryptography is a field of study that emphasizes the use of cryptographic primitives and protocols optimized for resource-constrained devices, such as those found in M2M networks. These devices often have limited computational power, memory, and energy resources [29].

The chapter begins by presenting an overview of state-of-the-art fault attacks. Fault attacks are a class of attacks where an adversary deliberately introduces faults or errors into a cryptographic system to exploit vulnerabilities and extract sensitive information. This section likely reviews the latest developments and techniques in fault attacks within the context of cryptographic research [30].

This chapter explores two distributed solutions for lightweight encryption in DABE and compares their performance. It finds that both approaches offer lightweight encryption properties, with secret sharing performing better in certain scenarios, especially with a small number of attributes. The choice between the two approaches may depend on the specific use case and attribute requirements [31].

15.9 CLOUD IoT AUTHENTICATION TECHNIQUES

In Cloud IoT, authentication techniques are used to verify the identity of devices, users, and other entities involved in the communication and data exchange processes. Here are some common authentication techniques used in Cloud IoT:

i. *Password-based Authentication:* This is the most common authentication method, where the user or device is required to provide a password or passphrase to authenticate themselves. However, passwords can be weak and vulnerable to brute-force attacks, so it's recommended to use strong, unique passwords and multi-factor authentication.

ii. *Certificate-based Authentication:* In this method, each device or user is issued a digital certificate that contains a public key and other information. The certificate is signed by a trusted certificate authority (CA) and can be used for authentication purposes.

iii. *Biometric Authentication:* This method uses physical or behavioral characteristics, such as fingerprints, facial recognition, or voice recognition, to authenticate users. Biometric authentication can be more secure than password-based authentication, but it may not be practical for IoT devices with limited processing power.

iv. *Token-based Authentication:* This method involves the use of tokens, such as smart cards or USB keys, to authenticate users or devices. The token contains a unique identifier and a digital signature, which are used to authenticate the device or user.

v. *OAuth Authentication:* OAuth is an open standard for authorization and authentication, commonly used in cloud-based services. In OAuth authentication, the user or device is authenticated using an access token, which is issued by the authorization server and used to access protected resources.

These authentication techniques can be combined to provide a multilayered security approach, depending on the specific requirements and constraints of the IoT deployment. It's important to choose the appropriate authentication technique based on the level of security needed, the resources available on the device, and the usability requirements.

15.10 STATIC AND DYNAMIC AUTHENTICATION FOR CLOUD IoT

Static authentication and dynamic authentication are two different approaches to verify the identity of an IoT device trying to access a system or resource.

Static authentication is a method of authentication that uses fixed or unchanging credentials, such as a username and password, to verify the identity of the IoT device. Once the credentials have been verified, the IoT device is granted access to the system or resource. Static authentication is widely used because it is simple to implement and manage, but it is also vulnerable to various security threats, such as password cracking and phishing attacks.

Dynamic authentication, on the other hand, is a method of authentication that uses a combination of various factors to verify the identity of the user. These factors may include biometric data (such as fingerprints or facial recognition), one-time passwords, and security tokens. Dynamic authentication is considered more secure than static authentication because it requires the user to provide multiple pieces of information, making it much harder for an attacker to impersonate the user.

Here are some key differences between static and dynamic authentication:

i. *Security:* Dynamic authentication is considered more secure than static authentication because it requires multiple factors to verify the identity of the user. Static authentication, on the other hand, can be vulnerable to various security threats, such as password cracking and phishing attacks.

ii. *Complexity:* Dynamic authentication is typically more complex than static authentication because it requires multiple factors to be used. Static authentication, on the other hand, is simple to implement and manage.

iii. *Usability:* Static authentication is generally more user-friendly than dynamic authentication because it only requires the user to remember one or two credentials. Dynamic authentication, on the other hand, may require the user to carry a security token or use a biometric scanner, which can be inconvenient.

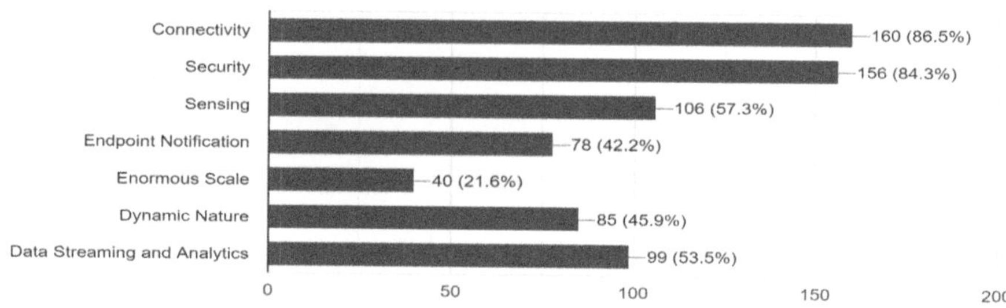

Figure 15.2 Factors to be considered for developing IoT solutions.

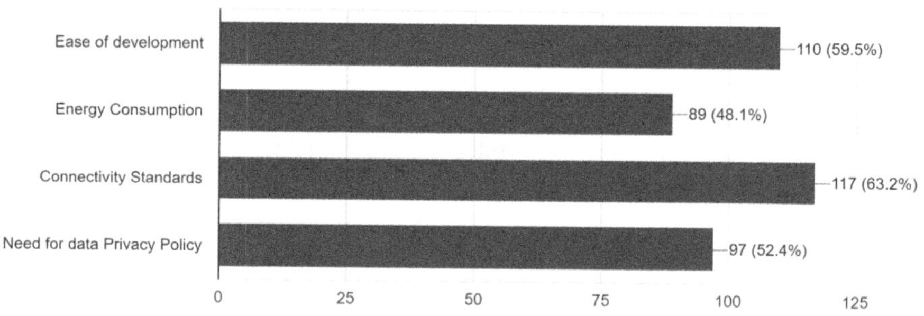

Figure 15.3 Impact of speeding up the benefits of IoT.

Our survey for Cloud IoT shows that connectivity, security, and sensing are important factors to be considered for developing IoT solutions (Figure 15.2).

Figure 15.3 shows survey of greatest impact in speeding up the benefits of the IoT

Figure 15.4 highlights the programming languages used in Cloud IoT

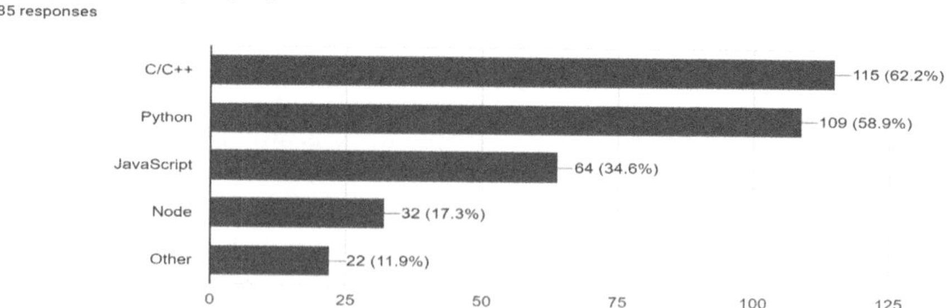

Figure 15.4 Programming language used in Cloud IoT.

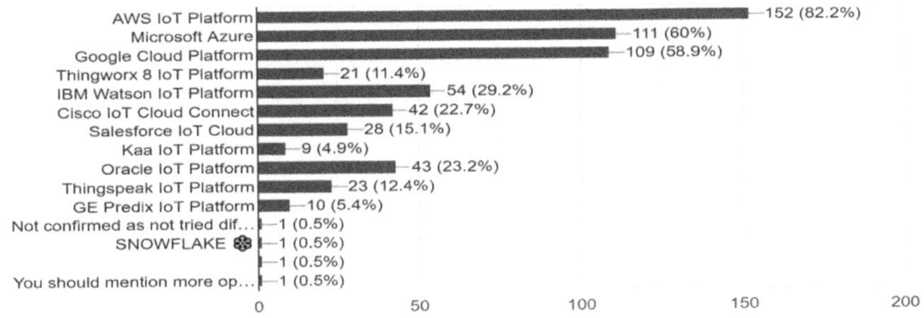

Figure 15.5 CSP in Cloud IoT.

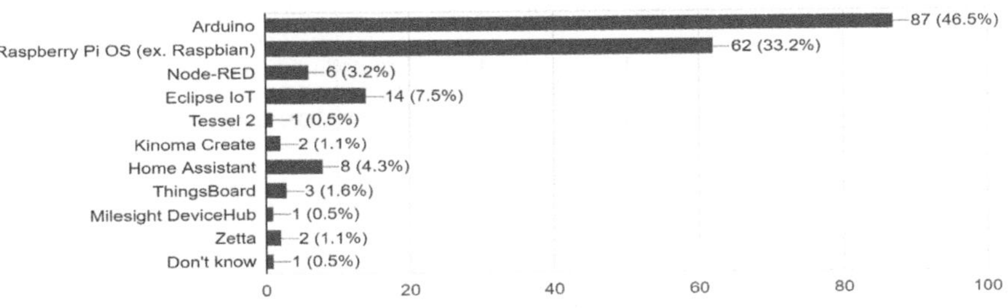

Figure 15.6 IoT tools and platforms.

Figure 15.5 displays the CSP for IoT solution.

Figure 15.6 displays the frequently used IoT tools and platforms for IoT development and developers.

Figure 15.7 shows the most commonly type of sensor technology used.

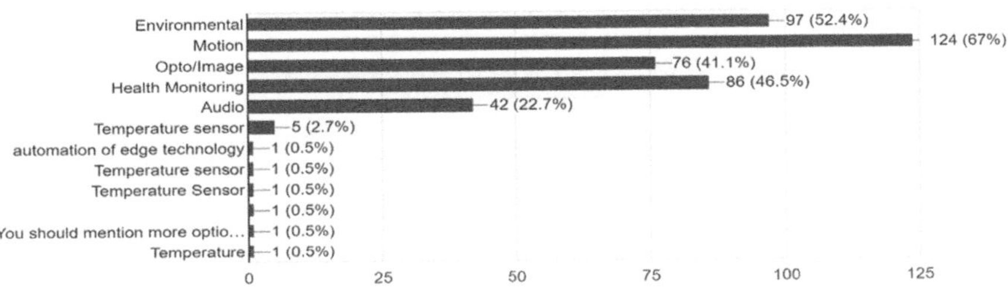

Figure 15.7 IoT tools and platforms.

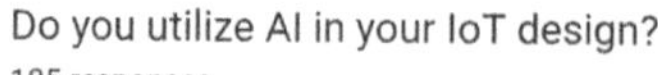
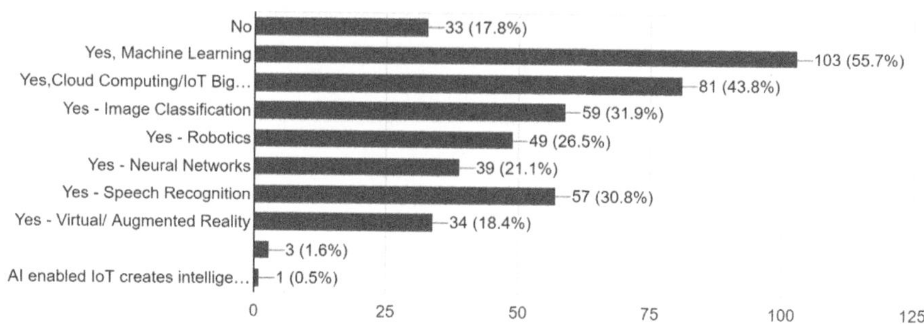

Figure 15.8 AI utilization in IoT design.

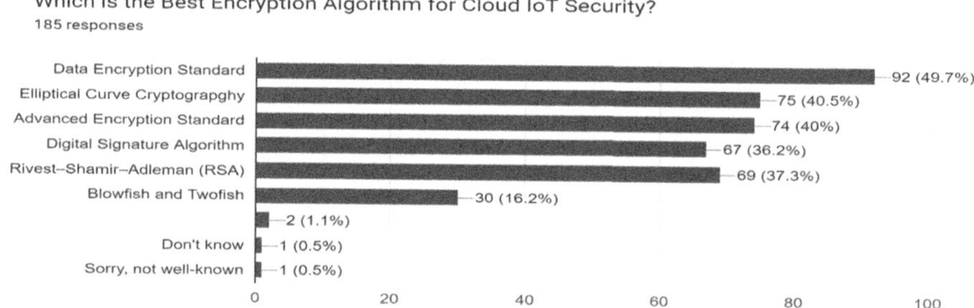

Figure 15.9 Best encryption algorithm for Cloud IoT.

Figure 15.8 shows how AI is utilized in IoT design.

Figure 15.9 shows best encryption algorithm for Cloud IoT security.

Figure 15.10 displays the challenges faced by people for implementing lightweight cryptography in resource-constrained IoT devices.

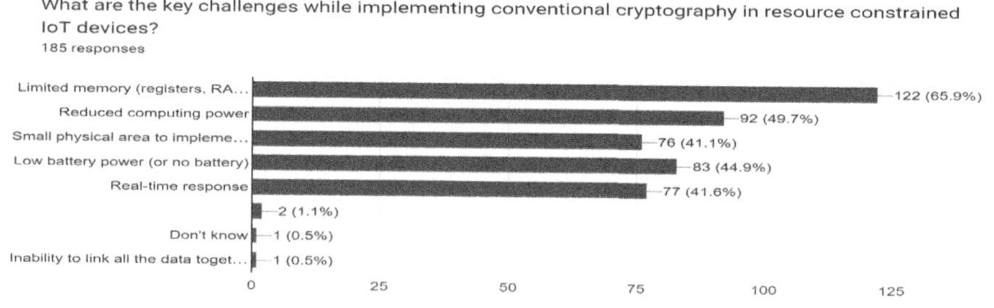

Figure 15.10 Challenges in implementing conventional cryptography in resource-constrained IoT devices.

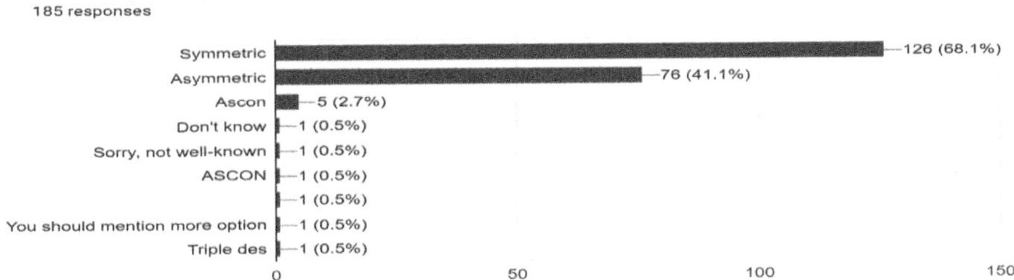

Figure 15.11 Cryptographic algorithms more secure for Cloud IoT.

Figure 15.11 displays the survey for more secure cryptographic algorithm for Cloud IoT.

15.11 CONCLUSION

Cloud-based IoT has emerged as a powerful technology for connecting physical devices and systems to the cloud. It offers many benefits, such as scalability, flexibility, and cost-effectiveness. However, there are also several challenges in implementing Cloud IoT, such as security, privacy, and interoperability. Attacks on Cloud IoT systems are becoming more frequent, making it crucial to emphasize the use of lightweight cryptography in securing these systems. Lightweight cryptography is preferred for Cloud IoT because it offers high security with low computational and power resources. Therefore, the above survey states that organizations implementing Cloud IoT must prioritize security and invest in lightweight cryptography to mitigate potential risks. Overall, Cloud IoT has great potential, but careful consideration must be given to security and privacy concerns to ensure its success in the long run. Lightweight cryptography plays a crucial role in securing cloud-based IoT systems. These systems frequently use devices with finite resources, including processing speed, memory, and energy. The chapter highlights the comparison of symmetric and asymmetric cryptography. It also focuses on Cloud IoT authentication techniques, by considering the differences in static and dynamic authentication. At the last, we conclude by the survey for Cloud IoT by considering the factors like connectivity, security, and sensing as important factors to be considered for developing IoT solutions.

REFERENCES

1. Zhou, L., Su, C., Yeh, K.-H. (2019). A Lightweight Cryptographic Protocol with Certificateless Signature for the Internet of Things. ACM Transactions on Embedded Computing Systems, vol. 18, No. 3, pp. 1–10. https://doi.org/10.1145/3301306

2. Bakhtiar, F. A., Pramukantoro, E. S., Nihri, H. (2019). "A Lightweight IDS Based on J48 Algorithm for Detecting DoS Attacks on IoT Middleware," 2019 IEEE 1st Global Conference on Life Sciences and Technologies (LifeTech), Osaka, Japan, pp. 41–42. doi: 10.1109/LifeTech.2019.8884057

3. Bala, D. Q., Maity, S., Jena, S. K. (2017). "A lightweight remote user authentication protocol for smart E-health networking environment," 2017 International Conference on I-SMAC (IoT in Social, Mobile, Analytics and Cloud) (I-SMAC), Palladam, India, pp. 10–15. doi: 10.1109/I-SMAC.2017.8058330

4. Choudhury, T., Gupta, A., Pradhan, S., Kumar, P., Rathore, Y. S. (2017). "Privacy and Security of Cloud-based Internet of Things (IoT)," 2017 3rd International Conference on Computational Intelligence and Networks (CINE), Odisha, India, pp. 40–45. doi: 10.1109/CINE.2017.28

5. Massonet, P., et al. (2017). "Security in Lightweight Network Function Virtualisation for Federated Cloud and IoT," 2017 IEEE 5th International Conference on Future Internet of Things and Cloud (FiCloud), Prague, Czech Republic, pp. 148–154. doi: 10.1109/FiCloud.2017.43

6. Patil, A., Banerjee, S., Borkar, G. (2002). A Survey on Securing Smart Gadgets Using Lightweight Cryptography. In: Proceedings of International Conference on Wireless Communication. https://doi.org/10.1007/978-981-15-1002-1_51

7. Pallavi, K. N., Kumar, V. R., Srikrishna, S. (2020). "Comparative Study of Various Lightweight Cryptographic Algorithms for Data Security between IoT and Cloud," 2020 5th International Conference on Communication and Electronics Systems (ICCES), Coimbatore, India, pp. 589–593. doi: 10.1109/ICCES48766.2020.9137984

8. Schaumont, P. (2017). "Security in the Internet of Things: A Challenge of Scale," Design, Automation & Test in Europe Conference & Exhibition (DATE), 2017, Lausanne, Switzerland, 2017, pp. 674–679. doi: 10.23919/DATE.2017.7927075

9. Singh, S., Sharma, P. K., Moon, S. Y., et al. (2017). Advanced Lightweight Encryption Algorithms for IoT Devices: Survey, Challenges and Solutions. Journal of Ambient Intelligence and Humanized Computing, vol. 15, pp. 1625–1642. https://doi.org/10.1007/s12652-017-0494-4

10. Boussada, R., Elhdhili, M. E., Saidane, L. A. (2017). "Privacy Preserving Solution for Internet of Things with Application to eHealth," 2017 IEEE/ACS 14th International Conference on Computer Systems and Applications (AICCSA), Hammamet, Tunisia, pp. 384–391. doi: 10.1109/AICCSA.2017.75

11. Prasad, Gudapati, Gaikwad, Vidya. (2018). A Survey on User Awareness of Cloud Security. International Journal of Engineering and Technology(UAE), vol. 7, pp. 131–135. doi: 10.14419/ijet.v7i2.32.15386

12. Gudapati, S.P., Gaikwad, V. (2021). Light-Weight Key Establishment Mechanism for Secure Communication between IoT Devices and Cloud. In: Satapathy, S., Bhateja, V., Janakiramaiah, B., Chen, Y. W. (eds) Intelligent System Design: Advances in Intelligent Systems and Computing, vol 1171. Springer, Singapore. https://doi.org/10.1007/978-981-15-5400-1_55

13. Wankhede, D.S. (2021). Analysis and Prediction of Soil Nutrients pH, N, P, K for Crop Using Machine Learning Classifier: A Review. In: Raj J. S. (ed.) International Conference on Mobile Computing and Sustainable Informatics. ICMCSI 2020. EAI/Springer Innovations in Communication and Computing. Springer, Cham. https://doi.org/10.1007/978-3-030-49795-8_10

14. Bhattacharjee, K., et al. (2020). "Survey and Gap Analysis of Word Sense Disambiguation Approaches on Unstructured Texts," 2020 International Conference on Electronics and Sustainable Communication Systems (ICESC), pp. 323–327. doi: 10.1109/ICESC48915.2020.9155947

15. Shetty, A., Thorat, A., Singru, R., Shigawan, M., Gaikwad, V. (2020). "Predict Socio-Economic Status of an Area from Satellite Image Using Deep Learning," 2020 International Conference on Electronics and Sustainable Communication Systems (ICESC), pp. 177–182. doi: 10.1109/ICESC48915.2020.9155696

16. Wankhede, D. S., Rangasamy, S. (2021). Review on Deep Learning Approach for Brain Tumor Glioma Analysis. Journal of Information Technology in Industry, vol. 9, No. 1, pp. 395–408. https://doi.org/10.17762/itii.v9i1.144

17. Wankhede, D. S., Selvarani, R. (2022). Dynamic Architecture Based Deep Learning Approach for Glioblastoma Brain Tumor Survival Prediction. Neuroscience Informatics, vol. 2, No. 4, p. 100062. https://doi.org/10.1016/j.neuri.2022.100062.

18. Wankhede, D.S., Gamot, A., Motwani, K., Kayande, S., Agrawal, V., Chinchulkar, C. (2022). A Study on Identification of Plant Diseases Using Image Processing. In: Pandian, A. P., Fernando, X., Haoxiang W. (eds) Computer Networks, Big Data and IoT. Lecture Notes on Data Engineering and Communications Technologies, vol. 117. Springer, Singapore. https://doi.org/10.1007/978-981-19-0898-9_36

19. Wankhede, D. S., Pandit, S., Metangale, N., Patre, R., Kulkarni, S., Minaj, K. A. (2022). Survey on Analyzing Tongue Images to Predict the Organ Affected. In: Abraham, A., et al. Hybrid Intelligent Systems. HIS 2021. Lecture Notes in Networks and Systems, vol. 420. Springer, Cham. https://doi.org/10.1007/978-3-030-96305-7_56

20. Dikondkar, S., Mishra, V., Gaikwad, V. (2014). Cloud Computing System Based on Wireless Sensor Network. ERCICA 2014. Elsevier.

21. Railkar, P. N., Mahalle, P. N., Shinde, G. R., & Sable, N. P. (2022). Policy-aware Distributed and Dynamic Trust Based Access Control Scheme for Internet of Things. International Journal on Recent and Innovation Trends in Computing and Communication, vol. 10, pp. 155–165.

22. Sable, N., Gadekar, D. (2019). Exploring Data Security Scheme into Cloud Using Encryption Algorithms. International Journal of Recent Technology and Engineering, vol. 8, pp. 2277–3878. doi: 10.35940/ijrte.B2504.078219

23. Malpure, H., Maniyar, C., Shinde, S., Pingat, A., Mishra, V. (2020). Automatic Measurement of Gear Parameters Using IoT & Image Processing. International Journal of Creative Research Thoughts, vol. 8, pp. 2988–2992.

24. Gritti, C. (2020). Publicly Verifiable Proofs of Data Replication and Retrievability for Cloud Storage. *2020 International Computer Symposium (ICS)*, Tainan, Taiwan, pp. 431–436. doi: 10.1109/ICS51289.2020.00091

25. Li, H. (2022). Implementation and Evaluation of Publicly Verifiable Proofs of Data Replication and Retrievability for Cloud Storage.

26. Jovanovic, A., Milic, P. (2020). Towards Creating Methodology for Security Assessment of Cloud Containers: An Overview of Available Tools.

27. Nalajala, S., Thanvi, G.N., Kiran, D.K., Pranitha, B., Rachana, T., Laxmi, N. (2022). Secured Student Portal Using Cloud. In: Jeena Jacob, I., Gonzalez-Longatt, F.M., Kolandapalayam Shanmugam, S., Izonin, I. (eds) Expert Clouds and Applications. Lecture Notes in Networks and Systems, vol. 209. Springer, Singapore. https://doi.org/10.1007/978-981-16-2126-0_35

28. Sanger, A. K. S., Johari, R. Survey of Security Issues in Cloud. *2022 International Mobile and Embedded Technology Conference (MECON)*, Noida, India, 2022, pp. 490–493. doi: 10.1109/MECON53876.2022.9751959

29. Ullah, S., Radzi, R. Z., Yazdani, T. M., Alshehri, A., Khan, I. (2022). Types of Lightweight Cryptographies in Current Developments for Resource Constrained Machine Type Communication Devices: Challenges and Opportunities. IEEE Access, vol. 10, pp. 35589–35604. doi: 10.1109/ACCESS.2022.3160000

30. Karl, P., Gruber, M. (2021). A Survey on the Application of Fault Analysis on Lightweight Cryptography. 2021 11th IFIP International Conference on New Technologies, Mobility and Security (NTMS), Paris, France, 2021, pp. 1–3. doi: 10.1109/NTMS49979.2021.9432667
31. Kamel, M. B. M., Van Oosterhout, J., Ligeti, P., Reich, C. (2022). Distributed Cryptography for Lightweight Encryption in Decentralized CP-ABE. *2023 19th International Conference on Wireless and Mobile Computing, Networking and Communications (WiMob)*, Montreal, QC, Canada, 2023, pp. 476–480. doi: 10.1109/WiMob58348.2023.10187882

Security and privacy in the Internet of Medical Things (IoMT)-based healthcare

Ensuring trust and safety

Deepali Vashistha, Dhairya Mehta, Pranav Vashistha, Pranjal Mairal, Malaram Kumhar, and Jitendra Bhatia

16.1 INTRODUCTION

The bounds of creativity are constantly being pushed in an era of fast advancement in technology, radically transforming industries and completely changing how we connect with the outside world. Nowhere is this change more readily apparent than in the healthcare industry, where Internet of Medical Things (IoMT) was created through the fusion of cutting-edge technologies and medical procedures. This chapter sets forth an intriguing journey into the heart of IoMT, illuminating its existing issues, complexities, and the revolutionary potential it holds for healthcare ecosystems around the world.

IoMT, an aspect of the broader Internet of Things (IoT), is a network of connected sensors, software initiatives, and systems that work collectively to enhance patient care, expedite medical processes, and promote data-driven decision-making [1]. IoMT is emerging as a crucial catalyst, poised to address some of the most significant challenges that the healthcare industry is currently facing as the lines between the physical and digital worlds continue to blur. The IoMT ecosystem offers a wide range of opportunities to increase the efficacy and efficiency of healthcare delivery, from real-time health data collecting and remote patient monitoring to predictive analytics and personalized treatment methods.

16.1.1 Overview of IoMT

The concept of IoMT, which is growing rapidly, involves integrating medical instruments, sensors, software programs, and healthcare infrastructure into the wider IoT ecosystem. By connecting them to the internet and enabling them to communicate, receive data, and interact with other devices, systems, and stakeholders, IoMT expands the capabilities of standard medical instruments. The delivery of healthcare, patient monitoring, diagnoses, treatment, and overall management of the healthcare industry all could be revolutionized

DOI: 10.1201/9781003487647-16

by this integrated network of medical equipment and data [2]. Major aspects of IoMT are as follows:

Device Connectivity: The seamless linking of numerous medical devices and sensors to the internet or other communication technologies is referred to as device connectivity in IoMT. These gadgets, healthcare providers, and healthcare systems all can communicate health-related data continuously and in real time because of this connectedness. IoMT gadgets exist in a variety of shapes and sizes – wearable fitness trackers, implantable medical sensors, smart monitoring gear, and mobile health applications [3]. These devices gather a variety of health metrics, including vital signs, medication compliance, and activity levels, and securely communicate the information to regional healthcare systems or to healthcare professionals.

Enhanced Diagnostics: By giving medical professionals access to real-time data and visuals, connected medical devices can enhance diagnosis. For instance, radiologists can remotely assess the results of medical imaging, facilitating speedier and more precise diagnosis. Enabling earlier, more precise, and tailored diagnoses, improved diagnostics in IoMT harness the power of real-time data, analytics, and networking to revolutionize healthcare [4]. Along with enhancing patient outcomes, this has the ability to increase healthcare's effectiveness and efficiency while upholding the greatest levels of patient privacy and data security.

Improved Patient Outcomes: Remote monitoring of patients, early warning sign detection, and rapid intervention can enhance patient outcomes, lower the number of readmissions to the hospital, and boost the general standard of care. Therefore, the potential of IoMT to deliver tailored care, real-time data, and early intervention dramatically improves patient outcomes. It encourages patients to take charge of their health, makes the best use of available resources for healthcare, and ultimately improves people's health, reduces complications, and improves their quality of life [5].

Data Collection and Analysis: Real-time data, such as patient vitals, diagnostic pictures, information on medication adherence, activity levels, and other pertinent health metrics, are collected and transmitted via connected medical devices. Healthcare practitioners can make informed judgments by processing this data using advanced analytic and machine learning algorithms to uncover insights and patterns. IoMT devices cover a broad range of medical instruments, including implanted devices, wearable sensors, remote monitoring systems, and mobile health apps. IoMT devices generate an enormous amount of data, which calls for complex analysis. In conclusion, IoMT's transformational potential lies at the core of data collection and analysis. They make it possible to provide personalized care, identify health problems early, and make data-driven decisions, all of which improve patient outcomes, lower healthcare costs, and advance medical research and public health initiatives [6]. In the IoMT ecosystem, however, maintaining data security, privacy, and interoperability is essential.

16.1.2 Benefits of IoMT

IoMT, which has the potential to improve the results for patients and simplify healthcare processes, has the promise of transforming healthcare. In this section, we examine the several advantages that IoMT offers to the healthcare industry. We also explore the numerous difficulties associated with implementing IoMT in addition to these game-changing benefits [7]. We can successfully negotiate the IoMT landscape and ensure its safe and successful incorporation into contemporary healthcare by knowing its benefits. The key benefits of IoMT are shown in Figure 16.1 and discussed as follows:

Remote Patient Monitoring: IoMT devices continually gather patient data, including vital signs like heart rate, blood pressure, and glucose levels. These devices include wearable sensors and remote monitoring systems. It is especially useful for patients with chronic conditions like diabetes, hypertension, or heart disease as it enables early detection of issues and

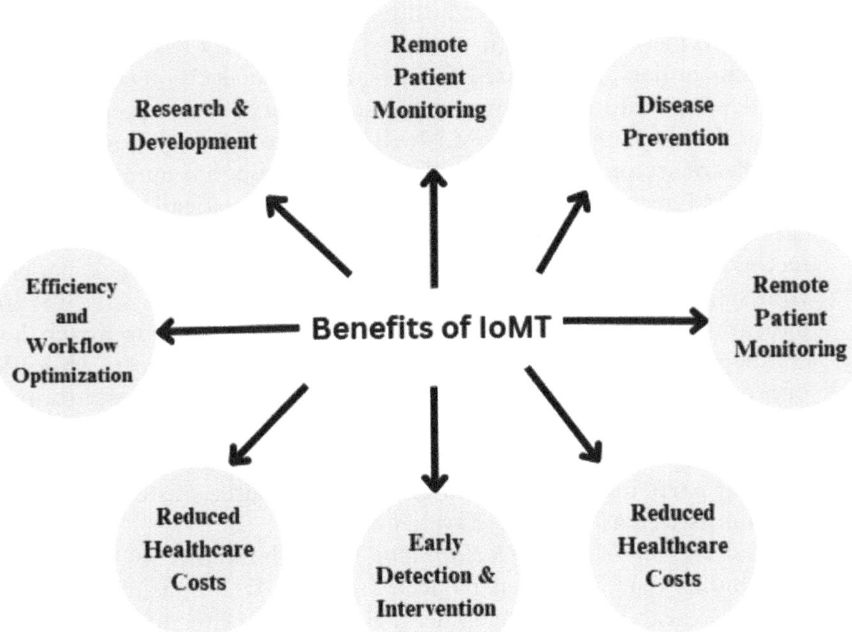

Figure 16.1 Advantages of IoMT.

prompt intervention [8]. This data is transmitted securely to healthcare providers, allowing them to monitor patients' conditions without the need for frequent in-person visits.

Early Detection and Intervention: Healthcare practitioners can monitor patients remotely and receive real-time data, thanks to connected medical devices that are part of the IoMT ecosystem. Vital signs, diagnostics, and other crucial health factors are included in this data. With this continuous data stream, it becomes possible to identify anomalies or warning indicators early. Healthcare professionals can take early action by quickly identifying variations from baseline health metrics. For instance, a wearable device may inform medical professionals if it detects abnormal cardiac rhythms or high blood sugar levels. Rapid medical measures are made possible by this instant notice, possibly averting catastrophic problems or even saving lives [9].

Efficiency and Workflow Optimization: IoMT has the potential to revolutionize the healthcare industry by improving efficiency and streamlining procedures. The automation of routine duties, such as data gathering and appointment scheduling, is a major advantage. The administrative tasks can be delegated to connected devices and systems, freeing up medical staff to focus on more crucial patient care activities. In addition to reducing the administrative burden, this automation improves workflow inside healthcare organizations. Devices that are part of IoMT can easily collect patient data, update electronic health records, and transmit critical information to medical experts in real time. Because they have access to current patient data, healthcare providers may make decisions more quickly and develop treatment plans and diagnoses that are more precise.

Reduced Healthcare Costs: IoMT will revolutionize cost control in the healthcare sector when it is implemented. Through a number of methods, IoMT technologies have the potential to drastically lower healthcare expenses. The avoidance of hospital readmissions is one significant factor that reduces costs. IoMT devices continuously track patients' vital signs and health metrics, enabling the detection of early warning indications and prompt management. This preventive approach lowers the risk of readmission, which decreases healthcare costs while also improving patient outcomes [10]. IoMT also makes it easier to avoid pointless medical procedures and examinations. Real-time data allows healthcare professionals to make more informed choices regarding the need for particular interventions, reducing resource waste and costs for patients as well as healthcare systems.

Enhanced Research and Development: The abundance of aggregated, anonymous data produced by IoMT devices is a treasure source for medical research and development. Researchers can make use of this gold mine to gain knowledge, spot patterns, and hasten the development of novel medications, medical devices, and therapies. Clinical studies benefit most from this data-driven methodology since it enables more focused and effective research. Additionally, it promotes the development of customized medicine, in which medical interventions are modified for particular patients in light of their particular health information [11]. As a result, IoMT expedites healthcare research and paves the road for better, more accurate, and patient-centered medical solutions. It signifies a paradigm shift in the way healthcare innovations are developed, evaluated, and provided, ultimately proving advantageous to patients and the medical profession.

Telemedicine and Virtual Consultations: Through telemedicine and virtual consultations, IoMT transforms healthcare accessible in a significant way. By bridging geographic distances, this groundbreaking method enables patients to consult medical experts from any location. People who live in distant or underserved locations, where access to healthcare services is frequently restricted, are significantly impacted by this. Now, patients can have video conversations with medical professionals, get prompt medical advice, and even have remote diagnostic procedures performed on them. Telemedicine supported by the IoMT improves patient access while also lightening the load on healthcare facilities, especially in times of public health emergencies [12]. It provides a versatile and practical healthcare solution that encourages early intervention and enhances all patient outcomes.

Personalized Medication: A new era of individualized treatment is made possible by the convergence of IoMT in healthcare. IoMT enables medical providers to design personalized treatment plans that would specifically cater to the needs of each patient by continuously gathering and evaluating personal health data. This change goes beyond a universally applicable healthcare model. It enables the personalization of treatments, drug schedules, and lifestyle advice based on current patient-specific data [13]. For instance, drug dosages can be changed to better suit shifting biomarker levels or vital signs. The effectiveness of therapies is increased through personalized medicine, which also reduces the possibility of negative side effects. Patients get care that is specifically tailored to their health state and changing situations, which encourages better adherence to medical guidance.

Disease Prevention: By enabling early disease and trend detection, IoMT plays a crucial part in disease prevention. IoMT devices continuously monitor vital signs, health metrics, and data analytics to provide insightful information that can lead to proactive healthcare interventions and public health initiatives. The prevention of illness development depends heavily on early identification. Healthcare systems can take rapid action in response to anomalies or worrying trends in patient health data, potentially delaying the onset of more serious illnesses. Additionally, IoMT supports public health initiatives by compiling anonymized data from a broad population. To locate illness outbreaks, monitor the transmission of infectious diseases, and guide vaccination campaigns, this data can be examined. Authorities can take preventive measures, such as issuing health advisories or allocating resources to restrict the spread of diseases, by identifying early health trends [14].

16.1.3 Objective and scope

This chapter delves into the pressing issue of security and privacy in the IoMT ecosystem. With a heightened emphasis on the medical field, the chapter illuminates the urgency of addressing these concerns due to the inherent sensitivity of healthcare data. Because of the distinctive characteristics of the IoMT, both the potential benefits and the hazards associated with employing it are amplified, requiring a thorough awareness of the security and privacy landscape. In order to accomplish this, the chapter aims to teach various stakeholders, such as healthcare professionals, device makers, and patients, with the knowledge to recognize, evaluate, and reduce potential risks in the context of IoMT.

Through providing readers a comprehensive overview of the privacy and security concerns raised by the IoMT, the chapter aims to provide readers an in-depth knowledge of the numerous issues. It analyzes the technical solutions, privacy-preserving technologies, and growing legal frameworks and standards that may improve the security posture of the IoMT. The study also emphasizes the importance of creating a cooperative ecosystem in which all parties actively participate in developing a culture of security awareness and best practices.

This chapter contributes to the accumulation of knowledge as the IoMT keeps influencing the future of healthcare by providing the spotlight on the delicate equilibrium required between innovation and preserving personal medical data. It imagines an environment where IoMT potential is realized while pre-serving the integrity, privacy, and security of healthcare data through increased awareness and education.

16.1.4 Evolution of IoMT in healthcare

Significant advances in technology and their integration into numerous aspects of healthcare delivery and management have led to the evolution of IoMT in the realm of healthcare, as shown in Figure 16.2.

> *e-Health (Electronic Health):* e-Health is a concept that first came into being in the late twentieth century. It primarily focuses on the electronic administration of health information and the digitization of healthcare operations. The following are the e-Health's essential components:
>   - *Electronic Health Records (EHRs):* Converting paper records to electronic records let healthcare providers organize and retrieve patient data more easily. This improved care coordination and decreased errors.

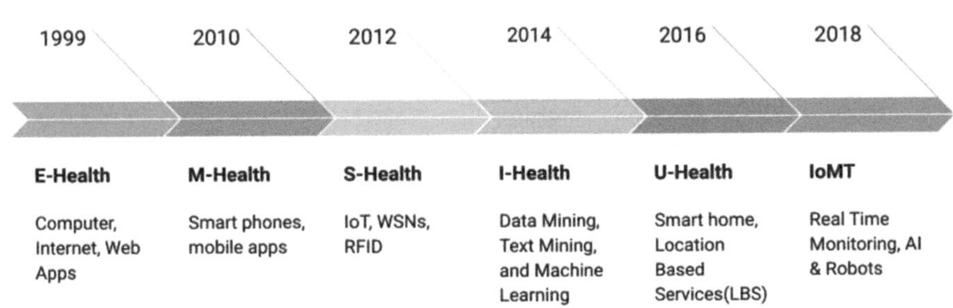

Figure 16.2 Evolution of IoMT.

- *Telemedicine:* e-Health pioneered telemedicine, allowing patients and medical professionals to consult over the internet using tools like video conferencing. This made healthcare more accessible, especially in isolated or underdeveloped areas.

m-Health: IoMT, often known as "m-Health," is a crucial element. It refers to using mobile devices, including smartphones, tablets, and wearable technology, for tasks linked to healthcare, such as monitoring, diagnosing, treating, and managing health information. m-Health is a crucial subset of IoMT because it makes use of the connection and mobility of mobile devices to provide healthcare services and information remotely [15].

S-Health: Samsung Electronics created the comprehensive health and fitness platform known as S-Health, or Samsung Health. Using Samsung smartphones, wearables, and other compatible devices, it is intended to assist people in managing many aspects of their health and well-being. S-Health provides a variety of features and capabilities that encourage leading a healthy lifestyle and allow users to monitor their physical activity, dietary intake, and general health. While S-Health is a useful tool for encouraging a healthy lifestyle and tracking different health metrics, it shouldn't be used in place of expert medical advice or diagnosis. Users who have particular health problems should consult medical professionals for individualized advice and care.

IoMT: A component of the larger IoT idea, IoMT focuses on the internet-based integration of medical equipment, healthcare systems, and software applications [16]. By facilitating the seamless sharing of healthcare data and information between diverse devices and systems, IoMT seeks to revolutionize healthcare by enhancing patient care, treatment outcomes, and healthcare effectiveness.

16.1.5 Architecture and components of IoMT

The architecture of IoMT is an advanced structure that brings together a number of components and technologies to promote seamless exchange of data, communication, and decision-making within the healthcare ecosystem.

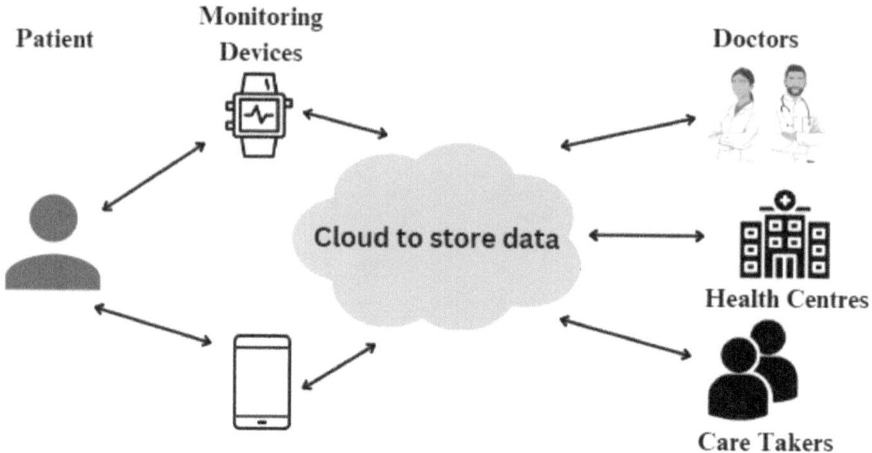

Figure 16.3 Components of IoMT.

Hardware, software, communication protocols, data management systems, security precautions, and interoperability standards all are included in IoMT layout. This complicated framework makes effective use of data and technology to improve patient care, streamline healthcare operations, and promote medical research. The fundamental components of IoMT architecture, as shown in Figure 16.3, are as follows:

Sensors and Medical Devices: Sensors and medical devices are at the heart of IoMT architecture, serving as the essential building blocks that power its transformative potential. Wearable technology, implantable sensors, medical devices, and monitoring tools are just a few of the many different types of sensors that are included in this technological ecosystem. These sensors are essential to IoMT because they continuously gather real-time information about patients' vital signs and health status. Smartwatches and fitness trackers are two examples of wearable technology that provide a noninvasive way to monitor several health factors like heart rate, activity levels, and sleep patterns. Implantable sensors, on the other hand, have the ability to keep track of internal biological processes, offering priceless information on ailments like blood glucose levels for diabetics or cardiac activity for heart patients medical technology.

Connectivity: IoMT adapts its strategy to meet different needs by relying on a wide range of connectivity techniques to enable communication among systems and devices. These connectivity choices, which include Bluetooth, Wi-Fi, cellular networks, and Low-Power Wide-Area Networks (LPWANs), are made depending on a number of important factors. In localized settings like hospitals or clinics, Wi-Fi offers high-speed data transfer ideal for applications requiring rapid information interchange. Cellular networks are the best choice for remote patient monitoring since they provide extensive coverage and guarantee connectivity even in isolated locations. Short- range connections are where Bluetooth shines, frequently linking wearables to smartphones or other devices for real-time data transfer. Remote IoMT devices can use LPWANs because they are designed for long-distance communication and consume little energy [17].

Gateway Devices: IoMT ecosystem's intermediates serve as an essential link between the cloud infrastructure and the countless sensors. Their main responsibility is to gather data from a variety of devices, a task that is frequently started at the network's edge where these sensors are placed. Then, in order to retrieve relevant information, these intermediaries perform preprocessing operations, filtering, and data aggregation. These middle-men permit the transport of this refined dataset to either cloud-based servers or nearby data centers after the pertinent data has been extracted. This transfer accomplishes two key goals. First of all, it spares sensors the time-consuming duty of transmitting unprocessed, raw data, preserving their energy and extending their lifespan. Second, it makes data centers and the cloud possible.

Regulatory Compliance: Systems using IoMT must abide by strict rules specific to the healthcare industry. Data integrity, patient safety, and moral behavior are all guaranteed by adherence to these criteria. It is essential to abide by international and national legal frameworks, such as HIPAA (Health Insurance Portability and Accountability Act) in the United States. These laws require the confidentiality and privacy of patients' private health information to be maintained. Additionally, they create ethical standards for the creation and application of IoMT technologies, guaranteeing that patients' needs continue to be at the forefront of these advancements. In order to maintain the highest standards of healthcare delivery and protect the confidence of patients and healthcare stakeholders, regulatory compliance is crucial in IoMT [18].

16.1.6 Security and privacy issues in IoMT-based healthcare

The crucial problems of security and privacy are highlighted as IoMT revolutionizes healthcare by seamlessly integrating devices and systems [19]. This section dives deep into the complex issues surrounding cybersecurity threats, the types of attacks that target IoMT devices and systems, the critical role that patient privacy plays in the IoMT ecosystem, and the nuanced ethical and legal issues that influence the safeguarding of patient data.

Cybersecurity Threats in Healthcare: Rapid adoption of IoMT has increased the risk of cyberattacks while also bringing about previously unheard-of potential for innovation and patient care. Healthcare businesses are at the forefront of a growing conflict against a wide range of cybersecurity threats. Attackers effectively impair healthcare operations by encrypting private medical records and requesting ransom payments, which causes patient care disruptions and financial strain [20]. In parallel, phishing attempts use false emails to target healthcare workers, deceiving them into disclosing passwords or unintentionally downloading malware. These attacks are getting more and more complex, including social engineering strategies to take advantage of human weaknesses [21].

IoT botnets and distributed denial-of-service (DDoS) assaults add a new level of risk to these more common risks brought on by the IoT. These attacks are planned by taking control of weak IoMT devices and converting them into nefarious network nodes. As a result of these infected devices amplifying attacks, vital infrastructure and networks are overloaded, potentially putting patient care services in peril. Because networked systems are increasingly used in healthcare, robust cybersecurity policies that include both staff training and technology fortification are needed to mitigate these threats [20].

Types of Attacks on IoMT Devices and Systems: The IoMT paradigm's integration of healthcare and technology has revealed a variety of attack vectors that target IoMT systems and devices, highlighting the seriousness of the security challenge. IoMT devices have developed into highly sought-after targets for bad actors looking for illegal access since they act as life-sustaining medical equipment and serve as warehouses of sensitive patient data [20]. The threat of illegal control over medical equipment or the falsification of patient data is posed by device tampering and hijacking. These assaults threaten patient safety and erode faith in medical interventions, undermining the entire foundation of healthcare.

Another dangerous trend is the theft of medical identities [22], which preys on the high value of medical documents in the dark web. Patients are exposed to inappropriate treatments and expensive consequences when attackers steal patient information to use medical services or pharmaceuticals.

The importance of data protection is underscored by the rise of man-in-the-middle attacks within IoMT networks. Given the prevalence of wireless connection in IoMT, adversaries have the ability to intercept and manipulate data transfers, resulting in privacy violations and illegal access. Unauthorized entry is made more likely by flaws in device firmware and unsafe software updates. Additionally, while IoMT ecosystems frequently depend on components from several sources, the rising frequency of supply chain assaults emphasizes the significance of carefully inspecting third-party vendors for security vulnerabilities.

Importance of Patient Privacy in IoMT: Even while IoMT has the potential to revolutionize healthcare, protecting patient privacy is still of utmost importance. In order to guard against malicious intent and unauthorized access, it is essential that networked systems that collect patient data, including medical histories and treatment plans, include strict security measures. In addition to being required by law, maintaining patient privacy is morally necessary to sustain patient confidence and uphold ethical norms.

   Sensitive patient data is collected and transmitted by IoMT devices, making strong security measures necessary. End-to-end encryption is used to ensure that data is kept private while being transmitted, preventing unauthorized access and maintaining data integrity. Patients must be able to make informed decisions about the use of their data, thanks to transparent consent methods. To provide consistency across multiple IoMT devices and networks and to boost patient confidence in the changing healthcare environment, standardizing privacy measures is crucial.

Legal and Ethical Considerations for Patient Privacy: Healthcare organizations need to be skilled at navigating the complex environment of legal and ethical problems introduced by the intersection of IoMT and patient privacy. Strict criteria for the protection of patient data are mandated by regulatory frameworks like the HIPAA in the United States and the General Data Protection Regulation (GDPR) in Europe [20]. Compliance with these rules is crucial since failure to do so not only have legal ramifications but also damages patient confidence.

However, ethical considerations go beyond merely following the law. Healthcare providers need to make sure that patient data is only used for legal purposes and that patients are informed about how their data is used. Patient trust in the IoMT ecosystem must be fostered by open communication about data-sharing procedures. With the development of blockchain technology, patients now have access to exciting new ways to manage their data and can grant and withdraw access while yet remaining anonymous [23]. Securing patient privacy emerges as a fundamental obligation for conscientious healthcare providers in an environment where data breaches are no longer merely operational disruptions but also ethical breaches.

In conclusion, to address the security and privacy issues that arise in IoMT-based healthcare, complete methods that take organizational vigilance, technical fortification, and ethical consideration into account are required. As technology transforms healthcare paradigms, it is essential to accept these difficulties and come up with creative solutions while maintaining an ethical awareness and patient-centric ideals. IoMT can reach its transformative potential to improve patient care and medical advancements by protecting patient data and maintaining their trust.

16.1.7 Secure communication protocols for IoMT devices

It is imperative to develop secure communication protocols, as shown in Figure 16.4, in the rapidly evolving IoMT-based healthcare environment. The integrity and trust of the entire ecosystem is built on top of these protocols. A growing number of threats to patient's data privacy and the general dependability of IoMT systems highlight the need of implementing communication protocols that are equipped with strict security measures.

Transport Layer Security (TLS): In the context of IoMT, the cryptographic protocol TLS is essential for protecting sensitive patient data during transmission across networks. TLS establishes a secure channel that ensures data exchange is done in an environment that is legitimate, confidential, and secure [24]. It works as an overlay protocol over traditional transport layer protocols like Transmission Control Protocol (TCP), encrypting data during transmission and only decrypting it at the desired location to prevent malicious parties from intercepting it. TLS excels at authenticating users via digital certificates, which serve as sender's and recipient's virtual identities. These certificates, which are issued by trusted Certificate Authorities, offer cryptographic evidence of authenticity and protect against man-in-the-middle and impersonation attacks. TLS also uses symmetric and asymmetric ways to guarantee data confidentiality. As the healthcare industry utilizes the revolutionary potential of IoMT, adopting TLS is essential. It takes on the issue of safeguarding communication between IoMT devices and healthcare systems with encryption, authentication, and data integrity. TLS promotes a future in which patient privacy and innovation coexist peacefully in

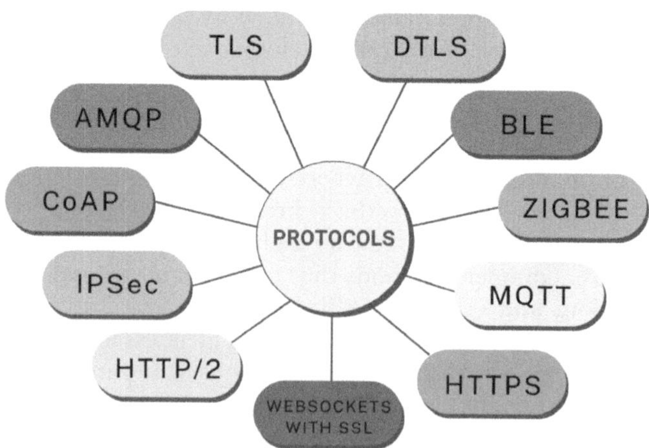

Figure 16.4 Communication protocols for IoMT.

the world of IoMT-based healthcare by supporting secure and unaltered data transport.

Datagram Transport Layer Security (DTLS): In the dynamic IoMT scenario, where secure and real-time device-to-system communication is important, DTLS emerges as a key protection. It offers a specialized solution that addresses the particular difficulties of rapid data sharing while ensuring strong security. DTLS, which is derived from TLS, is designed to move data quickly without sacrificing encryption and authentication for applications like audio and video communication. DTLS is designed for User Datagram Protocol (UDP) as opposed to TLS, which uses TCP and adds latency to real-time communication [25]. By integrating TLS security measures, using encryption, digital certificates, and cryptographic handshakes, DTLS reduces the shortcomings of UDP. DTLS places a strong emphasis on authentication, using public–private key pairs and digital certificates to confirm identities. These certificates, which are issued by reliable Certificate Authorities, build trust and deter unwanted access, data breaches, and possible man-in-the-middle attacks. The IoMT ecosystem places a high value on data integrity, hence DTLS uses cryptographic hash functions to provide distinct checksums for each data packet, maintaining the data's original state during transit. IoMT is able to offer accurate patient vitals, medical reports, and diagnostic data, thanks to its optimization for quick transmission, encryption, and authentication. This supports wise medical judgments in the constantly changing healthcare environment.

MQTT (Message Queuing Telemetry Transport): MQTT develops as a crucial communication protocol, enabling effective data sharing between devices and systems, inside the vast IoMT space. Its simplicity and dependability are ideal for IoMT, where seamless communication is essential. IoMT devices can publish data to a central broker using MQTT's publish–subscribe functionality, which subscribers can then access. Scalability is encouraged by this architecture, which is important for healthcare applications like remote monitoring. Its compact design is suitable for IoMT devices with limited computational and power capabilities [26]. Security is a top priority for MQTT, which frequently uses TLS for encryption and end-to-end confidentiality. To prevent data modification and illegal access, authentication techniques further ensure that only authorized devices communicate. MQTT stands out for real-time, secure, and effective communication in the IoMT environment. Because of its resource-friendly architecture and strong security features, MQTT is a key instrument for achieving the revolutionary promise of IoMT. MQTT's crucial role in fusing technology and security is crucial as IoMT improves patient care.

CoAP (Constrained Application Protocol): Due to the ever rising concerns in the field of security in IoMT healthcare, the issues created by resource-constrained IoMT devices have a specific answer in the form of CoAP. Medical wearables, remote monitoring sensors, and other devices requiring energy-efficient connectivity are well suited to CoAP's lightweight architecture. CoAP is perfect for real-time, low-bandwidth settings since it runs over UDP (User Datagram Protocol), which lowers overhead and delay [26]. It adheres to the processing and memory limitations of devices, allowing for a seamless integration into the IoMT network. CoAP allows for efficient data sharing by letting IoMT devices make requests and central servers answer, thereby following a client–server architecture. The use of DTLS for encrypted communication and authentication by CoAP which protects patient data in transmission addresses security concerns. CoAP's low latency shines for healthcare applications that require quick responses based on data readings. Its effectiveness increases reliability while simultaneously conserving device energy. CoAP becomes a crucial tool in IoMT by providing secure, effective, and lightweight communication, resulting in better patient outcomes and game-changing developments in healthcare.

AMQP (Advanced Message Queuing Protocol): For efficient patient care in the complex IoMT environment, enabling seamless communication between devices and systems is essential, AMQP emerges as a cutting-edge answer created to handle the intricate communication needs of IoMT. AMQP's design perfectly satisfies changing IoMT requirements with a focus on effectiveness, security, and scalability. AMQP is a flexible messaging protocol that makes it easier for IoMT devices and backend systems to exchange messages. Because of its adaptability, it can support a range of communication styles, including publish–subscribe and point-to-point, to meet different IoMT message needs. AMQP, which utilizes a client–server architecture, allows for effective and asynchronous communication [27]. It guarantees the timely data interchange necessary for wise medical judgments. An important feature of AMQP is that it provides trustworthy message delivery mechanisms with acknowledgments, preventing data loss during disruptions. High message flow can be handled by its scalability characteristics, which are essential for real-time monitoring and diagnosis in healthcare applications. AMQP is a flexible protocol designed to handle the unique challenges of IoMT. It is a key facilitator for effective communication due to its dependability, security, and scalability. AMQP is essential in enabling smooth data sharing that improves medical results and patient well-being as IoMT transforms patient-centric care.

IPSec (Internet Protocol Security): In order to improve the security of communication between IoMT devices, healthcare systems, and data repositories, IPSec emerges as a key framework. IPSec establishes a solid foundation for IoMT security by focusing on data integrity and confidentiality. Using encrypted data exchange, IPSec, which is part of the Internet Protocol (IP) suite, ensures secure connection [28]. IPSec serves as a sentinel to guard against unauthorized access and eavesdropping as

IoMT devices send sensitive medical data. Transport Mode and Tunnel Mode are the two operating modes for IPSec [29]. The former is best for same-network device communication because it merely encrypts the data payload. Healthcare businesses are able to customize security setups to data sensitivity and device capabilities by using a variety of cryptographic techniques, such as encryption, authentication, and key exchange protocols. No matter the network infrastructure, end-to-end security is IPSec's strongest point. This is essential for IoMT devices to ensure data protection regardless of the network type while communicating across it. IPSec's encryption, authentication, and secure key exchange support patient privacy while supporting the transformational potential of medical technology in an IoMT environment where data security is crucial.

Zigbee Security: IoMT device communication is facilitated via the low-power wireless protocol ZigBee. Zigbee contains a number of security measures, ensuring thorough defense against potential attackers. This is done to address the specific security difficulties faced by IoMT. Medical wearables and sensors that run on batteries are ideal match for Zigbee's energy-efficient design. Data security while transmission is ensured by its symmetric encryption using AES. This stops unauthorized devices from gaining access to sensitive data across the network. Administrators are given the ability to control network communication through access control, improving overall security. Secure key creation, which is essential for setting up a network, and key updates are supported by Zigbee, reducing the effects of compromised keys [30]. For real-time data accuracy in patient care, it prevents replay attacks and message tampering. Secure commissioning enables secure device joining, and OTA updates remotely correct security holes to keep the network secure. Zigbee is a good option for IoMT communication because of its security features. A strong framework is provided by its low power consumption, symmetric encryption, authentication, and secure key management capabilities. The healthcare industry can securely progress networked medical technologies while protecting patient information, privacy, and network integrity by using Zigbee.

BLE Security (Bluetooth Low-energy Security): A crucial communication method for IoMT devices like wearables and sensors is BLE. Through encryption, secure pairing, and access management, BLE places a high priority on data privacy and security [31]. BLE's security is designed to address IoMT issues by using AES–CCM encryption to protect data privacy while in transit. Sharing encryption keys is created during secure pairing, creating device trust. Passkey entry and out-of-band authentication are two techniques that verify the identification of the device and prevent unwanted access. Message authentication codes (MAC), which confirm the validity of sent data, are used to ensure data integrity. By allowing administrators to choose device and user access levels, role-based access control adds another layer of security by lowering the likelihood of unwanted activities. BLE uses private or public device addresses to solve issues regarding device privacy. Private addresses frequently change, reducing tracking hazards, which is essential for healthcare wearables that monitor patient's health. BLE's security mechanism in IoMT protects patient information and privacy, device security is aided by its encryption, secure pairing, data integrity, and access control. By embracing BLE security, healthcare may use connected devices for better patient care while maintaining high standards for data security and privacy.

WebSockets with SSL: Within the dynamic world of IoMT, WebSocket's with SSL (Secure Sockets Layer) emerge as a crucial communication method. WebSocket's fulfill the demand for prompt data transmission in the healthcare industry by providing real-time, bidirectional connection between devices and servers. This protocol addresses evolving issues in networked medical equipment by combining SSL encryption with efficiency and security. For situations requiring constant monitoring and quick responses, persistent connections from WebSocket's are essential. Due to the reduced connection overhead caused by this bidirectional communication, data is transmitted effectively and with less latency [28]. The addition of SSL improves security in the transfer of healthcare data. During data communication, SSL/TLS encrypts it to protect it from interception and unauthorized access. Data confidentiality and integrity are protected during transmission between IoMT devices and backend servers. Additionally, WebSocket's with SSL address identity confirmation and authentication. IoMT devices and servers are authenticated by SSL/TLS certificates, avoiding man-in-the-middle attacks and guaranteeing safe data transfer between authorized entities. Real-time monitoring, remote diagnosis, telemedicine, and communication between patients and providers all are supported by this technology combo. WebSocket's with SSL fill the gap between real-time data sharing and improved security as IoMT-driven healthcare gets traction. This technology helps to enhance patient outcomes and healthcare efficiency by enabling secure, effective, and timely communication.

HTTPS (Hypertext Transfer Protocol Secure): Through the incorporation of TLS or SSL, HTTPS adds a vital layer of security to standard HTTP. By converting transmitted data into an unintelligible format, this encryption ensures data's secrecy and integrity as it is shared in IoMT ecosystem. Applications for the IoT benefit greatly from HTTPS integration. It prioritizes maintaining data integrity by creating distinctive checksums that authenticate data packets using cryptographic hash functions. This dependability is essential for the accurate sharing of medical data, which supports individualized patient treatment. In addition to providing authentication security, HTTPS also defends against man-in-the-middle attacks [32]. Both IoMT devices and servers are verified using digital certificates from reputable Certificate Authorities, eliminating the possibility of impersonation and unwanted access. In the IoMT space, HTTPS takes on the role of a privacy protector for patients, especially when it comes to remote patient monitoring, telemedicine, and diagnostics. Encryption keeps private health information out of the hands of unauthorized individuals, enhancing patient confidence and adhering to rules like HIPAA. Additionally, HTTPS improves overall IoMT security, protecting against online threats in a connected healthcare environment. Network resilience is improved by encryption's strong shielding against potential threats. HTTPS protects patient information in a dynamic healthcare environment that embraces linked devices, promoting innovation, patient care, and data security.

HTTP/2: In the evolving IoMT environment, HTTP/2 emerges as a protocol that meets the rapid communication needs of linked medical devices. In addition to improving communication speed, HTTP/2 introduces multiplexing, which enables many requests and responses on a single connection. It deals with head-of-line blockage and prioritizes the delivery of crucial data for quick access in IoMT applications. Additionally, HTTP/2 uses HPACK header compression to lighten the computational load and conserve bandwidth which is essential for IoMT devices with limited resources. TLS, which is required and encrypts data to safeguard patient information, upholds security. The multiplexing of HTTP/2 decreases the number of TCP connections, lowering overhead and network congestion [32]. This efficiency lengthens device battery life in IoMT applications that need low energy consumption. In the IoMT ecosystem, HTTP/2 dramatically increases communication speed, efficiency, and security by integrating optimizations, including multiplexing, prioritization, header compression, and required TLS, enabling fast and secure data transmission for improved patient care.

16.1.8 Securing data transmission in IoMT networks

The emphasis on data security that is currently prevalent has prompted the development of multiple encryption schemes and cutting-edge anonymization techniques, as depicted in Figure 16.5, all with the goal of enhancing the privacy and integrity of patient information within this dynamic ecosystem.

End-to-End Encryption: Among IoMT networks' data security measures, end-to-end encryption is at the forefront. In order to protect patient information as it travels from IoMT devices to backend servers, this cryptographic approach acts as a sentinel. Encoding data at the source and only decoding it at the intended destination is the fundamental idea behind end-to-end encryption. This makes sure that data is encrypted the entire way and is therefore protected against breaches and illegal access.

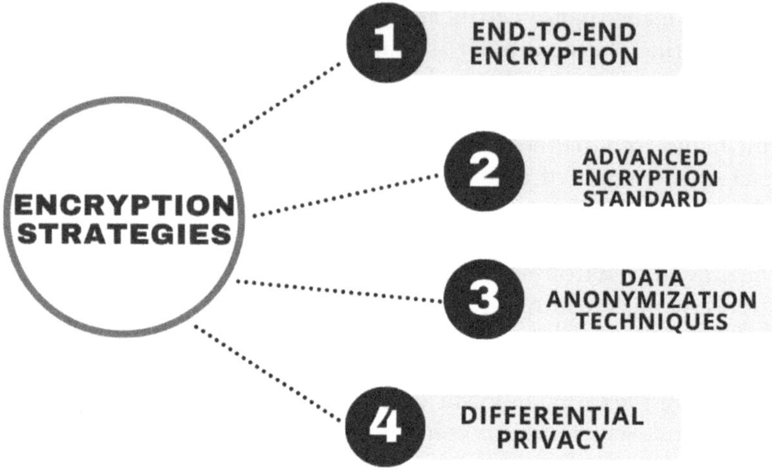

Figure 16.5 Securing data transmission in IoMT networks.

Advanced Encryption Standard (AES): A widely used encryption technology, AES is essential for protecting IoMT data transmissions. AES uses symmetric-key cryptography, which is well-known for its dependability and effectiveness, to encrypt and decrypt data blocks. This encryption method assures that even if data packets are intercepted during transit, the encrypted content remains unreadable without the decryption key. Patient health data is kept secure from unauthorized access when in transit or storage via the use of AES and the end-to-end encryption paradigm. This strengthened security structure maintains patient privacy while also preserving the data integrity, which is crucial for precise medical diagnosis and well-informed treatment choices.

Data Anonymization Techniques: Modern advances in safeguarding data transmission within IoMT networks involve advanced anonymization methods in addition to encryption. These techniques deal with the conundrum of protecting patient privacy while allowing for the extraction of useful information from aggregated data.

Differential Privacy: Applying controlled noise to the data prior to transmission, this technique effectively masks individual identities while preserving the dataset's general statistical characteristics. This means that any attempts to trace data back to specific individuals are pointless since even as IoMT systems capture and transmit data, the specifics of each patient's information remain hidden. In circumstances where IoMT systems share aggregated data for research and analysis, differential privacy is particularly relevant. The approach assures that any future attempts at reidentification provide inconclusive findings by calibrating noise to the data. Because people are assured that their involvement in data-sharing programs does not threaten their privacy, this fosters an atmosphere of trust between healthcare practitioners and patients.

A solid foundation for safeguarding data transmission within IoMT networks is laid by the convergence of end-to-end encryption and data anonymization algorithms. The GDPR and the HIPAA, which require strict data protection and patient privacy, are just two examples of the evolving regulatory frameworks that are aligned with this multifaceted approach.

In a nutshell, protecting data transmission inside IoMT networks is a crucial component of the design of contemporary healthcare systems. A robust barrier against potential breaches and unwanted access is created by the coordination of end-to-end encryption, strengthened by the AES, and cutting-edge anonymization techniques like Differential Privacy. These trends highlight a future in which patients can comfortably interact with technology, secure in the knowledge that their health information will be protected without sacrificing the breakthroughs that IoMT brings to the field of patient care, as IoMT continues to reshape healthcare paradigms.

16.1.9 IoMT security monitoring tools and techniques

In the rapidly evolving world of IoMT-based healthcare, maintaining these networked systems' security and dependability is essential, where the fusion of connectivity and medical devices is reshaping the patient-care's paradigm. The issues brought on by potential security flaws and vulnerabilities grow along with the IoMT ecosystem. The monitoring tools and techniques discussed in this section are shown in Figure 16.6.

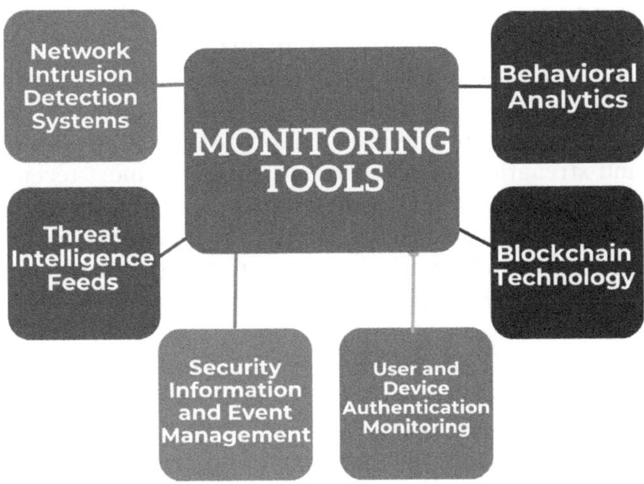

Figure 16.6 Monitoring tools and techniques.

Network Intrusion Detection Systems (NIDS): The deployment of NIDS has emerged as a fundamental technique to safeguard the integrity of IoMT systems in light of the persistent evolution of cyber threats. NIDS serve as watchful sentinels, always observing network traffic to spot anomalies or patterns that differ from accepted standards [33]. NIDS may quickly discover and notify administrators about potential breaches or illegal activity by examining data packets in real time, enabling quick response and mitigation. Advanced algorithms and signature-based detection techniques that recognize well-known attack patterns are included in NIDS, along with anomaly-based detection that alerts to any changes from normal network behavior. An additional layer of security is created by the incorporation of NIDS within IoMT networks, which actively wards off dangers that can jeopardize patient privacy and system functionality.

Behavioral Analytics: Behavioral analytics emerges as a cutting-edge method to strengthen IoMT security in a time dominated by machine learning and artificial intelligence. This strategy involves developing baseline behavior profiles for IoMT users and devices, as well as ongoing inspection for deviations from these patterns. Using machine learning algorithms, behavioral analytics can instantly spot anomalies like irregular data transmission or illicit device access and send out alarms for more thorough inquiry [34]. The advantage of behavioral analytics is its capacity to identify cutting-edge dangers that could elude conventional security procedures. These systems adapt to new threat vectors by continuously learning from ongoing data patterns, which makes them essential for securing the complex IoMT landscape.

Threat Intelligence Feeds: Real-time updates on newly discovered vulnerabilities and attack vectors are required due to the dynamic nature of the cyber threat landscape [35]. Organizations can receive timely and pertinent information from threat intelligence feeds regarding developing threats, malicious IP addresses, malware strains, and exploit methodologies. Healthcare providers can proactively keep ahead of potential risks and strengthen their defenses against the most recent attack tactics by incorporating these feeds into IoMT security monitoring systems. Threat intelligence feeds are used by healthcare organizations to respond quickly and effectively to threats as they emerge, narrowing the window of vulnerability and boosting the overall resilience of IoMT-based systems.

Blockchain for IoMT Security: A revolutionary method for boosting IoMT security has been developed with the rise of blockchain technology. Blockchain is the perfect technology for safeguarding IoMT data because of its inherent decentralized and tamper-proof architecture. Data cannot be changed or removed after it has been recorded because of the distributed ledger technology used by blockchain [36]. This immutability and transparency can be used in the context of IoMT-based healthcare systems to uphold the accuracy of patient data. On the blockchain, every interaction with IoMT devices, data transfer, and update can be tracked, establishing an unchangeable chain of custody.

Security Information and Event Management (SIEM): Effective data analysis is crucial for security monitoring as the IoMT landscape creates an unparalleled volume of data. Through the consolidation of data from numerous sources, such as IoMT devices and network logs, SIEM systems provide a comprehensive solution [37]. The data is then examined by these systems for security incidents, irregularities, and potential risks. A command center for ensuring the security of IoMT environments, SIEM systems offer real-time monitoring, threat detection, and response coordination. SIEM systems give healthcare companies the ability to detect complex threats and act quickly to minimize any breaches by combining data from several sources.

User and Device Authentication Monitoring: Monitoring user and device authentication activity carefully is crucial for IoMT security [38]. Monitoring login attempts, device connections, and access requests entails constant observation of user and device authentication. With the help of this proactive strategy, it is possible to spot suspicious activity, such as repeatedly failed login attempts or strange device connections, and take quick action to stop unwanted access. Patient data is protected from potential breaches by user and device authentication monitoring, which also acts as a disincentive to unwanted access attempts.

Therefore, the integration of strong security monitoring tools and approaches is crucial to preserve data privacy, uphold trust, and minimize potential dangers as IoMT-based healthcare systems continue to improve patient care. A strong defense against emerging cyber threats is provided by the integration of Network Intrusion Detection Systems (NIDS), behavioral analytics, threat intelligence feeds, blockchain technology, Security Information and Event Management (SIEM), and user/device authentication monitoring. By adopting these trends, the healthcare sector may successfully negotiate the complex problems presented by the evolving IoMT landscape and promote an atmosphere that values innovation, safety, and patient-centered care.

16.1.10 Compliance and legal considerations for IoMT security

IoMT has become a huge part in our lives over the past decade. Everyone who is concerned about their health and want to track various indicators of a healthy body such as oxygen levels is using IoMT devices on a regular basis. Most of the healthcare sector in the past decade has adopted IoMT infrastructure for its benefits such as fast data transmission, cost-cutting, and many more. But the concern arises when the sensitive data of a person or patient can be misused or may be stolen. As there are many doubts and shortcomings even today looking at the security and privacy of a smart IoMT device, a set of rules and regulations are issued by the competent authorities on how this data should be collected, used, shared, and about the overall usage of a smart healthcare device such that it does not invade and harm the privacy and integrity of an individual.

NIST Cybersecurity Framework: NIST CSF provides a structured framework for managing cybersecurity risk which is common to all and is flexible and adaptable. This NIST CSF should be adopted in the healthcare sector by the organizations to improve the IoMT functioning [39]. The NIST CSF is organized in five core functions:
- *Identify:* Identification of physical and information assets and establish the strategies accordingly.
- *Protect:* Protect the data from intrusions and attacks.
- *Detect:* Detect the anomalous behavior in the networks and IoMT devices.
- *Respond:* Respond to the attacks or attempts made to hinder the privacy and security of the data.
- *Recover:* Restructure the system after the attack, learn from the mistakes, and adjust the security and strategies accordingly.

The HIPAA Privacy Rule: HIPAA protects medical records and other health-related information (collectively referred to as "protected health information") in the United States and establishes national standards for doing so. It applies to health plans, healthcare organizations, and those healthcare providers who engage in specific electronic healthcare transactions [40].

The whole set of HIPAA Administrative Simplification Regulations is available at 45 CFR Parts 160, 162, and 164 and consists of the following:
- Transactions and Code Set Standards
- Identifier Standards
- Privacy Rule
- Security Rule
- Enforcement Rule
- Breach Notification Rule

Data Protection and GDPR: The European Union passed this legislation. The following roles in a user's data protection are defined by the GDPR's 99 articles, which are divided into 11 chapters:
- The data subject is the one who's data is collected, used, and processed.
- The data processor lays the guidelines of how to use the data.
- The data controller analyzes and controls the data.
- Data protection officers pays attention toward securing the data.
- The supervisory authority audits GDPR compliance.

Six data processing principles are outlined in the GDPR. A controller should adhere to these standards when gathering, storing, and processing personal data [41]:

- Personal information must be managed properly by following regulations and with transparency.
- The information should be relevant and limited.
- The data should be updated time to time and its accuracy should also be high.
- Information of an individual should be stored only till the time it is needed, otherwise it should be deleted.
- Information or data must be handled with integrity.
- Purpose for collecting the information should be adequate and reasonable.

Every country has their own set of rules and regulations for security and privacy of IoMT devices and healthcare in general. These include HIPAA in the United States, the IT Act in India, the Privacy Protection Act in Australia, Canada's Personal Information Protection Act, etc. Some of the Regulation frameworks which are broader in scope and more comprehensive to protect personal identifiable information are discussed here.

16.2 CONCLUSION

This chapter explores in depth the crucial concerns relating to security and privacy within the IoMT ecosystem, especially in the context of the healthcare industry. The significance of addressing these issues is stressed by the chapter, given the private nature of healthcare information. The IoMT's special qualities magnify both its potential advantages and threats, so it is essential to have a thorough awareness of the security and privacy situation. The main goal of the chapter is to arm different stakeholders like healthcare professionals, device manufacturers, and patients, with the knowledge they need to recognize, evaluate, and reduce any risks that can arise from the implementation of IoMT. The work offers a detailed grasp of these complicated concerns by providing a thorough analysis of privacy and security challenges in the IoMT space. It looks at technical fixes, privacy-protecting innovations, and developing legal frameworks and standards that could improve IoMT security.

The chapter, in particular, emphasizes the value of building an interactive ecosystem in which all stakeholders actively participate to develop a culture of security awareness and best practices. This strategy strives to establish a setting where the advantages of IoMT can be fully realized while also maintaining the security and privacy of healthcare data.

This study offers insightful contributions to the IoMT landscape, highlighting the delicate balance between innovation and protecting patient's privacy.

The study imagines a future in which the potential of IoMT is realized without compromising the security and privacy of healthcare by focusing on increasing awareness and education.

REFERENCES

1. Internet of Medical Things (IoMT) or healthcare IoT, 2022 (accessed 30 August 2023).
2. The rise of artificial intelligence in healthcare applications, 2020 (accessed 30 August 2023).
3. Artificial intelligence (AI) and Internet of Medical Things (IoMT) assisted biomedical systems for intelligent healthcare, 2022 (accessed 23 September 2023).
4. Internet of Medical Things and trending converged technologies: A comprehensive review on real-time applications, 2022 (accessed 23 September 2023).
5. The role of nurses in improving health care access and quality, 2022 (accessed 23 September 2023).
6. Big data analytics in healthcare: Promise and potential, 2014 (accessed 23 September 2023).
7. Embracing the future of healthcare: Exploring the Internet of Medical Things (IoMT), 2020 (accessed 23 September 2023).
8. Early detection and management of the high-risk patient with elevated blood pressure, 2008 (accessed 23 September 2023).
9. Medical error reduction and prevention, 2023 (accessed 30 August 2023).
10. Strategies to reduce hospital readmission rates in a non-Medicaid-expansion state, 2019.
11. Personalized medicine could transform healthcare, 2017 (accessed 23 September 2023).
12. Telemedicine for healthcare: Capabilities, features, barriers, and applications, 2024 (accessed 23 September 2023).
13. Security and privacy of Internet of Medical Things: A contemporary review in the age of surveillance, botnets, and adversarial ML, 2022 (accessed 23 September 2023).
14. Confidentiality and privacy of personal data, 1994 (accessed 23 September 2023).
15. M. Kumhar and J. Bhatia. Emerging communication technologies for 5G-enabled Internet of Things applications. *Blockchain for 5G-enabled IoT: The New Wave for Industrial Automation* (pp. 133–158), 2021.
16. M. Kumhar and J. Bhatia. Edge computing in SDN-enabled IoT-based healthcare frameworks: Challenges and future research directions. *International Journal of Reliable and Quality E-Healthcare (IJRQEH)*, 11(4):1–15, 2022.
17. Security and privacy management in Internet of Medical Things (IoMT): A synthesis, 2022 (accessed 30 August 2023).
18. Security in IoMT communications: A survey, 2020 (accessed 30 August 2023).
19. Potential of Internet of Medical Things (IoMT) applications in building a smart healthcare system: A systematic review, 2021 (accessed 30 August 2023).
20. B. Mago, N. Shingari, S. Verma and M. S. Javeid. A review of cybersecurity challenges and recommendations in the healthcare sector (pp. 1–8), 2023.
21. J. Obuhuma and Z. Shingai. Social engineering based cyber-attacks in Kenya. In *2020 IST-Africa Conference (IST-Africa)* (pp. 1–9), 2020.
22. A. H. W. Brandon and D. Pottas. Best practices to address medical identity theft awareness. In 2021 IST-Africa Conference (IST-Africa) (pp. 1–9), 2021.

23. A. A. Jolfaei, S. F. Aghili, and D. Singelee. A survey on blockchain-based IoMT systems: Towards scalability. *IEEE Access*, 9:148948–148975, 2021.
24. What is transport layer security (TLS)?, 2022 (accessed 31 August 2023).
25. DTLS – datagram transport layer security, 2023 (accessed 31 August 2023).
26. Study paper on security and privacy in the Internet of Medical Things (IoMT). (accessed 31 August 2023).
27. MQTT vs AMQP for IoT, 2022 (accessed 31 August 2023).
28. A comprehensive guide to IoT protocols, 2022 (accessed 31 August 2023).
29. What is IPSec? Internet protocol security explained, 2022 (accessed 31 August 2023).
30. Zigbee security: Basics (Part 2), 2017 (accessed 31 August 2023).
31. Internet of medical threats? Exploring Bluetooth low energy vulnerabilities in medical devices, 2021 (accessed 31 August 2023).
32. Why you should migrate to https and http/2, 2016 (accessed 31 August 2023).
33. 8 ways to secure the Internet of Medical Things (IoMT), 2021 (accessed 31 August 2023).
34. Solving IoT security challenges with behavioral analytics, 2022 (accessed 31 August 2023).
35. State of cybersecurity report, 2019 (accessed 31 August 2023).
36. J. Elhachmi and A. Kobbane. Blockchain-based security mechanisms for Internet of Medical Things (IoMT). *International Journal of Computer Networks & Communications*, 14(6): 115–136, 2022.
37. Best practices for securing medical IoT devices, 2023 (accessed 31 August 2023).
38. N. Alsaeed and F. Nadeem. Authentication in the Internet of Medical Things: Taxonomy, review, and open issues. *Applied Sciences*, 12(15): 7487, 2022.
39. National Institute of Standards and Technology, 2023 (accessed 31 August 2023).
40. HIPPA rules, 2003 (accessed 31 August 2023).
41. General data protection regulation (GDPR), 2018 (accessed 31 August 2023).

Chapter 17

A comprehensive study of the problem and challenges associated with machine learning–enabled IoT in biomedical applications

Sandeep Bhatia, Basetty Mallikarjun, Neha Goel, Amit Kumar Goel, Bharat Bhushan Naib, and Soniya Verma

17.1 INTRODUCTION

Wireless sensor networks (WSNs) have grown in a way that has never been seen before in terms of applications, interfaces, scalability, interoperability, and data processing. The Internet of Things (IoT) has a strong basis, thanks to these technological advancements as well as advancements in RFID, wireless networks, and cellular technology. In the context of supply chain management, Kevin Ashton first used the phrase "Internet of Things" in 1999. It alludes to a more intelligent universe of things where everything is wired onto the Internet. All these things, sometimes referred to as entities in the IoT, have digital identities, may be remotely organized, managed, and controlled, and have a range beyond what is physically possible. IoT has improved practically every area of our everyday lives because of the expansion in the development of smart items, and it continues to do so with a variety of fresh, creative, and intelligent applications. Figure 17.1 illustrates a few of these applications, such as smart healthcare, smart cities, smart agriculture, crowd sensing, and crowd sourcing (Li et al., 2021).

By connecting common things and devices to the Internet, IoT is transforming how we interact with the physical world. It has a wide range of applications across numerous industries. The following are a few noteworthy IoT applications:

1. *Smart Houses:* IoT gadgets like smart thermostats, lighting controls, and security cameras let homeowners monitor and control their houses remotely, improve security, and increase energy efficiency.
2. *Healthcare:* Wearable fitness trackers, remote patient monitoring, and intelligent medical equipment like insulin pumps are examples of IoT devices in the healthcare industry. For real-time monitoring and intervention, these devices collect and transmit patient data to healthcare professionals.

DOI: 10.1201/9781003487647-17

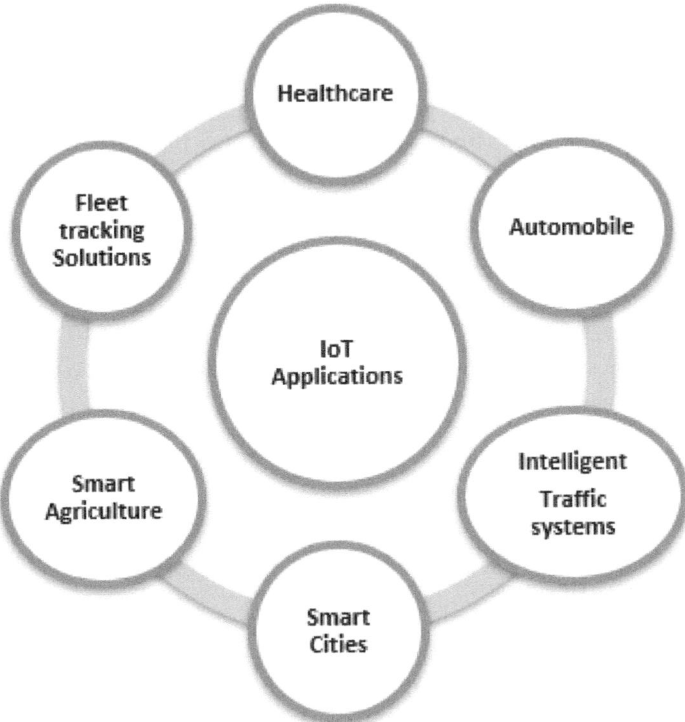

Figure 17.1 IoT applications (Li et al. 2021).

3. *Smart Cities:* IoT technology is employed in "smart cities" to effectively manage urban infrastructure. Smart trash management, street lighting, and environmental monitoring for ozone and noise pollution are a few examples.
4. *Industrial IoT (IIoT):* IoT is revolutionizing companies through predictive maintenance, asset tracking, and process optimization, or IIoT. IoT sensors are used by manufacturers to track the condition of their equipment and boost productivity.
5. *Agriculture:* Precision agriculture uses the IoT to analyze soil, manage irrigation, and track livestock. Crop yields are improved, and resource waste is decreased.
6. *Retail:* Retailers can use IoT to better manage their supply chains, personalize customer experiences by using beacons and sensors, and watch inventory levels in real time.
7. *Logistics and Supply Chain:* IoT sensors on cars, warehouses, and shipping containers offer real-time visibility into the movement and condition of goods, improving logistics and lowering theft and waste.

8. *Energy Management:* IoT devices monitor and regulate how much energy is used in factories and buildings, which helps to cut expenses and consumption.

9. *Environmental Monitoring:* Environmental variables, including temperature, humidity, and pollution levels are measured by IoT sensors. For predicting disasters, doing climate research, and designing cities, this information is essential.

10. *Connected Vehicles:* The development of autonomous cars and vehicle-to-vehicle (V2V) communication for safer and more effective transportation depends on the IoT.

11. *Smart Grids:* Intelligent power grids are built using IoT technology to control electricity supply and demand dynamically, resulting in more dependable and effective energy distribution.

12. *Water Management:* In order to maintain this precious resource, IoT sensors and devices monitor water quality, identify leaks, and improve water distribution systems.

13. *Security and Surveillance:* Smart locks, access control systems, and surveillance cameras driven by IoT improve security and enable remote monitoring of residences and commercial buildings.

14. *Wearable Technology:* Wearable IoT devices, such as fitness trackers and smartwatches, track health parameters, send notifications, and allow easy access to data and services.

15. *Consumer Electronics:* Smart appliances, voice-activated speakers, and smart TVs are becoming more and more prevalent in homes for their improved functionality and convenience.

16. *Education:* Campus security, asset tracking, and interactive learning all are made possible by IoT in educational settings.

17. *Sports and Fitness:* IoT devices monitor vital signs while exercising, track sports performance, and offer athletes and fitness aficionados information.

18. *Aerospace and Defense:* For better situational awareness and mission accomplishment, IoT sensors and systems are used in military logistics, battlefield communication, and aircraft maintenance.

These are just a few examples of IoT applications, and the list continues to grow as technology evolves and industries find innovative ways to leverage IoT for efficiency, safety, and convenience.

IoT applications for health and biomedicine are significant research fields. Applications of the IoT include the hospital management system, remote patient monitoring, medical waste management, robotic nursing assistants, cancer detection by body scanning, Parkinson patient monitoring, dementia patient monitoring by GPS smart soles, depression monitoring by smartwatches, glucose monitoring, effective drug management, and hand hygiene monitoring. Ingestible sensors, smart pills, connected inhalers, connected contact lenses, integrated hearing aids, and other integrated devices pave the way for integrated biomedical applications (Bzai et al., 2022).

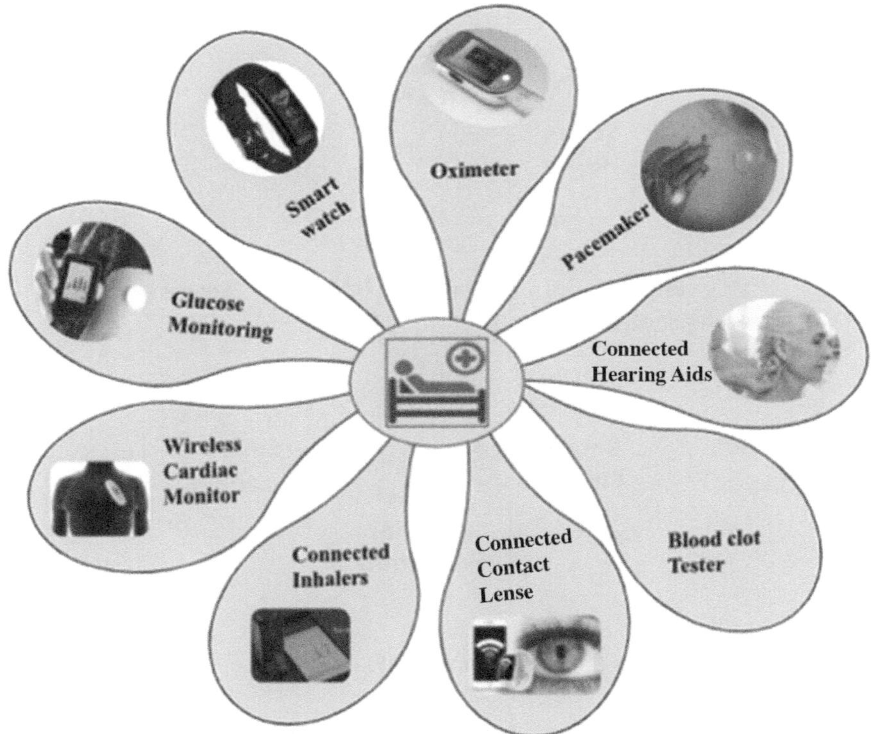

Figure 17.2 IoT in biomedical applications (Neeta et al., 2020).

It is comprehensive research related to technical factors, including interoperability across all platforms, devices and technologies, data security, privacy concerns, and related laws, as shown in Figure 17.2.

Machine learning (ML) is a branch of artificial intelligence (AI) that focuses on creating statistical models and algorithms that let computers get better over time at a given activity without being explicitly taught. In other words, ML enables computers to gain knowledge from data and enhance their capacity to forecast the future or make judgments based on it (Bhatia et al., 2023c).

Applications for ML include audio and picture recognition, natural language processing, recommendation engines, self-driving cars, medical diagnostics, and many more by Mohapatra and Panda (2019), as shown in Figure 17.3.

Utilizing ML, IoT in biomedical applications has the potential to improve healthcare by giving patients and healthcare professionals individualized and effective solutions. Huge volumes of data are produced by IoT devices, including connected medical equipment, wearable sensors, and health monitoring equipment (Sandeep et al., 2023). This data can be processed and analyzed by ML algorithms to yield insightful results, better patient outcomes, and expedite medical procedures (Bhatia et al. 2023f).

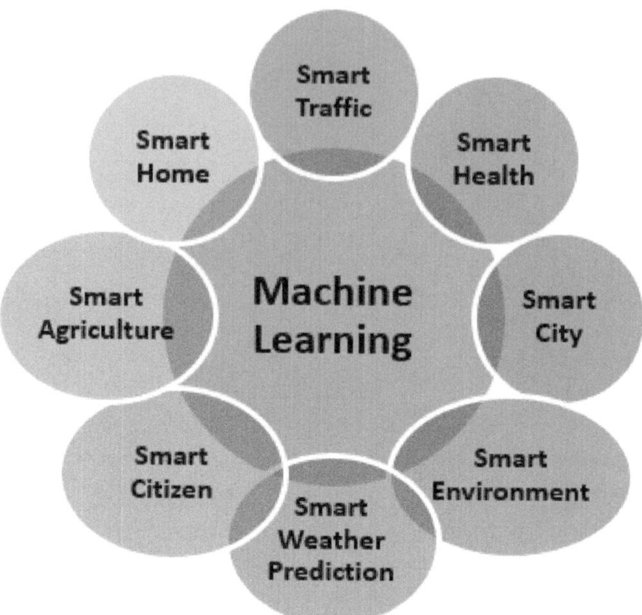

Figure 17.3 ML applications (Mohapatra et al., 2019).

Powered by ML, IoT in biomedical applications has the power to completely change the healthcare industry by delivering individualized, data-driven, and effective solutions. To maximize the advantages of new technologies for patients and healthcare professionals, it will be crucial to resolve issues and ensure their ethical use (Sandeep et al., 2023e).

17.2 LITERATURE REVIEW

IoT is a rapidly expanding concept that makes use of a network of connected devices with integrated sensors to collect and exchange data. It is widely used for healthcare applications. The current epidemic highlights the flaws in the current healthcare system, yet there are numerous technologies that can support the current solutions, such as smart and linked wearables, as described in Munnangi et al. (2023) and Bzai et al. (2022).

IoT and ML have come together to produce amazing improvements in a variety of fields, including biomedical applications. The goal of this literature study is to give a thorough overview of how ML-enabled IoT is used in the biomedical industry. This review illustrates the substantial contributions, difficulties, and potential of this synergistic method by looking at pertinent research articles.

By enabling real-time monitoring and analysis of patient data, IoT-ML-based devices have revolutionized healthcare. In 2021, Bolhasani et al. (2021) introduced a wearable IoT device that continually monitors vital signs and uses ML algorithms to spot anomalies, enabling early intervention in life-threatening circumstances. To provide precise arrhythmia detection, Sworna et al. (2021) created a system that combines ML-driven electrocardiogram (ECG) analysis with IoT-enabled wearable devices.

A precise disease diagnosis is necessary for effective disease treatment. The capability of ML-enabled IoT has been demonstrated in this case. Aguayo et al.'s approach for precisely diagnosing neurodegenerative disorders in 2023 used IoT devices and ML algorithms to collect patient data. Additionally, using predictive analytics and ML algorithms, early diagnosis of diseases, including diabetes and cancer, has been accomplished (Khaleel & Al-Bakr, 2023).

With personalized medicine, patients receive therapies that are specifically tailored to their needs. ML systems that are IoT-enabled have proved crucial to this project. To offer tailored treatment regimens, Gao et al. (2021) created an IoT-driven platform that combines genetic data, patient history, and ML algorithms. These systems may increase therapy effectiveness while minimizing negative consequences.

Additionally, telemedicine and remote monitoring enabled by ML, along with NLP for electronic health records, promote patient engagement and individualized care. This investigation of ML's additional capabilities highlights the technology's potential to restructure the healthcare system and move it toward data-driven, patient-centered, and organized healthcare delivery.

There are difficulties in ML and IoT integration in biomedicine. The importance of data quality assurance, security and privacy issues, and regulatory compliance cannot be overstated. In addition, it is still difficult to evaluate ML models when used in medical decision-making (Obermeyer & Emanuel, 2016). To ensure the secure and efficient implementation of ML-enabled IoT systems in healthcare, it is imperative to address these concerns.

IoT with ML capabilities have a bright future in biomedicine. It is projected that more research will be done to create cutting-edge ML algorithms that can manage complicated and heterogeneous biomedical data. Furthermore, by combining edge computing and federated learning, it is possible to increase privacy while facilitating group analysis of distributed medical data (Chen et al., 2021). Furthermore, for the seamless integration of IoT devices into healthcare ecosystems, defined protocols for data exchange and interoperability must be established.

A new era of healthcare innovation has begun because of the integration of ML and IoT in biomedical applications. The impact of this synergy is clear in real-time monitoring, disease detection, and individualized treatment. Despite difficulties, current research and technological developments hold out hope for making healthcare a more effective, individualized, and patient-centered undertaking.

The sensitive nature of medical data makes it a prime target for cyberattacks, leading to privacy breaches and data theft. Nasiri et al. (2019) discuss security mechanisms and cryptographic techniques for securing IoT data in healthcare. Data curation and quality strategies are covered by Liaw et al. (2013) for enhancing the performance of ML models in the healthcare industry.

Sharma et al. (2023) propose a blockchain-based framework for ensuring data integrity and privacy in IoT-enabled healthcare systems.

For integrated chronic disease management (CDM) and population health, effective use of routine data depends on the underlying data quality (DQ) and, for cross-system data use, semantic interoperability. A potential remedy for DQ is an ontological approach, but there hasn't been much of it done (Liaw et al., 2013).

Strategies for dealing with imbalanced datasets in biomedical ML applications are presented Zhang et al. (2022).

Sandeep et al. (2023d) present ML algorithm to detect and predict diabetes and its cure. Sandeep et al. (2023) focus on the use of 5G, 6G, and 7G communication to felicitate IoT for data collection and processed in computer using ML algorithm.

Imran et al. (2021) discuss healthcare applications for elderly people using intelligent task mapping system, it is an efficient system for healthcare management. Sandeep et al. (2023b) show the automatic seat identification using hardware and ML-based algorithm.

Srinivasan et al. (2023) present the use of Python and OpenCV for the optimization of data using ML.

Ganai et al. (2022) mentioned the security issues and threats in IoT-based system while collecting data and optimize them using ML. Sandeep et al. (2023a) present the ML algorithm to detect Zomato restaurant sales analysis.

17.3 RESEARCH OBJECTIVES

A thorough investigation of the issues and difficulties posed by ML-enabled IoT in biomedical applications is intended to meet several important research goals. ML, IoT, and healthcare all are combined in one interdisciplinary sector, which presents both exciting prospects and substantial obstacles.

The following list summarizes this chapter's main research goals:

1. To study ML-enabled IoT in healthcare structure.
2. Survey on ML and its application to healthcare.
3. Investigating ML's complementary features to improve the organization in the healthcare system.
4. Successful IoT implementation strategy in the biomedical field.
5. To discuss list and talk about the key ML challenges in healthcare.
6. At the end, we will discuss conclusion and future scope.

The evolution of healthcare technology and patient care can be aided by a thorough study that addresses these research aims. Such a study can offer insightful information about the prospects and difficulties of applying ML-enabled IoT in biomedical applications.

17.4 HEALTHCARE STRUCTURE USING ML-ENABLED IoT

Figure 17.4 illustrates the range of shrewd and compassionate traits connected with the ML culture and its vast healthcare services. It also involves assistance from a variety of clever and digital tools, like cloud data performance and AI. The creation of electronic medical records, even at a low cost, further impressively benefits the healthcare industry. Other significant areas where ML principles investigate its quality services in the healthcare arena include smart produced reports, digital notes, records maintenance, etc.

ML-enabled IoT has the potential to revolutionize biomedical applications by enhancing data collection, analysis, and decision-making processes in healthcare and life sciences. More devices than ever will be online as we enter the 2020s, and this trend will continue. By 2020, there will be more than 21 billion linked devices worldwide, which is a tenfold increase from just four years ago (Kelly et al., 2020). At its most basic level, IoT is a network that connects

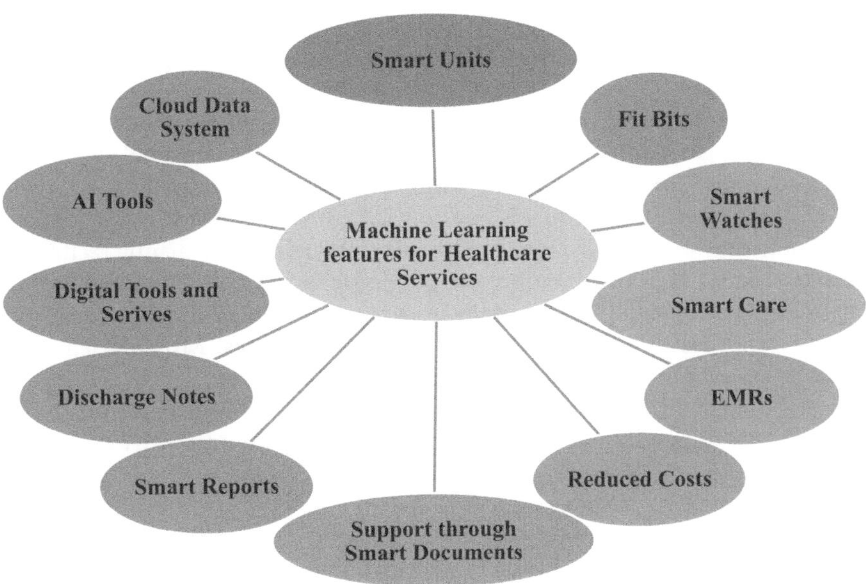

Figure 17.4 ML in perspective of biomedical applications (Javaid et al., 2022).

objects with identifiers to the Internet. They can send, store, and gather information via this. Any device that can gather patient health information falls within the definition of IoT in the context of healthcare. IoT technology has become more popular as because of a variety of health initiatives that aim to enhance population health. The many services and applications of IoT in healthcare, including mobile health (mHealth), eHealth, semantic devices, ambient assisted living, smartphones and wearables, and community-based healthcare, have been covered in recent reviews (Khaleel, 2023). These solutions have been thoroughly explained and can be used for a variety of single-condition and cluster-condition management tasks, including enabling healthcare professionals to remotely monitor and track patients' conditions, facilitating self-care for those with chronic conditions, assisting in the early detection of issues, identifying symptoms, and making clinical diagnoses more quickly, etc.

IoT is a complex network of "things" that are connected to a server that offers the necessary services and have individual identities. By exchanging pertinent data from the actual and virtual worlds, they can communicate with one another and with individuals in the real world. These entities have the capacity to respond autonomously to events occurring around them. Some of these processes can be initiated by either humans or machines conversing with one another. They are also able to offer services. The delivery of healthcare will soon shift because of IoT opportunities. The tele-monitoring of patients in hospitals and, more importantly, at home, will heavily rely on this technology Gao et al. (2021). Early detection of diseases and dangerous circumstances can help individuals avoid them.

The growth of biomedical systems in recent years has greatly increased employment and income. In the past, diagnosing diseases and bodily anomalies required a physical examination. Most patients had to stay in the hospital while receiving therapy. Prices for biomedical products have increased as a result, and biomedical institutes in remote and rural locations are now overworked. The development of technology has made it possible to monitor one's health and diagnose many illnesses using tiny, embedded sensors in wristbands (Sworna et al., 2021). Tercan and Meisen et al. (2022) mentioned predictive quality in manufacturing sector based on deep learning and machine learning techniques.

In recent years, the development of biological systems has significantly expanded employment and income. In the past, a physical examination was necessary to diagnose diseases and physical deformities. Most patients were required to remain in the hospital while receiving treatment. As a result, the cost of biomedical items has skyrocketed, and remote and rural biomedical institutes are currently overburdened. Using tiny, embedded sensors in wristbands, technology has made it feasible to track one's health and diagnose a variety of disorders (Zhang et al., 2022).

With its vast range of intelligent features and capabilities, ML has made tremendous improvements in the healthcare industry. By enhancing diagnosis, treatment, patient care, and administrative procedures, these smart features are revolutionizing healthcare.

17.5 SURVEY ON ML AND ITS APPLICATION TO HEALTHCARE

The following are some smart capabilities of ML in the healthcare industry:

- ML algorithms can examine patient data to forecast the likelihood that particular diseases, such as diabetes, cardiovascular conditions, and cancer, will manifest in the future. Early intervention and specialized preventive actions are made possible by this.
- ML algorithms can examine medical images like X-rays, MRIs, and CT scans to help identify abnormalities, tumors, fractures, and other conditions. This improves diagnostic precision and expedites the analysis of medical images.
- ML algorithms can examine large datasets to find prospective drug candidates and forecast how well they will work to treat ailments. This lowers expenses and speeds up the drug discovery process.
- To suggest tailored treatment regimens, ML models can examine patient data, including genetic data. This guarantees that therapies are personalized for every patient for better results.
- Clinical decision support: By assessing patient data and recommending the best treatment options based on the most recent scientific findings and recommendations, ML systems can offer real-time decision support to healthcare clinicians.
- NLP approaches can extract useful data from unstructured EHRs, facilitating access to patient histories, spotting trends, and enhancing patient care for healthcare professionals.
- ML algorithms can continually monitor patient data, such as vital signs and data from wearable devices, to spot anomalies and provide early warnings for deteriorating health, enabling remote patient monitoring and telemedicine.
- ML can be used to identify erroneous healthcare billing and fraudulent insurance claims, which will assist to cut expenses and assure fair billing procedures.
- ML models can forecast patient admission and discharge rates, enabling hospitals to more effectively allocate resources and cut down on patient wait times.
- ML can evaluate information from a variety of sources, including social media and search engines, to track health trends and monitor disease outbreaks in real-time, assisting in the early detection of public health concerns.
- ML algorithms can analyze genomic data to identify genetic mutations associated with diseases, enabling genomic medicine uses ML algorithms to find genetic variants linked to disease-causing conditions, enabling tailored treatments and precision medicine.

- ML can examine medical databases to find and keep track of negative side effects related to drugs, enhancing drug safety.
- ML-powered chatbots and virtual mental health assistants can offer timely support and resources to people who are struggling with mental health difficulties.
- ML can help researchers create more efficient trials by identifying candidates for clinical trials, streamlining the patient recruiting process, and more.
- ML can anticipate patient admissions, optimize staff schedules, and better allocate hospital resources, all of which lower costs and enhance patient care.

These smart characteristics of ML in healthcare highlight its potential to improve patient outcomes, streamline healthcare processes, and spur medical research and innovation. However, it is crucial to make sure that these technologies are created and implemented with a strong focus on data privacy, morality, and legal compliance.

17.6 EXAMINING ML'S SUPPLEMENTAL CAPABILITIES TO ENHANCE THE STRUCTURE OF THE HEALTHCARE SYSTEM

The important areas where ML can supplement and enhance the structure of the healthcare system are shown in Figure 17.5.

A disruptive potential for healthcare delivery is shown by looking at the supplementary capabilities of ML to improve the structure of the healthcare system. For healthcare professionals, administrators, and politicians, the ability of ML to process and analyze enormous volumes of healthcare data provides priceless insights. ML improves the accuracy and effectiveness of healthcare decision-making, from predictive analytics that predict disease outbreaks and patient readmissions to clinical decision support systems that provide healthcare workers with real-time information. Additionally, ML supports the interpretation of medical imaging by quicker and more precisely spotting irregularities in X-rays and MRI data. The use of ML to stratify patient risk profiles, improve medication discovery, and streamline supply chains ensures that resources are allocated in a way that is both effective and economical.

Additionally, telemedicine and remote monitoring enabled by ML, along with NLP for electronic health records, promote patient engagement and individualized care. This investigation of ML's additional capabilities highlights the technology's potential to restructure the healthcare system and move it toward data-driven, patient-centered, and organized healthcare delivery.

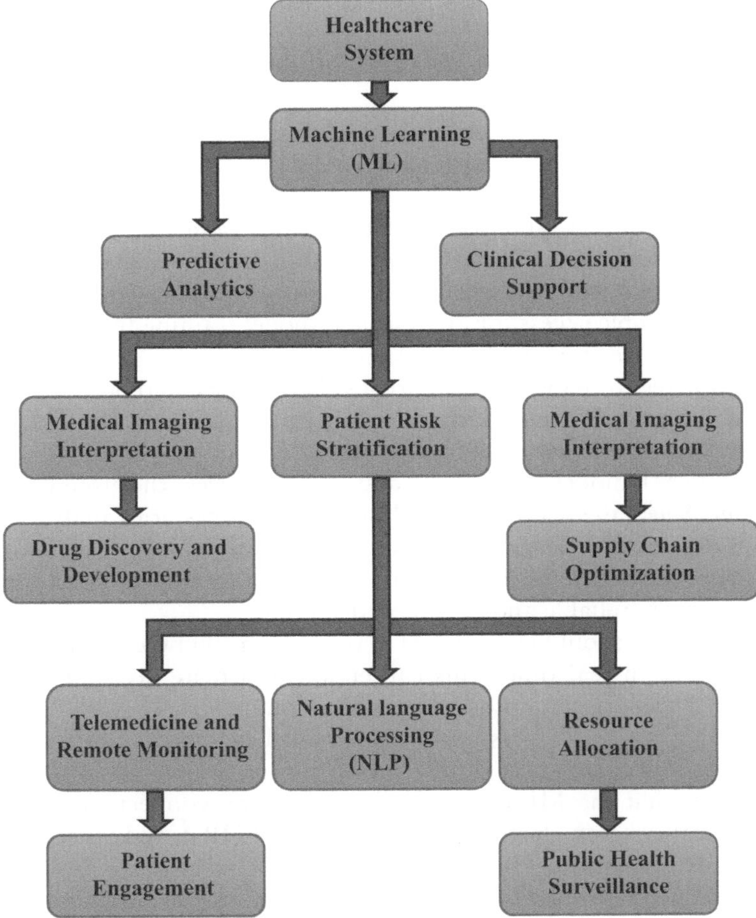

Figure 17.5 Diagram on investigating ML's complementary features to improve the organization of the healthcare system.

17.7 SUCCESSFUL IoT IMPLEMENTATION STRATEGY IN THE BIOMEDICAL FIELD

In order to ensure efficacy, accuracy, and compliance with regulatory norms, the deployment of ML-enabled IoT solutions in the biomedical industry requires careful planning and consideration of numerous elements. Here is a successful IoT deployment methodology for biomedical applications:

- Clearly state the exact issue you're trying to tackle or the precise goals you hope to accomplish with ML-enabled IoT. It might be early disease identification, patient monitoring, or drug discovery, for instance.

- Assemble and prepare top-notch biomedical data. This could consist of genomic information, patient records, sensor readings, and medical imaging. Ensure data protection and conformity with legal specifications like HIPAA.
- Select IoT gadgets and sensors that can gather the necessary data. Think about elements like precision, dependability, connectivity, and battery usage.
- Use trustworthy and secure data transmission methods to transfer information from IoT devices to cloud or local servers. To safeguard data while it is in transit, use the necessary encryption techniques.
- Ensure simple access for analysis and model training by storing data in a scalable, secure, and legal manner.
- Decide regarding whether to process ML in the cloud or at the edge (on IoT devices). When making this choice, consider elements like latency, processing capacity, and data privacy.
- Create ML models specifically designed to address the given biomedical issue. Select the relevant algorithms, such as time-series analysis for sensor data or deep learning for picture analysis.
- Utilize labeled data to train and improve the models. Make sure the models are reliable and easy to understand.
- ML models should be deployed to the chosen computer environment for inference in real time. This can entail immediate decision-making by edge devices or data processing in the cloud.
- Put in place procedures for ongoing model evaluation and retraining to preserve accuracy over time.
- Ensure that the ML-powered IoT system can connect to current biomedical systems, electronic health records (EHRs), and other healthcare IT infrastructure.
- To make interoperability easier, use standardized data formats and communication protocols.
- Put in place strong security measures to safeguard data while it is in transit and at rest.
- Obey laws governing the protection of patient data, such as the GDPR in Europe or the HIPAA in the United States.
- Ensure that your ML-enabled IoT solution conforms with applicable laws, standards, and guidelines for medical devices and data protection by working with regulatory specialists.
- To prove the efficacy and safety of your ML-enabled biomedical IoT solution, carry out extensive testing, validation, and clinical trials.
- Create a system that can scale to accommodate growing data volumes and device deployments.
- Create a maintenance schedule that considers regular model upgrades, security patches, and hardware and software changes.
- Create user-friendly user interfaces so that patients and healthcare professionals can communicate with the system.

- Utilize monitoring tools to keep tabs on the system's functionality, data integrity, and security.
- Utilize analytics to glean insights from the gathered data and raise the efficiency of the system.
- Gather suggestions and make ongoing improvements to the user experience.
- Give administrators and users thorough documentation.
- Provide healthcare employees who will be using the system with training and assistance.
- Utilize monitoring tools to keep tabs on the system's functionality, data integrity, and security.
- Utilize analytics to glean insights from the gathered data and raise the efficiency of the system.
- Conduct compliance audits frequently to make sure the system keeps up with legal standards.
- Work together with regulatory organizations, patients, healthcare professionals, and other stakeholders to meet their needs and expectations.

This deployment methodology will help you successfully adopt ML-enabled IoT solutions in the biomedical sector while considering the particular difficulties and demands of healthcare and regulatory compliance. Table 17.1 illustrates the comparison analysis of ML-based IoT role in the healthcare sector by different authors.

Here is an overview of how ML and IoT intersect in the biomedical field:

- *Remote Patient Monitoring:* IoT sensors can collect continuous real-time data from patients, such as heart rate, blood pressure, glucose levels, and more. ML algorithms can analyze this data to detect anomalies and patterns, allowing healthcare providers to remotely monitor patients with chronic conditions and provide timely interventions.
- *Predictive Healthcare:* ML models can predict disease outbreaks and patient-specific health trends by analyzing data from IoT devices. For example, monitoring environmental data like air quality, weather, and pollen levels alongside patient health data can help predict and manage asthma or allergy-related conditions.
- *Wearable Health Devices:* Wearable IoT devices, like smartwatches and fitness trackers, collect a wide range of health-related data. ML can process this data to provide personalized health recommendations, early disease detection, and fitness tracking.
- *Drug Development and Discovery:* ML algorithms can analyze vast datasets generated during drug discovery, clinical trials, and genomics research. IoT devices can collect data on drug efficacy and patient response in real time, accelerating drug development processes.
- *Hospital and Clinic Operations:* IoT sensors can optimize the management of medical equipment, patient flow, and inventory in healthcare

Table 17.1 Comparison analysis of ML-based IoT role in healthcare sector

Author	Year	ML techniques	Research challenges	Conclusion	Applications
Li et al.	2021	Big data analytics	Highlighted	Suggest government agencies and healthcare persons to be up to date and well-equipped with current trends in ML	Healthcare
Awasthy & Nikhila	2021	Integrated devices approach	Highlighted	Discussed impact of IoT in healthcare	Biomedical
Kelly et al.	2020	-	Highlighted	Discussed potential issues, barriers, privacy and safety related to ML-based IoT	Healthcare delivery
Munnangi et al.	2023	Deep learning–based approach	Highlighted	Discussed data analytics based on deep learning in healthcare	Smart healthcare framework
Bzai et al.	2022	ML-based IoT	Highlighted	Author mentioned challenges in ML-based IoT using few parameters like individual, business, technology, and society	Industry
Sworna et al.	2021	IoT-ML	Highlighted	Author highlights future research direction in ML-based IoT	Healthcare
Aguayo et al.	2023	DNN	Highlighted	Survey on predicting neurodegenerative using ML	Neurodegenerative diseases
Sandeep et al.	2023	ML prediction algorithm	Highlighted	Author mentioned survey on ML-based success of Zomato	Zomato data analysis
Khaleel & Al-Bakr	2023	Predictive analysis	Highlighted	Author discussed ML applications in diabetes patient treatment	Clinical decision support system
Gao et al. 2021	Blockchain	Blockchain	Highlighted	Discussed role of blockchain in ML based IoT.	Smart healthcare
Obermeyer et al.	2016	Big Data	Highlighted	Discussed role of ML in big data and healthcare support	Clinical medicine

facilities. ML can help predict equipment maintenance needs and streamline operations to reduce costs and improve patient care.

- *Medical Imaging:* ML can enhance medical imaging by analyzing and interpreting data from MRI, CT scans, X-rays, and ultrasound images. IoT-connected devices can transmit these images securely, enabling remote diagnosis and consultation.
- *Healthcare Fraud Detection:* ML algorithms can be employed to detect fraudulent activities in healthcare billing and insurance claims, helping to reduce healthcare fraud and lower costs.
- *Genomic Analysis:* ML can analyze genetic data collected through IoT devices to identify disease risks, develop personalized treatment plans, and advance precision medicine.
- *Telemedicine and Telehealth:* IoT-connected devices can facilitate telemedicine consultations by transmitting vital signs and patient data to healthcare providers. ML can help interpret this data and support diagnostic decisions.
- *Epidemiological Surveillance:* ML algorithms can process data from IoT sensors to track the spread of diseases, such as COVID-19, and predict hotspots, enabling more effective public health responses.

17.8 KEY ML CHALLENGES IN HEALTHCARE

ML has emerged as a powerful tool in healthcare, promising to revolutionize diagnosis, treatment, and patient care. However, it also faces several significant challenges in this complex and sensitive domain.

- *Data Quality and Quantity:* One of the foremost challenges is the availability of high-quality, labeled healthcare data. Healthcare data is often fragmented, incomplete, and contains errors. Moreover, acquiring a sufficiently large and diverse dataset for training robust ML models can be challenging, especially while respecting patient privacy and data security regulations.
- *Interoperability:* The healthcare industry relies on a multitude of systems and platforms, often from different vendors, which struggle to communicate with each other seamlessly. ML models need access to data from various sources, and interoperability issues can hinder the integration and deployment of these models in clinical settings.
- *Ethical and Regulatory Compliance:* Healthcare ML models must adhere to strict ethical guidelines and regulations, such as patient privacy (HIPAA in the United States) and ethical considerations surrounding sensitive medical data. Ensuring that ML models are transparent, explainable, and unbiased is a constant challenge.
- *Clinical Validation and Adoption:* Transitioning from experimental ML models to real-world clinical use requires rigorous clinical validation to

ensure safety and efficacy. Convincing healthcare professionals to adopt these models into their practice and integrate them into existing workflows is another significant hurdle.

- *Generalization and Adaptation:* ML models that perform well in controlled research settings may struggle to generalize to diverse patient populations and adapt to changing healthcare conditions. The ability to make models robust, adaptable, and resilient to changes is crucial.
- *Interpretability and Explainability:* Understanding why an ML model makes a particular prediction is vital in healthcare to gain the trust of medical practitioners. The "black box" nature of some advanced ML techniques poses a challenge in this regard.
- *Bias and Fairness:* Bias in healthcare ML models can lead to disparities in healthcare outcomes, particularly for underrepresented groups. Addressing bias and ensuring fairness in ML algorithms is essential to avoid perpetuating healthcare inequalities.
- *Cost and Resource Constraints:* Developing, deploying, and maintaining ML systems in healthcare can be expensive. Healthcare organizations need to allocate resources effectively to support the integration and long-term sustainability of ML solutions.
- *Security and Privacy:* Protecting patient data from cyber threats and ensuring compliance with privacy regulations is paramount. ML models must be designed with robust security measures to safeguard sensitive information.

Despite these challenges, the potential benefits of ML in healthcare are substantial. Addressing these issues through collaborative efforts among healthcare professionals, data scientists, and policymakers can pave the way for more effective, efficient, and ethical healthcare solutions powered by ML.

17.9 CONCLUSION

This study will address both the opportunities and difficulties the industry is facing by examining the current state of ML in healthcare and its promise for the future. It will help to shape upcoming advancements and applications of ML in healthcare as well as add to the increasing body of knowledge in this quickly evolving sector.

In conclusion, ML-enabled IoT has the potential to revolutionize biomedical applications by enhancing patient care, expediting research, and streamlining administrative processes in the healthcare industry. However, it also raises issues with data privacy, rules, and ethics that need to be carefully addressed in order to be implemented.

The use of ML techniques for big data analysis in the healthcare industry has been thoroughly reviewed in this research. Additionally, the strengths and weaknesses of the currently used approaches as well as numerous research difficulties are emphasized. Our research will help government organizations and healthcare professionals stay up to date on the latest developments in ML-based big data analytics for smart healthcare.

Data science, healthcare, engineering, and ethical knowledge all are necessary for the successful adoption of ML-enabled IoT in biomedical domains. It is possible to fully utilize ML and IoT to alter healthcare and enhance patient outcomes by taking these factors into account.

This chapter intends to contribute to the knowledge and development of this revolutionary subject by performing an extensive investigation of the issues and difficulties related to ML-enabled IoT in biomedical applications. Researchers, practitioners, and policymakers can use the study's findings and insights to develop practical solutions and methods to deal with these problems, resulting in better healthcare outcomes and tailored treatments.

17.10 FUTURE SCOPE

The potential for ML-enabled IoT in the field of healthcare is enormous. The combination of ML and IoT in healthcare is anticipated to have a wide range of positive effects, alter patient care, and improve healthcare administration. Here are several crucial areas where important developments can be anticipated:

1. *Remote Patient Monitoring:* IoT devices with ML capabilities can continually track patients' vital signs, enabling the early identification of health problems. These gadgets can transmit real-time data to medical professionals, allowing for prompt actions. In the future, wearable technology and sensors for remote monitoring are projected to grow.
2. *Predictive Analytics:* ML algorithms can examine huge datasets produced by IoT devices to forecast disease outbreaks and health concerns. Healthcare practitioners will be able to manage resources effectively and take preventative action because of this predictive capability.
3. *Personalized Medicine:* ML algorithms may examine a person's genetic, lifestyle, and health information from IoT devices to provide personalized treatment regimens. This may result in treatments that are more efficient and have fewer negative effects.
4. *Medication Discovery:* By evaluating massive datasets to find prospective medication candidates and forecast their efficacy, ML helps speed up the drug discovery process. IoT gadgets can help by gathering actual information on drug usage and patient outcomes.
5. *Telemedicine:* By offering improved diagnostic support, the integration of IoT and ML will improve telemedicine. Medical photos and data can be collected by IoT devices, which ML algorithms can then analyze to help remote healthcare providers make precise diagnoses.
6. *Healthcare Operations Optimization:* By anticipating patient admissions, automating resource allocation, and improving the general effectiveness of healthcare facilities, ML-enabled IoT can enhance hospital operations.

7. *IoT-enabled Medical Devices:* More intelligent medical devices will be developed and integrated with IoT and ML. For instance, smart inhalers for asthmatics that send adherence reminders and real-time feedback.

8. *Data Security and Privacy:* Protecting the security and privacy of patient data will be a major problem as IoT in healthcare becomes more prevalent. Future innovations will emphasize strong security safeguards and adherence to laws like HIPAA.

9. *Explainable AI:* The necessity for explainable AI in the healthcare industry will increase as ML models get more complicated. Healthcare practitioners must be able to comprehend and rely on the decisions produced by ML algorithms.

10. *Cost Reduction:* By reducing readmissions, optimizing resource use, and raising the precision of diagnoses and treatment plans, ML-enabled IoT can help lower healthcare expenses.

11. *Healthcare Access:* By enabling telemedicine and remote monitoring, IoT and ML can assist in increasing access to healthcare, particularly in underserved or remote places.

12. *Collaborative Research:* IoT and ML will make it easier to do collaborative research in the field of medicine. Global data collection and analysis capabilities enable researchers to conduct more thorough research and make more significant discoveries.

13. *Patient Engagement:* By offering individualized health suggestions and feedback based on IoT-generated data, ML can help to boost patient engagement. Patients will feel more empowered to participate actively in their healthcare as a result.

In conclusion, the use of ML-enabled IoT in the healthcare industry has a very bright future. It might completely alter how patients are treated, diseases are managed, and how healthcare is delivered. But as these technologies advance, it will also present issues with data privacy, security, and ethical considerations, which will need to be properly handled.

This study will address both the opportunities and difficulties the industry is facing by examining the current state of ML in healthcare and its promise for the future. It will help to shape upcoming advancements and applications of ML in healthcare as well as add to the increasing body of knowledge in this quickly evolving sector.

REFERENCES

Aguayo, G. A., Zhang, L., Vaillant, M., Ngari, M., Perquin, M., Moran, V., & Fagherazzi, G (2023). Machine learning for predicting neurodegenerative diseases in the general older population: A cohort study. *BMC Med. Res. Methodol.*, 23(1), 1–13.

Awasthy, N., & Nikhila, V (2021). Impact of IoT in Biomedical Applications: Part II. In *Electronic Devices, Circuits, and Systems for Biomedical Applications* (pp. 441–460). Academic Press.

Bhatia, S., Arya, C., Verma, S., Gautam, D., Naib, B. B., & Kumar, A. (2023a). Predict Success of a Zomato Restaurant Using Machine Learning. In *2023 World Conference on Communication & Computing (WCONF)* (pp. 1–7). IEEE.

Bhatia, S., Gautam, D., Kumar, S., & Verma, S. (2023b). Automatic Seat Identification System in Smart Transport Using IoT and Image Processing. In *2023 3rd International Conference on Intelligent Communication and Computational Techniques (ICCT)* (pp. 1–6). IEEE.

Bhatia, S., Goel, N., Ahlawat, V., Naib, B. B., & Singh, K. (2023c). A Comprehensive Review of IoT Reliability and Its Measures: Perspective Analysis. In *Handbook of Research on Machine Learning–enabled IoT for Smart Applications across Industries* (pp. 365–384). IGI Global.

Bhatia, S., Goel, A. K., Naib, B. B., Singh, K., Yadav, M., & Saini, A., (2023d). Diabetes Prediction Using Machine Learning. In 2023 World Conference on Communication & Computing (WCONF), RAIPUR, India, pp. 1–6. doi: 10.1109/WCONF58270.2023.10235187

Bhatia, S., Jaffery, Z. A., & Mehfuz, S. (2023e, January). A Comparative Study of Wireless Communication Protocols for Use in Smart Farming Framework Development. In *2023 3rd International Conference on Intelligent Communication and Computational Techniques (ICCT)* (pp. 1–7). IEEE.

Bhatia, S., Jaffery, Z. A., & Mehfuz, S. (2023f, May). Development and Analysis of IoT based Smart Agriculture System for Heterogenous Nodes. In *2023 International Conference on Recent Advances in Electrical, Electronics & Digital Healthcare Technologies (REEDCON)* (pp. 62–67). IEEE.

Bhatia, S., Mallikarjuna, B., Gautam, D., Gupta, U., Kumar, S., & Verma, S. (2023g, March). The Future IoT: The Current Generation 5G and Next Generation 6G and 7G Technologies. In *2023 International Conference on Device Intelligence, Computing and Communication Technologies, (DICCT)* (pp. 212–217). IEEE.

Bhatia, S., Naib, B. B., Goel, A. K., Kumar, L., & Singh, K. (2023h, June). Drowsy Driver Alert System Using OpenCV. In *2023 3rd International Conference on Pervasive Computing and Social Networking (ICPCSN)* (pp. 614–619). IEEE.

Bolhasani, H., Mohseni, M., & Rahmani, A. M. (2021). Deep learning applications for IoT in health care: A systematic review. *Inform. Med. Unlocked*, 23, 100550.

Bzai, J., *et al.* (2022). "Machine learning-enabled Internet of Things (IoT): Data, applications, and industry perspective," *Electronics*, 11(17), 2676. doi: 10.3390/electronics11172676

Chen, R.J., Lu, M.Y., & Chen, T.Y., *et al.* (2021). Synthetic data in machine learning for medicine and healthcare. *Nat. Biomed. Eng. 5*, 493–497. https://doi.org/10.1038/s41551-021-00751-8

Ganai, P. T., Bag, A., Sable, A., Abdullah, K. H., Bhatia, S., & Pant, B. (2022). A Detailed Investigation of Implementation of Internet of Things (IoT) in Cyber Security in Healthcare Sector. In *2022 2nd International Conference on Advance Computing and Innovative Technologies in Engineering (ICACITE)* (pp. 1571–1575). IEEE.

Gao, Y., Wang, J., Yuan, Y., Jiang, Y. Z., & Yue, X. (2021). Machine learning and blockchain technology for smart healthcare and human health. *J. Healthc. Eng.*

Gautam, D., Bhatia, S., Goel, N., Mallikaijuna, B., Ganesha, H. S., & Naib, B. B. (2023). Development of IoT Enabled Framework for LPG Gas Leakage Detection and Weight Monitoring System. In *2023 International Conference on Device Intelligence, Computing and Communication Technologies,(DICCT)* (pp. 182–187). IEEE.

Imran, Iqbal N, Ahmad, S, & Kim, DH (2021). Health monitoring system for elderly patients using intelligent task mapping mechanism in closed loop healthcare environment. *Symmetry, 13*(2), 357. https://doi.org/10.3390/sym13020357

Kelly, J.T., Campbell, K.L., Gong, E., & Scuffam, P. (2020). The Internet of Things: Impact and implications for health care delivery. *J. Medical Internet Res.* 22: e20135. https://doi.org/10.2196/20135

Khaleel, F. A., & Al-Bakry, A. M. (2023). Diagnosis of diabetes using machine learning algorithms. *Mater. Today, 80*, 3200–3203.

Liaw, S. T., Rahimi, A., Ray, P., Taggart, J., Dennis, S., de Lusignan, S., & Talaei-Khoei, A (2013). Towards an ontology for data quality in integrated chronic disease management: A realist review of the literature. *Int. J. Med. Inform., 82*(1), 10–24.

Li, W., Chai, Y., & Khan, F. *et al.* (2021). A comprehensive survey on machine learning-based big data analytics for IoT-enabled smart healthcare system. *Mobile Netw Appl 26*, 234–252. https://doi.org/10.1007/s11036-020-01700-6

Mohapatra, B. N., & Panda, P. P (2019). Machine learning applications to smart city. *ACCENTS Trans. Image Process. Comput. Vision, 5*(14), 1.

Munnangi, A.K., UdhayaKumar, S., & Ravi, V. *et al.* (2023). Survival study on deep learning techniques for IoT enabled smart healthcare system. *Health Technol. 13*, 215–228. https://doi.org/10.1007/s12553-023-00736-4

Nasiri, S., Sadoughi, F., Tadayon, M. H., & Dehnad, A (2019). Security and privacy mechanisms of Internet of Things in healthcare and non-healthcare industry. *J. Health Admin., 22*(4), 86–105.

Obermeyer, Z., & Emanuel, E. J (2016). Predicting the future: Big data, machine learning, and clinical medicine. *New Engl. J. Med., 375*(13), 1216–1219.

Sharma, P., Namasudra, S., Chilamkurti, N., Kim, B. G., & Gonzalez Crespo, R (2023). Blockchain-based privacy preservation for IoT-enabled healthcare system. *ACM Trans. Sensor Netw., 19*(3), 1–17.

Srinivasan, R., Kavita, R., Kavitha, M., Mallikarjuna, B., Bhatia, S., Agarwal, B., & Goel, A. (2023). Python and Opencv for Sign Language Recognition. In *2023 International Conference on Device Intelligence, Computing and Communication Technologies, (DICCT)* (pp. 1–5). IEEE.

Sworna, N. S., Islam, A. M., Shatabda, S., & Islam, S. (2021). Towards development of IoT-ML driven healthcare systems: A survey. *J. Netw. Comput. Appl., 196*, 103244.

Tercan, H., & Meisen, T (2022). Machine learning and deep learning based predictive quality in manufacturing: A systematic review. *J. Intell. Manuf., 33*(7), 1879–1905.

Zhang, A., Xing, L., Zou, J., & Wu, J. C (2022). Shifting machine learning for healthcare from development to deployment and from models to data. *Nat. Biomed. Eng., 6*(12), 1330–1345.

A machine learning-enabled Internet of Things model for cloud-based biomedical applications

Palanivel Kuppusamy, Nandhu Palanivel, and Suresh Joseph K

18.1 INTRODUCTION

The rapid development of information and communication technology (ICT) impacts everyone's health and quality of life. Biomedical applications are the application of engineering to biological things, particularly in creating and using devices for healthcare purposes. The healthcare sector is changing due to the latest generation of networked biomedical sensors. ICT tools assist in keeping track of a person's condition and quickly offering helpful advice with numerous ways to examine patients and conduct monitoring procedures and clinics in the healthcare system. However, exchanging raw data of the healthcare system continues to have significant risks and difficulties.

Today, advanced technologies allow healthcare businesses to provide their customers various services, possibilities, and amenities. Incorporating artificial intelligence (AI) (Anichur et al., 2022) into a healthcare system and the progress of the Internet of Things (IoT), wearable technology, customized biosensors, and healthcare systems with body sensor networks (BSN) results from the continuous improvement communication technologies of contemporary innovative items.

18.1.1 Biomedical applications and their challenges

Technology-assisted precaution, avoidance, and disease control have become significant concerns for the biomedical and healthcare sectors.

- Patients now want greater control over their healthcare data and the actual value of their data.
- Patients want a unified method for their data to be dispersed among several healthcare providers.
- Healthcare providers and patients need integrated health records distributed among several locations (such as hospitals, pharmacies, clinical labs, etc.).
- The fragmented healthcare data increases budgets because of system inadequacies that cause the nonexistence of transparency, data traceability, and patient safety issues.

DOI: 10.1201/9781003487647-18

- Technical security and privacy threats, such as data breaches, data integrity issues, and data collaboration, have brought the issues to light.

With the above issues, more ethical and legal frameworks, operational procedures, prediction models, and resilience are required to implement Healthcare 5.0 (Saraswat et al., 2022). When communicating, traditional systems frequently provide security for patient health monitoring data. They often need assistance in handling complex attacks during data translation and transmission. According to Bhatia et al. (2022), the healthcare sector accounts for more than 10% of the GDP in several nations, leading to serious security issues in health monitoring (Tao et al., 2019). In the fast-expanding world of technology, it has become impossible to maintain a healthy lifestyle due to hectic job schedules. Many health concerns exist, including heart and breathing-related issues (Arora & Goel, 2020) and disease outbreaks and emergencies (Sujith et al., 2022).

Advanced healthcare technologies can enhance healthcare services, and integrating these technologies may present new opportunities in the healthcare industry (Mansour et al., 2021). With enabled technologies like AI, IoT, big data, and assisted networking channels, Healthcare 5.0 (Saraswat et al., 2022) motivates patient monitoring in real time, ambient control and well-being, and security amenability. AI has advanced valuable techniques for data processing and analysis (Wang et al., 2023). Recently, a smart health monitoring system (Shiva et al., 2022) addressed the pandemic better, which could result in remote healthcare monitoring.

The main issues with the current state of healthcare data are as follows:

a. The vast amounts of data can be exciting to determine which data and insights are worthwhile.
b. The individuals must be informed of the data insights and analysis to function logically.
c. The complexity of the healthcare data increases due to ambulatory locations and services.
d. Healthcare Apps like diagnosis support, reconstruction, restoration, and data analysis are challenges for biomedical signal processing and imaging.
e. Aged patients must have their health state periodically checked by a doctor.

As a result, Biomedical apps must be integrated with technological developments to overcome these issues.

18.1.2 Motivation

Biomedical sciences use tools and techniques for clinical diagnosis, patient management, and application-driven, helpful research. Advanced technologies are used in the biomedical field for digital-to-physical connectivity and for generating enormous amounts of data possible. Integrating biomedical signal and image processing has a wide range of applications, from diagnosis to therapy. For example, a Healthcare App (a Smartwatch) monitors the patient's pulse (biomedical data) and communicates information straight to the Cloud. Similarly, wearable fitness trackers can transmit patients' heart rate and physical activity to physicians and monitor their health in an emergency.

This has been motivated by the expanding application of ML in biology. The processing of biomedical signals and imaging difficulties can be solved using ML techniques. ML-enabled IoT (MIoT) can be developed to combine the most recent methodological and practical developments in machine learning (ML) for biomedical data.

18.1.3 MIoT model

IoT in healthcare enables data transfer, machine-to-machine communication, and information exchange. IoT-enabled sensors can detect every aspect of the patient, including their behavior, anatomy, and physiology (Taştan, 2018) in healthcare systems. IoT-based smart health monitoring systems (Bhardwaj et al., 2023) may trail a patient's blood pressure (BP), heart rate, oxygen capacity, and body temperature. They can then communicate with city hospitals about the patient's health problems and notify the doctor or physician as necessary. The Internet of Medical Things (IoMT) (Wagan et al., 2022) provides patients with affordable solutions and round-the-clock healthcare services and reliable real-time data to identify issues and find solutions immediately. Integrating IoT devices with ML can help us observe the contemporary climate of mechanical mechanization. The recent IoT medical treatment applications with ML capabilities can be implantable, portable IoT model devices that are studied for computing data transfer.

IoT and ML (IoTML or MIoT) offer insight for quicker, automatic responses, better decision-making, and predictive analytics. MIoT can gather and translate data into a standard format, construct an ML model, and disseminate the ML for the Healthcare cloud, edge, and devices. The smart health monitoring system based on MIoT can provide quicker, more affordable, and more dependable health monitoring services from remote places than traditional healthcare systems.

18.1.4 Objectives

The following are the objectives and key features of this chapter:

- To address the biomedical (i.e., healthcare) applications in a real-time background
- To highlight the latest modernizations, proposals, growths, and IoMT for healthcare data
- To provide an analytical solution to existing challenges in healthcare applications

- To discuss the MIoT-based remote healthcare monitoring systems
- To present case studies on the next-generation biomedical and health-care systems

18.1.5 Chapter organization

Section 18.2 discusses the resources and techniques used in this chapter, Section 18.3 presents the consequences and discussions as well as upcoming improvements, and Section 18.4 concludes this chapter.

18.2 MATERIALS AND METHODS

Biomedical applications may use technologies in the design and interaction of healthcare devices. Hence, this section describes smart healthcare systems, technologies, and data analytics. It outlines the architectural model, discusses the benefits, and illustrates examples.

18.2.1 Biomedical applications

Biomedical applications include medical transplants, dental supplies, anti-microbial agents, medication delivery systems, biomimetic actuators, wound dressings, scaffolds for enzyme immobilization, and safeguarding fabrics from biological and chemical dangers (Ghajarieh et al., 2021). Also, the critical biomedicine applications are genomics advancements, tissue engineering, organ-on-a-chip, nanotechnology, quantum dots, nanobots, etc.

Hence, biomedical research has evolved into a digital, data-intensive process dependent on scalable and smart networks, data storage, and smart computing infrastructure (Navale & Bourne, 2018). The data-intensive computing system (Lin et al., 2013) and cloud-based resources in bioinformatics can make the enormous diversity of data intelligible and useable.

18.2.2 Smart healthcare system

In biomedical applications, especially healthcare systems, there is an exponential increase in healthcare data intensifying human–machine interaction. Healthcare monitoring (Shalini, 2021) is a severe concern nowadays because, without adequate health monitoring, many people suffer the negative impacts of genuine medical conditions. Also, COVID-19 demonstrated that the healthcare system must accommodate the growing number of patients. Providing automated help systems, pervasive monitoring, and invisible diagnostics are key turning points in transforming healthcare applications using technology. Healthcare procedures (Trompert, 2020), Telehealth monitoring tools, and biosensors have improved sophistication, dependability, and accuracy.

Today, healthcare systems collect patient data, store it in a database, analyze it, and then offer remedies based on the findings using sensors, computers, and other technology. A smart healthcare information system is an intelligent healthcare network enabling information sharing between medical professionals, clinics, hospitals, pharmacies, research centers, and educational institutions. The design of smart healthcare systems incorporates *analytics*, *connectivity*, *security*, and *transparency*.

Innovative technologies can be used to design and implement smart healthcare monitoring devices for smart healthcare monitoring systems (Rahaman et al., 2019). Platforms and technologies for big data analytics, cloud storage, information sharing, integrated sensors, smart wearables, and sustainability computing are used in IoT-based digital health. Examples are IoT-based systems (Bhardwaj et al., 2023), IoT-based real-time healthcare monitoring systems (Khalaf et al., 2021), and GSM-based smart healthcare monitoring systems (Fathi Busedra et al., 2021). They may activate sensors, turn applications on or off, and monitor and gather patient data through sensors.

18.2.3 Healthcare technologies

The advent of Industry 4.0 and connected, robotic, and smart industries has led to their creation. The digital revolution (Borro et al., 2022) can interact closely with employees, smart machines, and smart products. Biotechnology and biomedical research can benefit from recent technical developments, the availability of the Internet, and the big data era. De Giovanni et al. (2013) discussed the openings for AI and edge or fog computing in smart biomedical sensors and the significant difficulties in designing wearable methods and healthcare monitoring. Technical advancements in ICT and AI, including virtual reality/augmented reality/extended reality (XR), can facilitate the diagnosis and prediction procedures. They predict the onset of sepsis and multiple organ failure. They increase the future robustness and prediction performance of systems like text analysis, generation, and image recognition. Various technologies used by healthcare systems are Cloud, IoT, ML, DL, predictive analytics, etc. Innovative technologies such as text analysis, creation, and picture recognition enhance future robustness and prediction performance. Over time, numerous methods and tools have been used to identify and manage these illnesses. Table 18.1 shows the diverse healthcare technologies and their applications.

ML: Healthcare institutions must provide services more effectively to contribute to the quality of life and stay relevant in business. ML has proved its efficacy in the healthcare sector and has much potential in this field. In the biomedical industry, ML enables academics and healthcare professionals to analyze and interpret massive volumes of complex data in previously impossible ways. ML technology may be supervised, semi-supervised, and unsupervised learning, as shown in Table 18.2, and used for prediction and classification purposes. They may be KNN, NB, DT, SVM, NN, RT (Gradient Boosted), and RF.

Table 18.1 Diverse healthcare technologies and their applications

S/N.	Technology	Purpose	Issues to be solved	Examples
1	Cloud computing (Sangfor Technologies, 2023)	Healthcare data storage	Share data, privacy, and security	Rackspace, AWS Cloud, Microsoft Cloud, and Google Cloud
2	Healthcare cloud (Mehrtak et al., 2021)	Data transfer	Data sharing, enhance patient privacy and high-quality care.	
3	Digital twin (Sura et al., 2023)	Sustainable medical science decisions	Sustainability	Healthcare simulation
4	Digital twin solution (Sun et al., 2023)	A solution for musculoskeletal system diseases	Real-time analysis and personalized medicine	–
5	Digital twin framework (Dimitris et al., 2021; Moztarzadeh et al. 2023)	Visualize (MRI) scans	The data-acquiring, AI-based investigation	AI
6	Digital twin model (Liinasuo et al., 2022)	Information model design	Data retrieval	XR
7	Medical twins (Chase et al., 2022)	Handle molecular/ time series data	Data analysis and simulation	–
8	Medical digital twins (Robert et al., 2022)	Computational model	Data analysis and simulation	Computing
9	Wearable technology (Wadhwa et al., 2022)	Supply chain management	Security and privacy	Management
0	Blockchain technology (Kuo Tsung-Ting, 2017)	Information sharing, with privacy preservation	Data management, supply chain management, pharma examination, monitoring, and payment systems	Secured transactions
11	Next-Gen AI and blockchain (Mamoshina et al., 2018)	Growing of data	Availability and scalability	Secured transactions
12	Blockchain platform (Kuo et al., 2021)	Sharing healthcare data		Secured transactions
13	e-Biomedical systems (Ahmed et al., 2019)	Sharing healthcare data	Improvement	Secured transactions
14	Blockchain-based healthcare (Khezr et al., 2019)	Review	Technologies and applications	Secured transactions

(Continued)

Table 18.1 (Continued)

S/N.	Technology	Purpose	Issues to be solved	Examples
15	Biomedical apps (George and Eleni, 2019).	Review	Technologies and applications	Secured transactions
16	Blockchain-based federated learning (Wadhwa et al., 2022)	Data acquisition and storage	Accuracy and security	Detecting COVID-19 patients
17	Secured healthcare apps (Arul & Prasanna, 2017)	Review	Attacks and countermeasures	Cybersecurity
18	Medical obstacles (Mamoshina et al., 2018)	Authority of healthcare data	Security of healthcare apps	
19	Big data in healthcare	Review	Handle huge volumes of data	Data analytics
20	Distributed ML model (Ed-daoudy & Maalmi, 2019)	Stream healthcare data procedures	Data steaming	Data flow
21	Big data analytical apps (Khanra et al., 2020; Batko & Ślęzak, 2022)	Data analytics	Data digest	Business view
22	Medical AI	Analysis of healthcare images	Intelligent data analysis and accuracy	Image analysis, CT scans, MRIs, X-rays, mammograms, etc.
23	Human-centric AI and XAI (Saraswat et al., 2022)	Study	Promotion of AI in healthcare research	AI apps
24	AI application (Alia et al., 2023)	Study	Promotion of AI in healthcare research	AI apps
25	Integrating XAI (Korica et al., 2021)	Application	Workflows, accountability, and safety	AI apps
26	XAI (Mohammed & Shehu, 2023)	Building of XAI systems	Trustworthiness	AI apps
27	XAI models (Amirian et al., 2023)	AI-powered predictive or descriptive models	Predive analysis	AI apps
28	AI model (Chaddad et al., 2023)	Make AI models trustworthy	Robustness, safety, confidentiality, management, openness, diversity, non-discrimination, justice, social, environmental, and transparency	AI apps

(Continued)

Table 18.1 (Continued)

S/N.	Technology	Purpose	Issues to be solved	Examples
29	ML approach (Kant et al., 2023)	Use cases	Complexity of data	Medical imaging, drug development, personalized medicine, EHRs, genomics, and wearable technology
30	Distributed ML model (Ed-daoudy & Maalmi, 2019)	Applications	Streaming health data events	Medical imaging, drug development, personalized medicine, EHRs, genomics, and wearable technology
31	DL-based smart solution (Arul & Prasanna, 2017)	Security	Securing healthcare systems	Safety

These models are employed in several cancer classification applications to diagnose cancer classifications accurately. To determine the patient's behavior patterns and clinical problems, they evaluate the data gathered from the monitoring device and additional data sources. Most ML models can use labeled and unlabeled datasets under specific conditions. Semi-supervised learning can make use of both labeled and unlabeled data. Labeled data are utilized in supervised learning, while unlabeled data are used in unsupervised learning.

Table 18.2 Classification of ML algorithms

ML		
Supervised learning (SL)	*Unsupervised learning (UL)*	*Semi-supervised learning (SSL)*
• Target variable (continuous and categorized)	• Target variable (categorized)	• Target variable (not available)
• Classification • Regression	• Clustering • Classification	• Associative rules • Clustering
• Decision trees (DT) • K-nearest neighbor (KNN) • Naive Bayes (NB) • Neural networks (NN) • Random forest (RF) • Regression tree (RT) • Support vector machine (SVM)	• Linear regressions • Logical regressions	• K-means clustering • Association rules

IoT: IoT improves biotechnological and biomedical research and its applications. The IoT is becoming a hot topic in healthcare systems due to the limited availability of medical resources, the aging population's need for remote monitoring due to chronic diseases, rising medical expenses, and the necessity for telemedicine in developing nations. The healthcare system, bioprocesses, and biomedical equipment technologies all may be enhanced by IoT. IoT-based technologies in healthcare (Vidhyalakshmi & Angelin, 2023), IoT-enabled biomedical applications (Aski et al., 2019), smart healthcare using IoT (Panchatcharam Shanmugasundaram, 2019), technological advances (Ali, 2019), WBAN (Akkaş et al., 2020), and IoT-enabled framework (Mir et al., 2022) can be effective in the early identification and prediction of the disease in a better way.

Also, IoMT-based BMS (Ahmed & Lanonaca, 2020) for various medical applications and the multiple directions in the healthcare sector (Akkaş et al., 2020) were presented in the development of Bio-IoT and Nano-IoT or Internet of Nano Things. The architecture (Akkaş et al., 2020) and HIoT systems (Mostafa et al., 2021) are identified and compared, and existing investigations are taxonomically classified in the IoT systems. Verma et al. (2021) focused on the biotechnological and biomedical aspects, and Katzis et al. (2022) identified the communication supplies for smart healthcare sensors and devices.

The IoT-enabled healthcare ecosystems may include hardware, software, physical objects, and computer devices to collect, share, and exchange data. However, the problem is that primary medical gadgets and sensors generate enormous volumes of data.

MIoT: MIoT can provide insights otherwise concealed in data for quicker, automatic reactions and better decision-making. Using MIoT, healthcare institutions may do predictive analytics on various use cases, giving the company new insights and cutting-edge automation capabilities. MIoT offers a range of remote healthcare facilities, disease prediction, and in-home diagnostics capabilities, which are increasingly accepted by the healthcare sectors. To help with disease diagnosis, prediction, and therapy recommendations, the MIoT links medical equipment, patient monitoring tools, and wearable devices and identifies diseases and diagnostics, medication discovery, tailored treatment, and smart health records. An MIoT (Kuppusamy et al., 2023) assists farmers in various smart agricultural activities. Similarly, designing an MIoT system for smart healthcare can assist stakeholders across multiple healthcare operations.

e-Healthcare Monitoring System (Godi et al., 2020), ML applications for IoT-based healthcare (Agarwal et al., 2021), MIoT-based healthcare apps (Chnar & Shavan, 2021), and AI and IoT convergence-based disease diagnosis model (Mansour et al., 2021) can identify conditions and diagnoses, drug discovery, personalized drug, and smart health records, significantly impacting healthcare delivery.

Healthcare Analytics: Healthcare analytics can potentially transform the management of patients' health on an individual and population level. These insights can predict and prevent disease outbreaks and improve patients' quality of care. Healthcare analytics (Batko & Ślęzak, 2022) can assist insurance firms with tracking current claims, clients, and premiums, monitoring open claims, adjusting policies, detecting fraud, and providing more impactful service pricing models. It falls under the descriptive, diagnostic, predictive, and prescriptive categories.

   i. *Descriptive analytics* may look at a virus's positive rate in a particular population over a specific period, which can assist in identifying how contagious a virus is.
   ii. *Diagnostic analytics* can determine if a patient has a sickness based on a patient's symptoms.
   iii. *Predictive analytics* can analyze historical data and estimate and forecast the prevalence of a seasonal disease like whooping cough.
   iv. *Prescriptive analytics* can forecast based on a patient's current health issues and adherence to medication guidelines.

With a better understanding of the hazards, healthcare professionals can develop unique, individual preventative treatment strategies. For healthcare analytics, the data is gathered from a variety of sources, including Electronic Health Records (EHRs), Personal Health Records (PHRs), Electronic Prescription Services (E-prescription), Patient data from the Healthcare Cloud, Master Patient Indexes (MPI), and Healthcare Apps.

18.2.4 Findings

Various technologies, sensing-equipped wearable devices, the Healthcare Cloud, and mobile apps produce vast amounts of data; increasing the speed of data collection, gathering, processing, and analyzing such vast quantities of data in real time, taking immediate action in an emergency, and uncovering hidden insights are challenging tasks in MIoT systems. They are utilizing limited and time-consuming conventional approaches. Substantial demand for real-time significant data stream processing (Ed-daoudy & Maalmi, 2019) can guarantee an efficient and scalable solution.

Improved architecture and models for real-time health analytics systems, leveraging advanced technologies and medical big data processing, are crucial to confirming an efficient and scalable solution. To address this problem, it suggests a novel architecture paradigm for real-time healthcare prediction and analytics systems utilizing MIoT technology.

18.3 RESULTS AND DISCUSSIONS

This section presents the results of the chapter, including the smart healthcare management system, the proposed model, case study, discussion, and future enhancements, with the conclusion.

18.3.1 Smart health management system

A typical Hospital Management System (HMS) communicates with the external world through different types of users or stakeholders. A Smart HMS (SHMS) can be integrated with the IoMT devices and connect with the homes, smart-assisted living, patients, and the patient's guardians. This seamless working from the device to a decision is the core working of SHMS. The stages of the MIoT model are data collection, pre-processing, categorization, and parameter adjustment. Wearables, sensors, and other IoT devices make it easy to collect data, and AI approaches use that data to diagnose diseases. Healthcare monitoring systems have been implemented to track patients' health via MIoT (Taştan, 2018). The healthcare system uploaded the EMRs, EHRs, and PHRs to the HealthCare Cloud server and immediately informed the concerned doctor.

Figure 18.1 shows the overall structure of the proposed MIoT-enabled Healthcare System. It includes the healthcare applications, storage, infrastructure, stakeholders, etc.

i. *Healthcare Applications:* The healthcare management/monitoring applications may be MIoT-enabled healthcare solutions, healthcare monitoring, remote healthcare monitoring, and healthcare management available in the Healthcare Cloud.
ii. *Healthcare Storage:* It includes healthcare data such as EMRs/EHRs, scanned data, etc.
iii. *Infrastructure:* It comprises 4G/5G, Bluetooth, Wireless/Wi-Fi/WBAN, Gateways, etc.
iv. *Stakeholders:* They are doctors, physicians, nurses, physiotherapists, patients with IMoTs, hospitals, primary health centers, medical labs, pharmacies, academic and research institutes, data display tools, Blood Banks, Mobile Apps, etc.

By connecting over the Internet and gaining access to information about their health state via wearable devices, they may provide more excellent medical assistance to patients even in the most distant areas without hospitals in their region.

18.3.2 Features

A smart health monitoring system (Kandhro et al., 2022) regularly manages patients' health with the help of a mobile health app.

i. The patient's real-time health parameters (heart rate, blood pressure, fasting glucose, random glucose, etc.) are sent to the Healthcare Cloud.
ii. The doctors and patients can view these details from anywhere/remote locations.

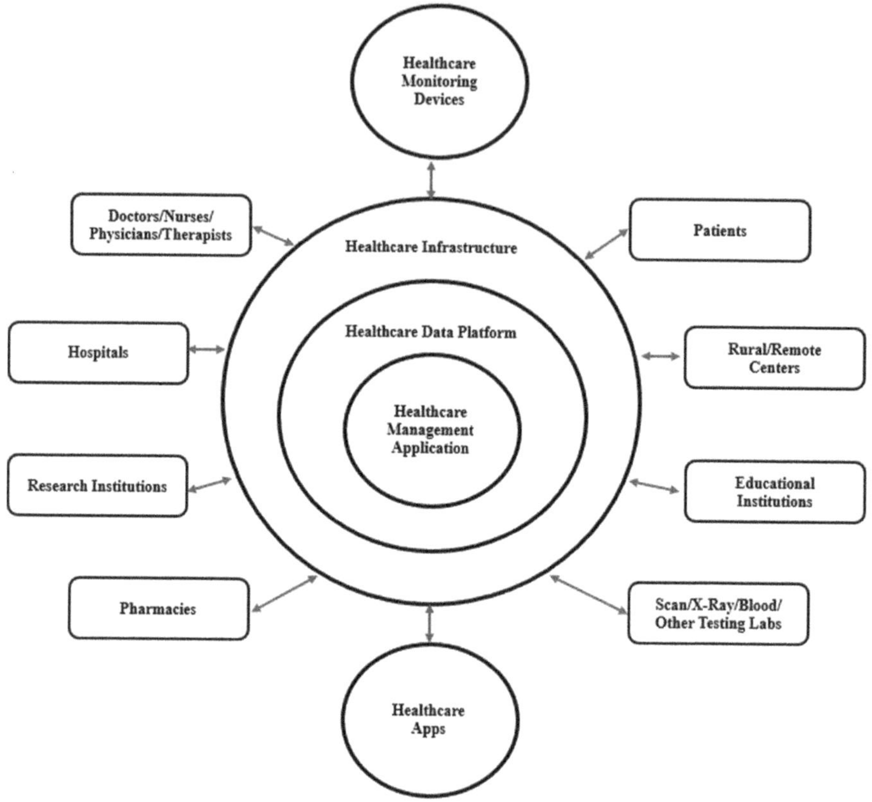

Figure 18.1 The structure of the proposed MIoT-enabled healthcare system.

   iii. Patients can store and later retrieve their medicines and medical records.

   iv. The patients can monitor their vital signs. The health parameters for GSM-based patient monitoring are supplied via SMS.

   v. The Mobile Apps illustrate nearby hospitals in case the patients want medical help.

   vi. Patients select the symptoms they wish to have predicted, and the application employs relevant algorithms to find specific diseases that match those symptoms in the symptoms-based disease identification technique.

   vii. It can provide an alert of a patient's critical condition sent to the doctor on the Internet.

   viii. The doctors can see patient health details by visiting a website/URL/Apps.

18.3.3 Design considerations

IMoT connectivity for medical equipment and sensors is crucial for healthcare monitoring systems. Hence, the design is considered scalability, interoperability, power management, cost, wireless capabilities, and secure storage.

a. *Cost:* It affords the cost of healthcare products with the newest technologies and updates.
b. *Interoperability:* It guarantees essential protection concerning interoperability concerns.
c. *Power Management:* It should be power-efficient by utilizing a long battery life.
d. *Scalability:* It has the scalability to accommodate the needs of expanding devices.
e. *Secure Storage:* It has a robust security mechanism that allows only authorized users to access it.
f. *Wireless Capabilities:* It provides a wireless facility that is widely accessible.

18.3.4 Healthcare services

With the above features, the proposed system can offer various services such as accounts and inventory management, drug management, garbage management, monitoring, rehabilitation, wheelchairs, etc.

- *Accounts and Inventory Management:* The accounting system manages the hospital's financial flow and ensures the right amounts of medications, critical supplies, and consumables. It maintains the hospitals' assets and repairing any damage.
- *Drug Management:* Drug management can track a patient's medicine; detect temperature, breathing, and heart rate; and show the patient's response to medications with the help of sensors.
- *Garbage Management:* The hospitals have Garbage full of germs and sharples. Hence, garbage management is responsible for carefully disposing of germs and sharples.
- *Monitoring Service:* It keeps track of conditions, including hypertension, heart arrhythmia, asthma, diabetes, dementia, and Alzheimer's, and the aged which is a significant task. Patients can check the availability of doctors without making a call by using sensors to track their health, raise the alarm (ambulance service), and monitor their condition.
- *Rehabilitation Management:* The IMoT devices collect data and send it to the Healthcare Cloud. The ML tools, coupled with the healthcare applications, provide feedback or warn clinicians regarding rehabilitation.
- *Wheelchair Management:* In hospitals, wheelchairs are crucial in supporting disabled people and toppling senior citizens from their chairs. Using the accelerometer and gyro-sensor, any jerk in the system can trigger the alarm.

MIoT model integrated with the sensors and devices allows people with disabilities to interact with the devices and offer the above services through a mobile app.

18.3.5 Architecture model for MIoT-enabled HMS

The MIoT healthcare system comprises numerous medical equipment that can communicate over a network to track and record patients' data in the Healthcare Cloud. The sensors and devices can collect heartbeat, body temperature, room temperature, and other data from the hospital environment and communicate the state of the patients to medical staff via a healthcare portal. The gathered data may be analyzed and utilized to forecast heart attacks and other ailments early, giving decision-makers an advantage and system notification to the doctor and family members.

Figure 18.2 depicts the architecture paradigm for the planned HMS utilizing MIoT. The model includes healthcare data presentation (visualization), medical data processing and storage, health monitoring/management applications, and medical data acquisition (medical devices and network layers). This system is made up of four layers: a data acquisition layer for gathering information from IMoT devices, a data layer for collecting the necessary information, an analytical layer for allowing connections between various data sources, processing the data, and performing calculations, and an application layer for creating and making the dashboard available to the user.

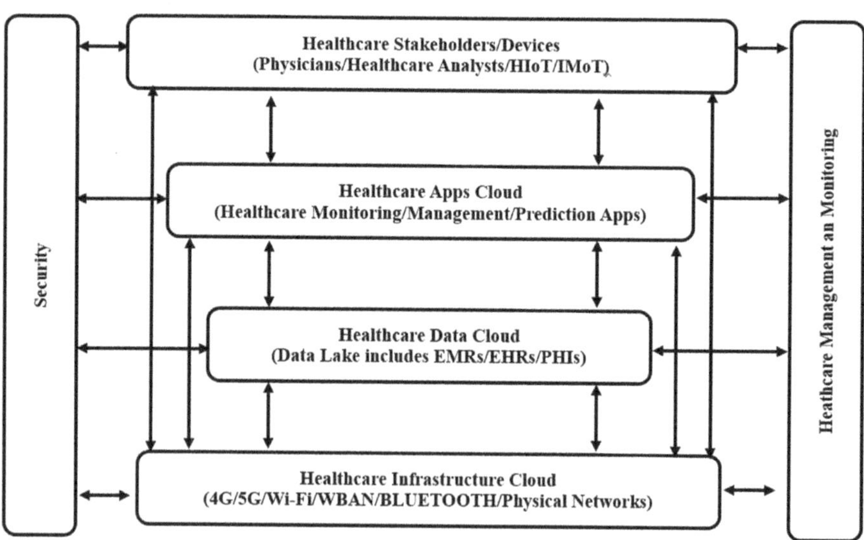

Figure 18.2 The architecture model of the proposed HMS using MIoT.

The IMoT environment (Islam et al., 2020) tracks a patient's vital signs and the state of the room in real time. It monitors patients' health in real time and alerts them in an emergency by employing healthcare bands (Chitra & Jayalakshm, 2022). In case of communication problems, ML-based analysis (regression analysis) of patients' sensory data (Alsareii et al., 2022) can obtain highly accurate predictions of the patients' sensory data.

Healthcare Data Acquisition Layer: It consists of three modules: *device*, *network*, and *Gateway*. In the *device model*, medical equipment and sensors can detect and gather health information from outside sources. These items could be gateways, actuators, sensor protocols, medical equipment, etc. The *network module* ensures that stakeholders and the data storage layer get data securely from devices with numerous communication protocols. Data must be sent as quickly as feasible when working with real-time data. The *Gateway* gathers all the data and transfers it to the storage layer. The Gateway can interpret and clean raw sensor data before sending it to the data storage layer. Devices integrated with healthcare applications and their functions are shown in Table 18.3.

The IoT devices and sensors may be used for patient monitoring, effective drug management, garbage management, tracking of depression, blood sugar levels, etc.

Table 18.3 Devices (d) and sensors (S) integrated with healthcare systems

S/No.	Name	Type	Functions
1	Accelerometer	D	Track body movement
2	Barometer pressure sensor	S	Measure changes in altitude
3	Blood clot tester	D	Send an alarm when the blood starts clotting and prevent brain strokes
4	Contact lenses	D	Monitor glucose levels
5	Glucose sensors	S	Monitor blood glucose
6	GPS-enabled smartwatches	D	Enable positioning, navigation, and timing
7	Gyroscopes	D	Measure rotation for many purposes
8	Hearing aids	D	Identify sounds in a noisy environment
9	Inhaler	S	Find a pattern of heavy breathing for asthmatic patients
10	Magnetometer	D	Improve tracking of patient movement
11	Optical blood flow sensor	S	Monitor heart rate and pulse
12	Pacemakers	D	Responds and monitors to heart activity
13	Pacemakers	D	Identify arrhythmia
14	Pulse rate sensor	S	Senses the amount of infrared light
15	Skin conductance sensor	S	Measure galvanic skin response
16	Temperature sensor	S	Determine exertion levels
17	Wireless cardiac monitor	S	Monitoring the heart patients

Healthcare Data Storage and Processing Layer: Healthcare Cloud servers receive the real-time data gathered from the medical equipment, pre-process it, and store it in the storage cloud for analysis. The storage cloud may offer a safe, scalable, and cost-effective solution.

Healthcare Data Analytical Layer: The analytical layer links various data sources, handles data processing, and runs computations to foretell the outcomes. This layer consists of several ML methods for data analysis and provides insightful results and forecasts using regression models. Based on the datasets, they deliver more accurate disease predictions – creating a decision tree that uses the datasets to produce regression models. For instance, the training and environment/weather information can predict the occurrence of an asthma condition.

Various ML algorithms (Aldahiri et al., 2021) such as ANN, association rule learning, Bayesian networks, clustering, DTs, inductive logic programming, K-means, KNNs, and computer vision, and DNNs provide intelligence to IoTML. Table 18.4 shows various IoTML algorithms (Aldahiri et al., 2021) and their corresponding healthcare applications that can be used in the proposed model.

Healthcare Data Presentation Layer: The healthcare application layer takes advantage of the data cloud's processed data. Healthcare management, monitoring, and healthcare applications could be found on the application layer. Doctors and patients receive application-specific services from the application layer. In this layer, the end users may access and see their solutions. Various tools are used to evaluate data for data visualization tools. Patients might use PCs, laptops, mobile phones, etc. to access the data.

18.3.6 Workflow of the model

The functioning of the proposed model is depicted in Figure 18.3a and 18.3b.

  i. Healthcare data can be captured with the help of medical sensors. The healthcare data sources include clinical text, electronic medical records (EMRs), electronic healthcare records (EHRs), public healthcare records (PHRs), hospital data, biomedical images, medical device readings, genomic data, biomedical signals, and sensing data.

  ii. The captured data are then directly forwarded to the healthcare cloud for storage and decision-making.

    a. The data platform performs the pre-processing and converts it into the datasets.

    b. The datasets are available in the scalable Data Lake or data cloud.

    c. The datasets made for information discourse can make better policy decisions.

Table 18.4 Various IoTML algorithms and the corresponding healthcare applications

S/No.	Healthcare applications	Methods/Algorithms	Type	Datasets	Remarks	Purpose/Remarks
1	Behavioral modification (or treatment)	BNC, DT, and SVM	SL and UL	Human behavior data	To evaluate each person's behavior and recommendations	Evaluation and recommendation
2	Clinical trials	ML	SL	Clinical and biomedical datasets/sensor data	To avoid harm to the patients	Assessment
3	Diagnosis of disease	SVM, DL, CNN, BPN	SL and UL	Image, time series, demographics, gene expression, symptoms	To improve diagnosis efficiency and accuracy	Diagonation
4	Drug management	(ML/DL) XGBOOST, pGBRT	SL	Pain, acne, anxiety, blood pressure	To recommend drugs	Data reliability, data transparency, and drug data flow
5	EHRs	ANN, LLR, & SVM	SL and UL	Sensor data	To offer quality care	To assess patient data, recommend treatment, and decision-making
6	Epidemic outbreak prediction	LSTM and DNN	SL	Clinical data and sensor data	To predict diseases	To predict future disease trends
7	Garbage management	(DL) CNN	UL	Moisture and garbage	Efficient garbage management	To save the environment
8	Health monitoring system	K-means, SVM, and NN	SL	Sensor data	To assess the technologies	To increase efficiency, decrease expenses, and improve the quality of care

(Continued)

Table 18.4 (Continued)

S/No.	Healthcare applications	Methods/Algorithms	Type	Datasets	Remarks	Purpose/Remarks
9	Heart disease prediction	NB, K-NN, SVM, DT, and decision tables	SL	Clinical datasets	To predict heart disease	To assess patient data and project the prevalence of heart disease
10	Medical imaging	ANN, CNN	SL	MRI, X-ray, and CT scans	To increase promptness of disease detection, diagnosis, and prediction	To aid in diagnosis and treatment
11	Personalized care	ML	SL	Clinical and sensor datasets	To review patient data, customized care, and action	To improve health services
12	Rehabilitation management	ML and DL	SL \and UL	Motion-capturing, activity-tracking, and social behaviors	To incorporate new digital technologies into rehabilitation	To optimize and reduce the disability of individuals
13	Wheelchair management	ML and DL	SL	GPS/GPRS	To enable monitoring and provide accessibility	To enable remote operations

Abbreviations: BNC – Bayes network classifier, BP – blood pressure, DT – decision trees, SVM – support vector machine, DL – deep learning, CNN – convolutional neural networks, BPN – backpropagation networks, LLR – linear and logistic regression, ANN – artificial neural networks, LSTM – long short-term memory, DNN – deep neural network, NB – naive Bayes, XGBOOST – extreme gradient boosting, pGBRT – parallel gradient boosting regression trees, GPS – Global Positioning System, GPRS – General Packet Radio Services, SL – supervised learning, UL – unsupervised learning, SSL – semi-supervised learning.

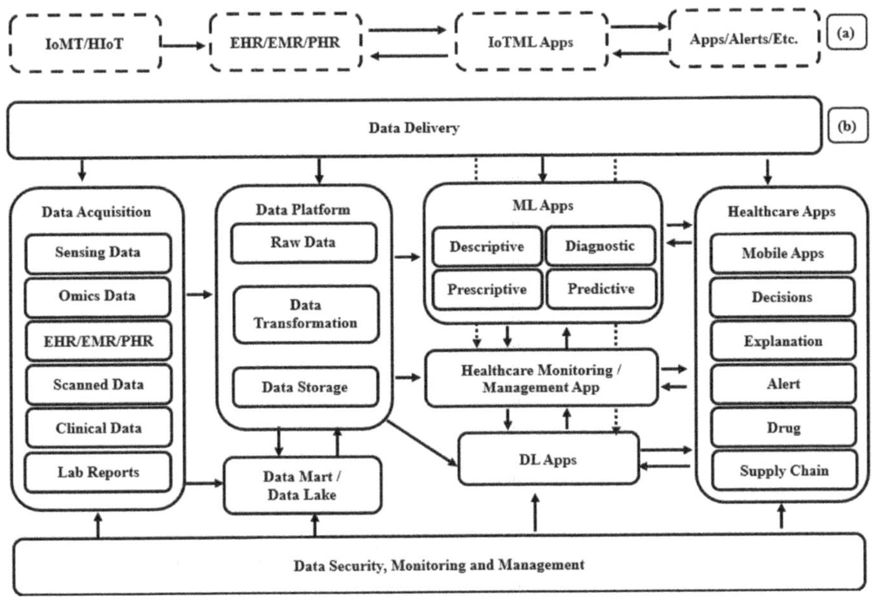

Figure 18.3 (a) Various modules and their functions in the proposed model. (b) The overall structure of the proposed model.

iii. With the arrival of data clouds or lake and their implicity, the automation of all clinical tests and medical histories in the healthcare systems has become a standard and extensively taken into practice today. For example, analyzing genomic data gives people a broader understanding of the connections among different inheritable labels and disease conditions.

iv. Clinical text mining converts data from clinical notes (unstructured format) into useful information. Information recovery and natural language processing (NLP) methods can uproot valuable data from large volumes of clinical text.

Figure 18.4 shows the multi-cloud structure of the proposed MIoT Healthcare mode. It comprises sensor data cloud, healthcare data storage, data analytical clouds (for ML and DL), healthcare apps cloud, and healthcare delivery cloud.

Medical Apps: Medical apps monitor activities, including walking and running, active energy, flights, workouts, meditation data, and sleep analysis. They can be integrated with smartphones to track the patients' daily activities. They provide everyone with constant access to medical records.

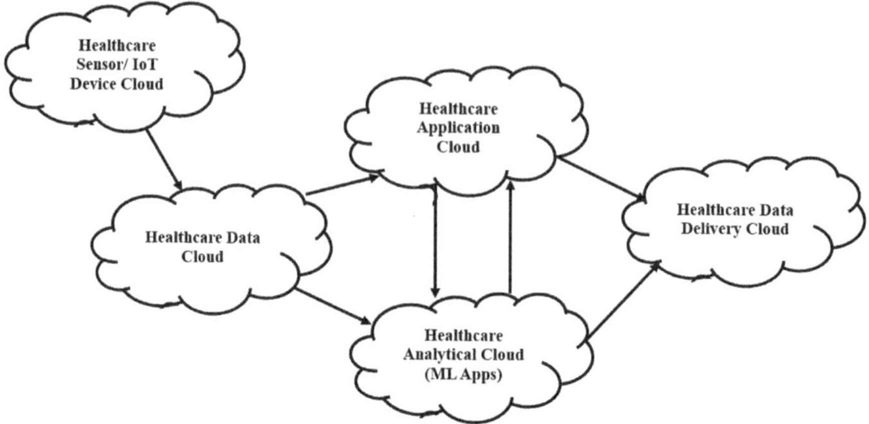

Figure 18.4 The multi-cloud structure of the proposed model.

Example: A smartwatch might continuously record the patient's heart-beat and pulse rate, and the mobile app records the measurement. The gathered information is subsequently uploaded to the Cloud, where the Healthcare app can display several visualization charts to highlight the data's progress. Additionally, it can provide us with security alerts if it notices abnormally high heartbeat rates. This can help users take safety steps in an emergency and even save their lives.

Advantages: The proposed model can reduce the time and expense of assistance by reducing the effort of experts. With this model, smart health monitoring apps (Hassan et al., 2023) can rapidly offer remote healthcare support and advanced developing technologies. The patient's data can be continually tracked by wearable technology and IMoT sensors, and the data can be controlled, tracked, and saved on a Healthcare Cloud server (Rahaman et al., 2019). This can facilitate effortless interaction among various healthcare modules. Automation, better patient care, flexibility, more efficiency, and fewer readmissions are some advantages of MIoT technology.

Challenges: There may be challenges with the large volume of data obtained from IMoT devices (Neeta, 2020). Some common challenges IoT faces may be battery limitations, computation speed, scalability, memory constraints, communication channels, and security. The security may attack devices, communication channels, and the healthcare cloud. The diverse challenges when applying technologies in healthcare (Chaddad et al., 2023) and wearable (Chowdhury et al., 2020) and implantable healthcare BAN may face several challenges (Chnar & Shavan, 2021).

18.4 FUTURE WORKS

Efficient healthcare systems can combine healthcare, data analytics, communication, embedded systems, and information security. Healthcare institutions must develop effective health forecasting systems using wearable technology and the IoT advance, and more data may become available. With this knowledge, healthcare organizations and marketers can use healthcare analytics to discover and keep patients most likely to need medical care. Sustaining a generic model and using the same platform to gather shared data from various devices can make the server prone to bias and failure, which makes storing data in a unified healthcare cloud problematic for ML. This could lead to an imprecise trained model and diminish the anticipated output's precision.

The developments in deep learning and neural networks (Kant et al., 2023), the advent of federated education, the integration of advanced technologies, and improved collaboration between ML and biomedical experts are nearly the future directions for ML in the biomedical field. Considering these variables, forthcoming 5G and IoT devices may relate to smart healthcare networks to improve network performance and cellular coverage while addressing security-related issues.

18.5 CONCLUSION

Biomedical involves using technology on living things, particularly in creating and using medical equipment. Biomedical and Health Informatics conveys incredible openings and addresses challenges due to ample accessible biomedical data. Healthcare is rapidly changing from a fragmented, patient-centric strategy to an antiquated hospital and specialist-focused one. Smart healthcare systems have excellently been accomplished in various areas of health informatics. The healthcare industry is rapidly changing due to advancements in communication and healthcare technologies, which also enable the provision of individualized and distant healthcare services.

Healthcare data supports the healthcare sector's ability to use data analytics in making strategic business decisions by enabling the digitalization of healthcare data and the emergence of value-based care. With cutting-edge breakthroughs in the biomedical and healthcare fields, MIoT is significantly improving. The healthcare system can gather, store, and analyze patient data and test results using cutting-edge technology to generate valuable insights. These advanced technologies and predictive analytics enable regular and frequent monitoring of the patient's health status – continuous patient monitoring made possible by MIoT results in vast data gathering in data lakes and warehouses. With the data repositories, healthcare organizations can combine healthcare insight to attract and keep patients by providing the best medical treatment.

18.5.1 Key terms

1. Cloud platforms may be Microsoft Azure, Thingworx, Google Cloud, AWS, IBM Watson, Salesforce, Cisco Cloud Connect, Oracle, and Kaa.
2. Communication protocols may include CoAP, DTLS, MQTT, IPv6, LPWAN, Zigbee, Bluetooth Low Energy, Z-Wave, RFID, NFC, Cellular, satellite, Wi-Fi, and Ethernet.
3. Patient-centered healthcare data include medical, dental, surgical, and behavioral data (diet), biometrics (BP), living conditions, etc.
4. Tissue engineering is restoring, maintaining, or improving damaged tissues or whole organs.

REFERENCES

Agarwal Neha, Singh Pushpa, et al. (2021). Machine Learning Applications for IoT Healthcare, Krishna Kant Singh, Akansha Singh, Sanjay Sharma (eds), Machine Learning Approaches for Convergence of IoT and Blockchain, Scrivener Publishing LLC. doi:10.1002/9781119761884.ch6

Ahmed Faeq Hussein, Abbas K Alszubaidi et al. (2019). An Adaptive Biomedical Data Managing Scheme Based on Blockchain Technique, *Applied Sciences*, 9, 2494. doi: 10.3390/app9122494

Ahmed Imran, Lanonaca Francesco (2020). Recent Development in IoMT-based Biomedical Measurement Systems: A Review, 24th International, Symposium & 22nd International Workshop on ADC and DAC Modelling and Testing, IMEKO TC-4, Italy.

Akkaş Mustafa Alper, Sokullu Radosveta, Ertürk Çetin Hüseyin (2020). Healthcare and Patient Monitoring Using IoT, *Internet of Things*, 11, 100173. doi: 10.1016/j.iot.2020.100173

Aldahiri Amani, Alrashed Bashair, Hussain Walayat. (2021). Trends in Using IoT with Machine Learning in Health Prediction Systems. *Forecasting*, 3, 181–206. doi: 10.3390/forecast3010012

Ali Mohammad Alqudah (2019). The Internet of Things in Healthcare: A Survey for Architecture, Current and Future Applications, Mobile Application, and Security, *International Journal on Informatics Visualization*, 3(2), 113–122.

Alia Omar, Abdelbaki Wiem, Shrestha Anup, et al. (2023). A Systematic Literature Review of Artificial Intelligence in the Healthcare Sector: Benefits, Challenges, Methodologies, and Functionalities, *Journal of Innovation & Knowledge*, 8 (2023), 100333.

Alsareii Saeed Ali, Raza Mohsin, Alamri Abdulrahman Manaa, et al. (2022). Machine Learning and Internet of Things Enabled Monitoring of Post-Surgery Patients: A Pilot Study, *Sensors*, 22(4):1420. doi: 10.3390/s22041420

Amirian Soheyla, Carlson Luke A, et al. (2023). Explainable AI in Orthopedics: Challenges, Opportunities, and Prospects. doi:10.48550/arXiv.2308.04696

Arora Shivam, Goel Amita (2020). IoT Smart Health Monitoring System. Proceedings of the International Conference on Innovative Computing & Communications. doi:10.2139/ssrn.3602545

Arul Treesa Mathew, Prasanna Mani (2017). Strength of Deep Learning-based Solutions to Secure Healthcare IoT: A Critical Review, *The Open Biomedical Engineering Journal*, 2023. doi: 10.2174/18741207-v17-e230505-2022-HT28-4371-2

Aski Vidyadhar Jaiput, Gupta Shashank, Sarkar Bharat. (2019). An Authentication-centric Multi-layered Security Model for Data Security in IoT-enabled Biomedical Applications. *IEEE 8th Global Conference on Consumer Electronics*, pp. 957–960.

Batko Kornelia, Ślęzak Andrzej. (2022). The Use of Big Data Analytics in Healthcare, *Journal of Big Data*, 9(1):3. doi: 10.1186/s40537-021-00553-4

Bhardwaj Vaneeta, Joshi Rajat, Gaur Anshu Mili. (2023). IoT-based Smart Health Monitoring System for COVID-19, *SN Computer Science*, 3(2):137. doi: 10.1007/s42979-022-01015-1

Bhatia Dinesh, Mishra Animesh, et al. (2022). Blockchain Technology for Biomedical Engineering Applications, Applications of Blockchain and Big IoT Systems, 1st edition, Imprint Apple Academic Press, p. 22

Borro Diego, Zachmann Gabriel, Giannini Franca, et al. (2022). Editorial: Digital Twin for Industry 4.0, *Frontiers in Virtual Reality*, 3:968054. doi: 10.3389/frvir.2022.968054

Chaddad Ahmad, Peng Jihao, Xu Jian, Bouridane Ahmad (2023). Survey of Explainable AI Techniques in Healthcare, *Sensors*, 23, 634. doi: 10.3390/s23020634

Chase Cockrell, Schobel-McHugh Seth, et al. (2022). Generating Synthetic Data with a Mechanism-based Critical Illness Digital Twin: Demonstration for Post Traumatic Acute Respiratory Distress Syndrome. doi: 10.1101/2022.11.22.517524

Chitra S, Jayalakshm V (2022). Smart Health Monitoring System of Patients through Internet of Things, *Journal of Algebraic Statistics*, 13(3), 424–432.

Chnar Mustafa, Shavan Askar (2021). Machine Learning for IoT HealthCare Applications: A Review. doi: 10.5281/zenodo.4496904

Chowdhury Muhamad EH, Khandakar Amit, Yazan Qibiawey, et al. (2020). Machine Learning in Wearable Biomedical Systems. IntechOpen. doi: 10.5772/intechopen.93228

De Giovanni Elisabetta, Forooghifar Farnaz, et al. (2013). Intelligent Edge Biomedical Sensors in the Internet of Things Era, MMS Aly and A. Chattopadhyay (eds.), Emerging Computing: From Devices to Systems, Computer Architecture and Design Methodologies, 407–433. doi: 10.1007/978-981-16-7487-7_13

Dimitris Mourtzis, John Angelopoulos, et al. (2021). A Smart IoT Platform for Oncology Patient Diagnosis based on AI: Towards the Human Digital Twin, *Procedia CIRP* 104(2), 1686–1691. doi: 10.1016/j.procir.2021.11.284

Ed-daoudy Abderrahmane, Maalmi Khalil (2019). A New Internet of Things Architecture for Real-time Prediction of Various Diseases Using Machine Learning on Big Data Environment. *Journal of Big Data* 6, 104. doi: 10.1186/s40537-019-0271-7

Fathi Busedra Hanan, Fathi Abusedra Lamia, et al. (2021). Smart Health Monitoring System Using GSM Technique. *7th International Conference on Engineering & MIS 2021*, 56, pp. 1–7. doi: 10.1145/3492547.3492636

George Drosatos, Eleni Kaldoudi (2019). Blockchain Applications in the Biomedical Domain: A Scoping Review, *Computational and Structural Biotechnology Journal*, Vol. 17, 229–240, https://doi.org/10.1016/j.csbj.2019.01.010.

Ghajarieh Amir, Habibi Sima, Talebian Aazam (2021). Biomedical Applications of Nanofibers. *Russian Journal of Applied Chemistry*, 94, 847–872. doi: 10.1134/S1070427221070016

Godi Brahmaji, Viswanadham Sangeetha, Muttipati AS, et al. (2020). e-Healthcare Monitoring System Using IoT with Machine Learning Approaches. *International Conference on Computer Science, Engineering and Applications*, pp. 1–5. doi: 10.1109/ICCSEA49143.2020.9132937

Hassan Mahedi, Rahman Lata Tuchi, et al. (2023). IoT-Based Smart Health Monitoring System for Efficient Service in the Medical Sector, *International Journal of Engineering Trends and Technology*, 71(4), 159–170. doi: 10.14445/22315381/IJETT-V71I4P215

Islam Md Milon, Rahaman Ashikur, Islam Md Rrashedul (2020). Development of Smart Healthcare Monitoring System in IoT Environment, *SN Computer Science* 1, 185. doi: 10.1007/s42979-020-00195-y

Kandhro Irfan Ali, Ali Fayyaz, Ashraf Syeda Nazia, et al. (2022). Smart Health Monitoring System (SHMS) an Enabling Technology for Patient Care, *Journal of Pharmaceutical Research International*, 34(27A), 19–30. doi: 10.9734/jpri/2022/v34i27A35990

Kant Rama, Singh Sanjiv Kumar, et al. (2023). Application of Machine Learning in Biomedical Field, *Scandinavian Journal of Information Systems*, 35(1). doi: 10.5281/zenodo.7808236

Katzis Konstaantinos, Berbakov Lazar, et al., (2022). Breaking Barriers in Emerging Biomedical Applications. *Entropy (Basel)*. 24(2):226. doi: 10.3390/e24020226

Khalaf Osamah Ibrahim, Khan Mohammad Monirujjaman, Antu Shaha, et al. (2021). IoT-based Smart Health Monitoring System for COVID-19 Patients, *Computational and Mathematical Methods in Medicine*. doi: 10.1155/2021/8591036

Khanra Sayantan, Dhir Amandeep, et al. (2020). Big Data Analytics in Healthcare: A Systematic Literature Review, *Enterprise Information Systems*, 14:7, 878–912, doi: 10.1080/17517575.2020.1812005

Khezr Seyednima, Moniruzzaman Md, et al. (2019). Blockchain Technology in Healthcare: A Comprehensive Review and Directions for Future Research, *Applied Sciences* 9 (9): 1736. doi: 10.3390/app9091736

Korica Petra, Elgayar Neamat, Pang Wei (2021). Explainable Artificial Intelligence in Healthcare: Opportunities, Gaps and Challenges and a Novel Way to Look at the Problem Space. In D. Camacho, P. Tino, and R, Allmendinger, et al. (eds), Intelligent Data Engineering and Automated Learning. L S in Computer Science, vol. 13113, pp. 333–342. doi: 10.1007/978-3-030-91608-4_33

Kuo Tsung-Ting (2017). Blockchain Distributed Ledger Technologies for Biomedical and Health Care Applications, *Journal of the American Medical Informatics Association*, 24(6), 1211–1220. doi:10.1093/jamia/ocx068

Kuo Tsung-Ting, Bath Tyler Ma Shuaicheng, Pattengale Nicholas, et al. (2021). Benchmarking Blockchain-based Gene–Drug Interaction Data Sharing Methods: A Case Study from the iDASH 2019 Secure Genome Analysis Competition Blockchain Track. *International Journal of Medical Informatics*, 154, 104559. doi: 10.1016/j.ijmedinf.2021.104559

Kuppusamy Palanivel, et al. (2023). Machine Learning-enabled Internet of Things Solution for Smart Agriculture Operations, Neha Goel and Ravindra Kumar Yadav (eds.), *Handbook of Research on Machine Learning-enabled IoT for Smart Applications across Industries*, IGI Global, pp. 84–115. doi: 10.4018/978-1-6684-8785-3.ch005

Liinasuo Marja, Timo Kuula, Goriachev *et al.* (2022). Building's Digital Twin Model Shown as First-Person and Third-Person Views, *IOP Conference Series: Earth and Environmental Science*, 1101, 082018. doi: 10.1088/1755-1315/1101/8/082018

Lin Chun-Yuan, Lin Ying-Chih, et al. (2013). Enabling Large-scale Biomedical Analysis in the Cloud, *BioMed Research International*, 85679, 6 pp. doi: 10.1155/2013/185679

Mamoshina Polina, Ojomoko Lucy, Yanovich Yury, et al. (2018). Converging Blockchain and Next-generation Artificial Intelligence Technologies to Decentralize and Accelerate Biomedical Research and Healthcare, *Oncotarget*, 9(5), 5665–5690.

Mansour Romany Fouad, Adnen El Amraoui, Issam Nouaouri, et al. (2021). Artificial Intelligence and Internet of Things Enabled Disease Diagnosis Model for Smart Healthcare Systems. *IEEE Access*, 9 (2021): 45137–45146.

Mehrtak Mohammad, SeyedAlinaghi SyedAhmad, et al. (2021). Security Challenges and Solutions Using Healthcare Cloud Computing. *Journal of Medicine and Life*, 14(4): 448–461. doi: 10.25122/jml-2021-0100

Mir Mahmood Hussain, Jamwal Sanjay, et al. (2022). IoT-enabled Framework for Early Detection and Prediction of COVID-19 Suspects by Leveraging Machine Learning in Cloud, *Journal of Healthcare Engineering.*, 2022, 7713939, 16 pp. doi: 10.1155/2022/7713939

Mohammed K, Shehu A. (2023). A Review of Artificial Intelligence Challenges and Future Prospects of Explainable AI in Major Fields: A Case Study of Nigeria, *Open Journal of Physical Science*, 4(1), 1–18. doi: 10.52417/ojps.v4i1.458

Mostafa Haghi Kashani, Madanipour Mona, et al. (2021). A Systematic Review of IoT in Healthcare: Applications, Techniques, and Trends, *Journal of Network and Computer Applications*, 192, 103164. doi: 10.1016/j.jnca.2021.103164

Moztarzadeh Omid, Jamshidi Mohammad, Saleh Sargozizaaei, et al. (2023). Metaverse and Healthcare: Machine Learning–enabled Digital Twins of Cancer. *Bioengineering.* 10(4), 455. doi: 10.3390/bioengineering10040455

Navale Vivek, Bourne PE. (2018). Cloud Computing Applications for Biomedical Science: A Perspective. *PLoS Computational Biology* 14(6): e1006144. doi: 10.1371/journal.pcbi.1006144

Panchatcharam Parthasarathy, Shanmugasundaram Vivekanandan (2019). Internet of Things (IoT) in Healthcare: Smart Health and Surveillance, Architectures, Security Analysis, and Data Transfer. *International Journal of Software Innovation*, 7(2), 21–40. doi: 10.4018/ijsi.2019040103

Rahaman Ashikur, Islam Md. Milon, Md. Rashedul Islam, et al. (2019). Developing IoT Based Smart Health Monitoring Systems: A Review. *Revue d'Intelligence Artificielle*, 33(6), 435–440. doi: 10.18280/ria.330605

Rahman Anichur, Hossain Md. Sazzad, Muhammad Ghulam, et al. (2022). Federated Learning-based AI Approaches in Smart Healthcare: Concepts, Taxonomies, Challenges, and Open Issues. *Cluster Computing*, 1–41. doi: 10.1007/s10586-022-03658-4

Sangfor Technologies (2023). Cloud Computing in the Healthcare Industry. https://www.sangfor.com/blog/cloud-and-infrastructure/cloud-computing-healthcare-industry

Saraswat Deepti, Bhattacharya Pronaya, Verma Ashwin, et al. (2022). Explainable AI for Healthcare 5.0: Opportunities and Challenges, *IEEE Access*, 10, 84486–84517. doi: 10.1109/ACCESS.2022.3197671

Shalini VB (2021). "Smart Health Care Monitoring System based on Internet of Things (IoT)," *2021 International Conference on Artificial Intelligence and Smart Systems (ICAIS)*, India, pp. 1449–1453, doi: 10.1109/ICAIS50930.2021.9396019.

Shiva Kumar V, Vinit K, et al. (2022). Smart Health Monitoring System, *International Journal of Advanced Research in Science, Communication and Technology*, 2(9), 384–388. doi: 10.48175/IJARSCT-5359

Sujith AVLN, Sajja Guna Sekhar, Mahalakshmi V et al. (2022). A Systematic Review of Smart Health Monitoring Using Deep Learning and Artificial Intelligence, *Neuroscience Informatics*, 2(3), 100028. doi: 10.1016/j.neuri.2021.100028

Sun Tianze, Wang Jinzuo, Suo Moran, et al. (2023). The Digital Twin: A Potential Solution for the Personalized Diagnosis and Treatment of Musculoskeletal System Diseases. *Bioengineering*, 10(6):627. doi: 10.3390/bioengineering10060627

Sura Hema Shreaya, Avesh Mohd, Mohapatra Swati (2023). Design and Modelling of Digital Twin Technology to Improve Freight Logistics, Transportation Energy and Dynamics, Springer Nature, Singapore.

Tao Hai, Bhuiyan Md Zhakirul, Abdalla AN, et al. (2019). Secured Data Collection with Hardware-based Ciphers for IoT-based Healthcare. *IEEE Internet of Things Journal*, 6, 410–420.

Taştan Mehmet (2018). IoT based Wearable Smart Health Monitoring System, *Celal Bayar University Journal of Science*, 14(3), 343–350.
Trompert Jack (2020). The Most Critical Biomedical Applications Now and in the Future. https://www.talent-101.com/blog/the-most-critical-biomedical-applications-now-and-in-the-future
Verma Vijay, Sharma Shreya, et al. (2021). Internet of Things: Frontier and Panorama for Biotechnology and Biomedical Applications, *International Journal of Biotech Trends and Technology*, 10(1):42–49. doi: 10.14445/22490183/IJBTT-V10I1P607
Vidhyalakshmi A, Angelin Jeba Malar J (2023). A Study on Internet of Things Based on Biomedical Applications, *European Chemical Bulletin*, 12(6), 4697–4711.
Wadhwa Shivani, Saluja Kamal, et al. (2022). Blockchain-based Federated Learning Approach for Detection of COVID-19 Using IoMT. doi: 10.2139/ssrn.4159195
Wagan Shiraz Ali, Koo Jahwan, et al. (2022). Internet of Medical Things and Trending Converged Technologies: A Comprehensive Review on Real-time Applications, *Journal of King Saud University – Computer and Information Sciences*, 34(10), 9228–9251. doi:10.1016/j.jksuci.2022.09.005
Wang Chan, He Tianyiyi, Zhou Hong, *et al.* (2023). Artificial Intelligence Enhanced Sensors: Enabling Technologies to Next-Generation Healthcare and Biomedical Platform, *Bioelectronic Medicine*, 9, 17. doi: 10.1186/s42234-023-00118-1

Machine learning–enabled IoT for biomedical applications

Problem and challenges

Hashmat Usmani and Renu Rani

19.1 INTRODUCTION

Recent years have seen a major expansion of the biomedical systems, which has increased employment and income. In the past, the only method available to diagnose illnesses and abnormalities in the human body was a physical examination. For the course of their therapy, the majority of patients had to remain in the hospital. Biomedical costs have increased as a result, and biomedical facilities in remote and rural locations are overworked. Thanks to technological breakthroughs, it is now possible to diagnose many illnesses and monitor health using tiny sensors placed in wristbands. Advancements in technology have completely transformed the biomedical system, shifting its focus from hospitals to patients [1]. Many medical tests, such as blood pressure and blood glucose levels, can be performed at home without the help of a biomedical specialist. Advanced computing technology can be used to deliver clinical data from remote places to biomedical centers. In the field of biomedicine, Internet of Things (IoT) and machine learning (ML) have immense potential to transform healthcare. It is also critical to understand the issues and difficulties with ML-enabled IoT in biomedical applications [2].

19.2 ML TECHNIQUES USED IN BIOMEDICAL APPLICATIONS

The most popular artificial intelligence (AI) technique for deriving predictions from patterns is ML.

ML may be further categorized into many types based on the learning method and algorithm structure (Figure 19.1).

There are three further categories for learning methods – supervised, unsupervised, and reinforced learning (Figure 19.1). The method is trained with input data in supervised learning. Applications where past data is accessible and may be utilized to forecast potential future events employ supervised learning. Because these algorithms are trained on historical data, the techniques are more precise and uncomplicated. Regression and classification algorithms are subsets

DOI: 10.1201/9781003487647-19

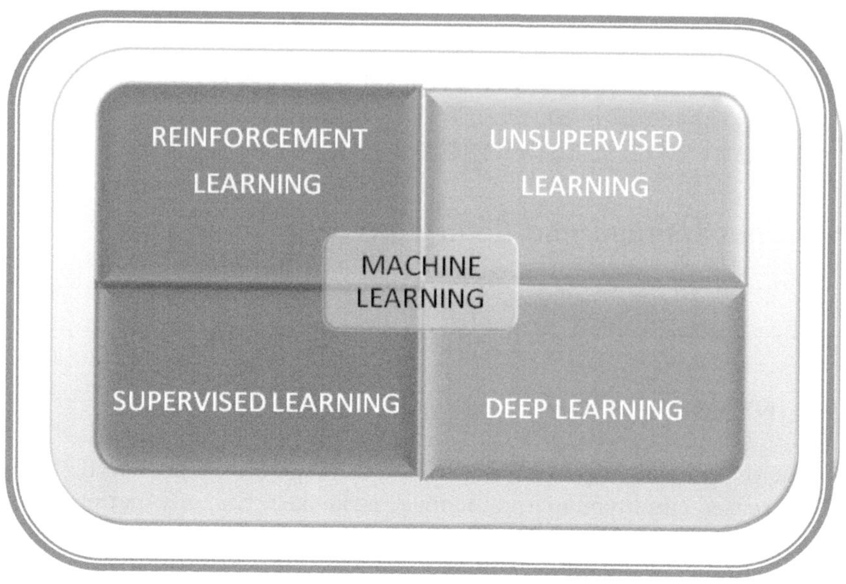

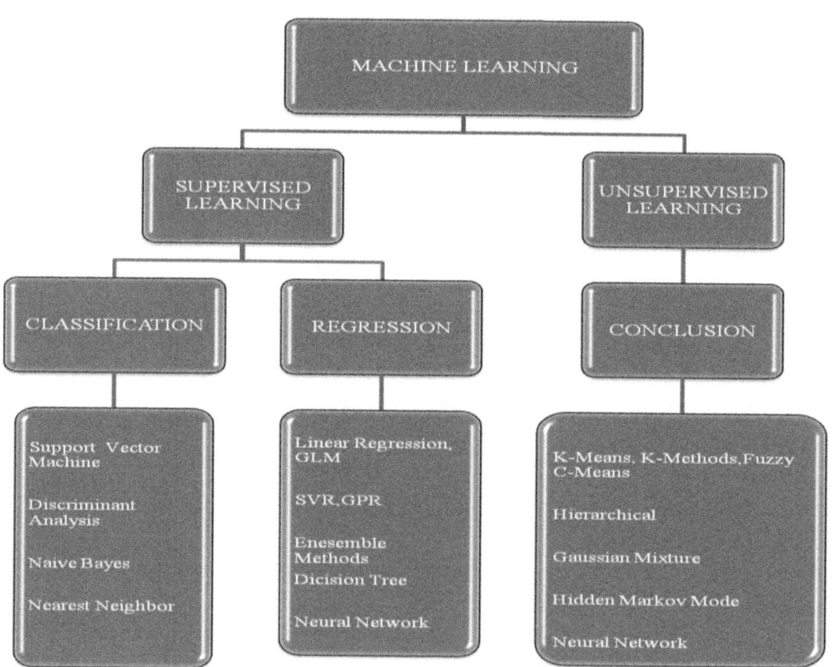

Figure 19.1 Schematic representation of relation between AI, ML, and DL and classification of ML algorithm.

of these methods. When there is a link between the input and output variables, like in weather forecasting, regression techniques can be applied. Regarding input variables, output variables in classification algorithms can be divided into classes like true–false and yes–no. These characteristics allow supervised learning to forecast the result based on available data and solve real-world problems. In each dataset, unsupervised learning techniques can find a pattern even in cases where the data are incorrectly categorized or labeled.

Algorithms become less accurate and more computationally complex in this direction. These algorithms are able to sort data according to the similarities and differences between the data. These fall into one of two categories – association (b) or clustering (a). Within the clustering algorithms group, product marketing is aided by data grouped according to commonalities, such as a consumer base's purchasing patterns. An association algorithm is a rule-learning algorithm that identifies links between variables in each dataset, such as individual customers' buying habits to provide product recommendations to customers. A reward-and penalty-based learning approach is called reinforced learning. Algorithms give unwanted effects a negative value and desired results a positive value. These algorithms require a lot of time and effort to train. One subset of ML that trains computers to imitate human behavior is called deep learning (DL). Neural networks (NN), which are used in DL, demand a lot of processing power to solve complex problems. But recent advances in data analytics and processing power have allowed DL algorithms to see, understand, and respond to challenging circumstances. Depending on the intended use, the DL algorithm can use supervised, unsupervised, or reinforced learning techniques. The best application example is email provider services, where AI is used to separate spam from essential emails, and with each new datum, its accuracy improves. Most of the current weather forecasts are based on ML model prediction [3].

Comparison of different applications along with advantages and disadvantages of support vector machines (SVMs), NNs, and other common AI/ML algorithms used in biomedical applications is provided in Table 19.1.

AIML has demonstrated the ability to completely transform IoMT-integrated medical devices as well as healthcare practices.

19.3 ML-ENABLED IoT HEALTHCARE PROBLEMS

The following are the list of numerous technological obstacles that must be overcome in order to realize the potential of commercialization and adaptability in clinics and society at large.

19.3.1 Data security

IoT in healthcare is a significant security issue. Because medical histories are private, the medical sector emphasizes data privacy. The company's software

Table 19.1 Comparison of applications

AI algorithms	Applications in medical sciences	Advantages	Disadvantages
SVM	Neurological and psychiatric disorders using biomarker imaging [4] Computer–human interaction [5] Diagnosis of cancer [6] Alzheimer's disease early detection [7] Cardiac observation [8] Forecasting infection at the surgical site [9] Monitoring blood sugar [10] Operation [11–13] Management of pandemic resources [14] Monitoring system for healthcare [15]	Highly precise quick convergence to a solution Adept in handling difficult issues Effective scalability for large-scale data Demanding a certain quantity of training samples	Choosing the right kernel function is crucial Longer training times are needed for large datasets with significant computing costs Difficulties in comprehending and evaluating the individual impacts and final model variable weights Issues with missing value management and propensity for overfitting
NN	Diagnosis of cancer [16–18] Recognizing Parkinson's illness [19] Cardiac monitoring based on images [14] The disease Alzheimer's [20,21] Operation [4–6] Applications of sensors [22,23] Prediction of diabetes [24] Computer–human interaction [25] Management of pandemic resources [15]	An effective, quick, and adaptable algorithm. Produces calculations without the need of programs. Continuously gains knowledge and gets better. Multitasking is useful in many situations. It is compatible with complicated and nonlinear databases	Large datasets and more training time are needed. High hardware costs and the need for protracted, complicated programming. Black box nature makes interpretation and customization impossible. Prone to being too tight. Results that are highly data dependent could be inaccurate
K-nearest neighbor (KNN)	Diabetes glucose monitoring [16] Management of pandemic resources [20] Prognosis of disease [25] Diagnoses made with a computer [26] Prediction of heart disease [27] System for monitoring healthcare [21]	Basic algorithm. No presumptions regarding the dataset's features or output. Efficient in handling big data and robust against noisy data. Steady performance, quick learning curve, and effective overfitting control	Time-consuming and dependent on local data. Moderate classification speed, moderate accuracy. Inadequate management of correlated data

may be accessed by malicious actors and anybody with access to sensitive data. A competent medical software developer, on the other hand, can successfully defend future IoT-enabled app from any unwanted behaviors. To prevent these problems, IoT in healthcare must prioritize data security. Undoubtedly, such a necessity entails additional costs. Patient data in IoT-connected healthcare applications is protected under the GDPR and the CCPA. In accordance with statutory standards, sensitive data will not only be avoided. Additionally, it will assist in avoiding paying expensive fines.

IoT security in healthcare has come to the public's attention in recent years. When developing IoT solutions for the healthcare industry, keep medical IoT security in mind. Medical device attacks are becoming more sophisticated. For example, in 2017, the Wanna Cry ransomware crippled numerous hospitals and clinics by prohibiting staff from accessing the infected devices, causing operations to stop [28]. During the COVID-19 epidemic in 2020, there were more IoT device assaults overall, with medical equipment emerging as the most popular target. IoT security is a crucial concern in healthcare, so why is that? The largest risk is undoubtedly to the safety of the patients, followed by concerns about the veracity of patient medical information and negative consequences for finances and reputation. Although there haven't been any examples when a hacker assault directly compromised a patient's safety, it is still possible. For instance, a small adjustment to the vital metrics measured by medical devices such as glucose or pulse oximeters may have a catastrophic impact on the administration of patient care and drug dosages. In addition, medical gadgets that are compromised by hackers may change how they function and become lethal weapons [29]. It's a bad but plausible situation for one device to break into a hospital network and gain access to other medical devices.

19.3.2 Integration of protocols

IoMT links a variety of IoT medical devices together. The healthcare sector relies on numerous technologies that use various procedures. As a result, it develops an adaptable environment. There is no one answer for communication standards and protocols. As a result, IoT integration in the healthcare sector is restricted and delayed [30].

When developing medical software, compliance with HIPAA and HITECH is essential. Processing patient personal information is subject to numerous laws and regulations. Such compliance can be facilitated and you can receive help from an IoT business with extensive experience [31].

19.3.3 Data overload

IoT medical devices process and collect a lot of data. For doctors, this might result in data overload and a lack of accuracy. Applications of IoT in healthcare have the potential to create a lot of data. Making treatment choices challenging is a benefit.

19.4 IoT HEALTHCARE CHALLENGES FOR ML

This section primarily enumerates and discusses the main drawbacks and difficulties with ML in IoT healthcare. Figure 19.2 shows the connection between personal healthcare (PH), ML, and IoT.

Figure 19.2 illustrates how IoT generates data for ML algorithms, which in turn produce solutions for Parkinson's disease (PH) such as disease diagnosis, patient behavior analysis, and recommendations for assistive care. The development of ML- and IoT-based assistive PH services have had, and will continue to have, a significant impact on people's lives. Nevertheless, assistive PH will need to deal with difficult problems like affordability and usability. Furthermore, issues with privacy and authentication on IoT devices can draw the attention of hackers and result in problems because they will be hacked if not controlled. Additional research reveals that we can use a predictive analysis approach to help patients who have been released from the hospital but may need to be readmitted by using an ML-based PH service [32–34]. Predictive analysis aims to develop a risk classification model that allows higher-risk patients to be managed with extra effort and supportive care, such as additional IoT devices and sensors for monitoring, constant (real-time) follow-up, and analysis. These models are heavily constructed using data and historical experience from the past [32]. In order to help with readmission avoidance efforts, the dynamic PH system must also make use of patient dynamic data, analyze it, forecast potential outcomes, and start an action plan to reduce likely complications.

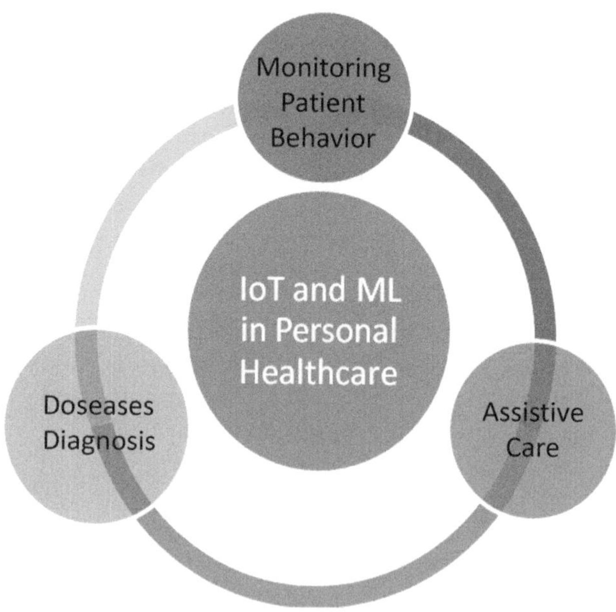

Figure 19.2 A general schema of IoT and ML applications in PH.

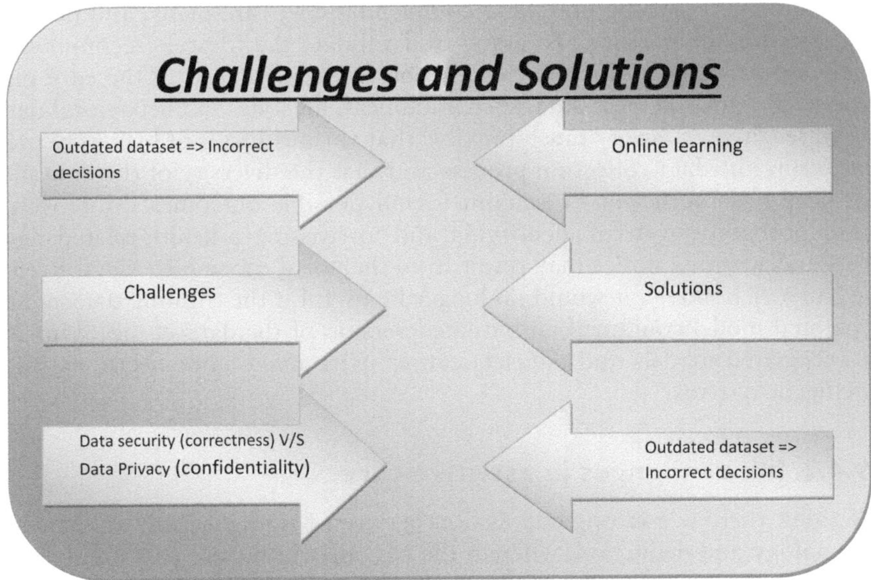

Figure 19.3 Challenges and solutions.

In Figure 19.3, two challenges are depicted which provides an abstract view of the problems and their solutions.

1. Outdated dataset, which causes us to make bad choices
2. Data privacy and security, which reduce IoT device dependability

However, the illustration offers us two related solutions:

1. Online education to continue learning about newly entered data.
2. Federated learning allows end users to learn from distributed data.

The first and second challenges are explained in this section along with possible scenarios for them.

19.4.1 Obsolete dataset

Numerous studies have examined the use of ML in IoT healthcare. The ML algorithms create analytical models that are incorporated into clinical smart systems and a variety of healthcare service applications. In order to identify behavioral patterns and various clinical conditions of the patients, such as recognizing the patient's improvements, habits, and anomalous actions in daily routine activities, as well as different sleeping, digestive, drinking, and eating patterns, these models are primarily evaluated on the data collected from IoT devices. With those patterns at hand, the intelligent decision-making systems suggest specific lifestyle recommendations, care plans, and targeted therapies for the patients. To assess and validate the lifestyle recommendations and care plans, doctors can also be further involved in the care plan process. Because medical data, such as clinical, lifestyle, and behavioral data, are so sensitive, it is very much possible that various forms of bias were present during the data collection process and that the diversity of the data may not have been sufficient to account for all possible outcomes. Moreover, a lower probability rate of identifying and forecasting a health-related diagnosis and warning notice may result from the noisy, incomplete data. Even if we had a rich model, it would no longer be useful if the training dataset and generated model contained an outdated version of the dataset [32]. Our use of antiquated models and datasets causes us to make poor decisions using intelligent systems.

19.4.2 ML challenges in assistive care

We think there is a strong connection between ML algorithms and statistical analogy and deduction, wherein the ML algorithms use past and current experience to predict and make decisions. When a patient is being watched over, the ML approach will keep an eye on things and evaluate them based on the training set. In order to find the current pattern and forecast the future trend of a particular new problem during a test phase, the training dataset is therefore essential. This dataset is not as diverse as it could be to cover a wide range of scenarios, and it is occasionally biased.

Let's take a look at a sleep monitoring scenario as an example. Everyone has different sleep patterns, from young children to the elderly, depending on their health. Because of this, there isn't a full dataset of all case studies available during training to monitor sleep patterns, which could result in an inaccurate PH estimation. Furthermore, using IoT and ML enables PH to make a decision for diagnosis and prediction. In certain cases, it is impossible to explain why a particular decision was made and ML-based decisions may not be accurate. For example, in the case of autonomous cars, a few accidents happened as a result of the vehicles' poor decision-making. The key question here is how to evaluate an AI machine's choice when it makes use of unsupervised ML algorithms. This could bring up moral issues such as who would be accountable for a false statement, how to identify or correct incompleteness in the decision-making process, and how unsupervised ML algorithms operate [34]. These difficulties would restrict the application of ML algorithms to sensitive applications (personalized medicine care, in particular).

19.4.3 Confidentiality and correctness

We may now have continuous PH monitoring anywhere, including at home, work, and hospitals, for a variety of applications like childcare and assisted living, thanks to the development of medical IoT devices and the enormous popularity of ubiquitous wearable gadgets. These gadgets gather electronic health measurements in real time from various items and sensors, then send the patient data to an application server where it is pre-processed and pre-analyzed before being restored on a data server.

ML algorithms are used in this processing and analysis to offer a variety of services, including motion tracking, displaying the number of steps taken, calories burned, tracking sleep, tracking distance traveled, and measuring vital signs like heart rate, electrocardiogram (ECG), skin temperature, and electroencephalogram (EEG). Therefore, processing the data produced by IoT devices and exchanging it with a server across a network connection raises concerns with confidentiality and trust. Both the communication networks and the data kept on a server are susceptible to hacking. Privacy and data security are so significant issues to address. By using encryption methods and keeping the data secure, there are simple ways available to boost data security. However, a hacker learns the decryption algorithm's key and discovers the data.

19.4.4 ML challenges in monitoring patient activities

Several research papers use data from motion sensors to define physical activity in real-world situations for a range of case studies in the context of monitoring patient behaviors. Studies have shown that the use of motion sensors is one of the most trustworthy methods for monitoring a patient's long-term physical activity while they are undergoing therapy. Data collection from medical IoT sensors and devices for healthcare applications is particularly sensitive due to the properties of IoT devices. Recent developments in wireless communication/transformation and web technologies improve data collection and remote real-time monitoring.

But during the many stages of data collection, including data collection, transmission, processing, and storage, the complex workflow for collecting medical data makes security problems and privacy hazards more likely. The difficulty lies in identifying the data that can protect user privacy while being relevant and crucial for ML jobs in the activity recognition process using mobile devices rather than wearable devices [35]. We might confront and respond to the following two questions to handle this difficult problem: First, does the data collection process use strong security measures or an encryption protocol to ensure that no one can access it? How can it be determined whether the protected data is being kept as accurately as it was originally captured?

The security, in particular the privacy of patient information in the ML analysis process, is one of the major difficulties in using IoT and ML for healthcare monitoring. Only users with valid accounts can access data and services, thanks to a strong user authentication system. Therefore, the issue is consumers' data accessibility, which leaves them open to sensitive hacker access. It will be difficult to share data from IoT devices as they currently exist.

19.5 CONCLUSION

The biomedical industry is one of the most challenging in terms of accountability and strict regulations, which makes it a vital and important area for innovation. The recent tremendous expansion of biomedical systems has resulted in a significant rise in employment and wealth. The accumulation of technical advances using small, in-built sensors in wristbands, advancements in technology have made it possible to diagnose various illnesses and monitor health. A patient-centered strategy has replaced the hospital-centered one in the biomedical system, thanks to this breakthrough. Additionally, a significant increase in biological data, such as genetic sequences, protein structures, and medical imaging, has been brought about by developments in high-throughput technology. To store, process, and understand this stream of enormous biological data, efficient and effective computing methods are required.

In the medical field, IoT has opened up a world of possibilities and may hold the key to various problems. In addition to strengthening independence, IoT has expanded the possibilities for interaction with the outside world. IoT uses futuristic technologies to facilitate worldwide connectivity, protocols, and algorithms. Among other things, telemedicine and remote patient status monitoring would be greatly enhanced by the use of the medical IoT. This may have to do with the ML framework sides [27, 36].

This chapter covered a survey of the widely used ML algorithms. IoT-based ML applications in the medical system have been explored along with problem and challenges in the biomedical area.

Computer-based intelligence, specifically DL, supports the development of dynamic IoT frameworks based on information analysis as well as on the communication foundation plan.

REFERENCES

1. Aiken, L.H.; Clarke, S.P.; Sloane, D.M. 2002. Hospital staffing, organization, and quality of care: Cross-national findings. *International Journal for Quality in Healthcare* 14(1):5–13.
2. Aiken, L.H.; Clarke, S.P.; Sloane, D.M.; Sochalski, J.A.; Busse, R.; Clarke, H.; Giovannetti, P.; Hunt, J.; Rafferty, A.M.; Shamian, J. 2001. Nurses reports on hospital care in five countries. *Health Affairs* 20(3):43–53.
3. Manickam, P.; Mariappan, S. A.; Murugesan, S. M.; Hansda, S.; Kaushik, A.; Shinde, R. and Thipperudraswamy, S. P. 2022. Artificial Intelligence (AI) and Internet of Medical Things (IoMT) assisted biomedical systems for intelligent healthcare. *Biosensors* 12(8):562.
4. Orru, G.; Pettersson-Yeo, W.; Marquand, A.F.; Sartori, G.; Mechelli, A. 2012. Using support vector machine to identify imaging biomarkers of neurological and psychiatric disease: A critical review. *Neuroscience and Biobehavioral Reviews* 36, 1140–1152.
5. Farina, D.; Vujaklija, I.; Sartori, M.; Kapelner, T.; Negro, F.; Jiang, N.; Bergmeister, K.; Andalib, A.; Principe, J.; Aszmann, O.C. 2017. Man/machine interface based on the discharge timings of spinal motor neurons after targeted muscle reinnervation. *Nature Biomedical Engineering* 1, 0025.

6. Sweilam, N.H.; Tharwat, A.A.; Moniem, N.K. 2010. Support vector machine for diagnosis cancer disease: A comparative study. *Egyptian Informatics Journal* 11, 81–92.
7. Khedher, L.; Ramírez, J.; Górriz, J.M.; Brahim, A.; Segovia, F. 2015. Early diagnosis of Alzheimer's disease based on partial least squares, principal component analysis and support vector machine using segmented MRI images. *Neurocomputing*, 151, 139–150.
8. Martin-Isla, C.; Campello, V.M.; Izquierdo, C.; Raisi-Estabragh, Z.; Baeßler, B.; Petersen, S.E.; Lekadir, K. 2020. Image-based cardiac diagnosis with machine learning: A review. *Frontiers in Cardiovascular Medicine* 7, 1.
9. Soguero-Ruiz, C.; Fei, W.M.E.; Jenssen, R.; Augestad, K.M.; Álvarez, J.-L.R.; Jiménez, I.M.; Lindsetmo, R.-O.; Skrøvseth, S.O. 2015. Data-driven temporal prediction of surgical site infection. In Proceedings of the AMIA Annual Symposium Proceedings, American Medical Informatics Association, San Francisco, CA, USA (vol. 2015, p. 1164). 14–18 November.
10. Shokrekhodaei, M.; Cistola, D.P.; Roberts, R.C.; Quinones, S. 2021. Non-invasive glucose monitoring using optical sensor and machine learning techniques for diabetes applications. *IEEE Access* 9, 73029–73045.
11. Hashimoto, D.A.; Rosman, G.; Rus, D.; Meireles, O.R. 2018. Artificial intelligence in surgery: Promises and perils. *Annals of Surgery* 268, 70–76.
12. Galbusera, F.; Casaroli, G.; Bassani, T. 2019. Artificial intelligence and machine learning in spine research. *JOR Spine* 2, e1044.
13. Chang, M.; Canseco, J.A.; Nicholson, K.J.; Patel, N.; Vaccaro, A.R. 2020. The role of machine learning in spine surgery: The future is now. *Frontiers in Surgery* 7, 54.
14. Goswami, M.; Sebastian, N.J. 2022. Performance Analysis of Logistic Regression, KNN, SVM, Naïve Bayes Classifier for Healthcare Application During COVID-19. In Raj, J.S., Kamel, K., Lafata, P. (eds.), *Innovative Data Communication Technologies and Application* (vol. 96, pp. 645–658). Springer Nature: Singapore. ISBN 9789811671661.
15. Kaur, P.; Kumar, R.; Kumar, M. 2019. A healthcare monitoring system using random forest and Internet of Things (IoT). *Multimedia Tools and Applications* 78, 19905–19916.
16. Khosravan, N.; Bagci, U. 2018. S4ND: Single-shot single-scale lung nodule detection. In Proceedings of the International Conference on Medical Image Computing and Computer-Assisted Intervention, Granada, Spain (pp. 794–802), 16–20 September.
17. Ardila, D.; Kiraly, A.P.; Bharadwaj, S.; Choi, B.; Reicher, J.J.; Peng, L.; Tse, D.; Etemadi, M.; Ye, W.; Corrado, G. 2019. End-to-end lung cancer screening with three-dimensional deep learning on low-dose chest computed tomography. *Nature Medicine* 25, 954–961.
18. Muhammad, W.; Hart, G.R.; Nartowt, B.; Farrell, J.J.; Johung, K.; Liang, Y.; Deng, J. 2019. Pancreatic cancer prediction through an artificial neural network. *Frontiers in Artificial Intelligence* 2, 2.
19. Hirschauer, T.J.; Adeli, H.; Buford, J.A. 2015. Computer-aided diagnosis of Parkinson's disease using enhanced probabilistic neural network. *Journal of Medical Systems* 39, 179.
20. Sarraf, S.; DeSouza, D.D.; Anderson, J.; Tofighi, G. 2017. DeepAD: Alzheimer's Disease Classification via Deep Convolutional Neural Networks Using MRI and fMRI. *BioRxiv*, 070441.
21. Ramzan, F.; Khan, M.U.G.; Rehmat, A.; Iqbal, S.; Saba, T.; Rehman, A.; Mehmood, Z. 2020. A deep learning approach for automated diagnosis and multi-class classification of Alzheimer's disease stages using resting-state fMRI and residual neural networks. *Journal of Medical Systems* 44, 37.

22. Pang, K.; Song, X.; Xu, Z.; Liu, X.; Liu, Y.; Zhong, L.; Peng, Y.; Wang, J.; Zhou, J.; Meng, F. 2020. Hydroplastic foaming of graphene aerogels and artificially intelligent tactile sensors. *Science Advances* 6, eabd4045.

23. Hayasaka, T.; Lin, A.; Copa, V.C.; Lopez, L.P.; Loberternos, R.A.; Ballesteros, L.I.M.; Kubota, Y.; Liu, Y.; Salvador, A.A.; Lin, L. 2020. An electronic nose using a single graphene FET and machine learning for water, methanol, and ethanol. *Microsystems & Nanoengineering* 6, 50.

24. Khanam, J.J.; Foo, S.Y. 2021. A comparison of machine learning algorithms for diabetes prediction. *ICT Express* 7, 432–439.

25. Kwon, Y.-T.; Kim, H.; Mahmood, M.; Kim, Y.-S.; Demolder, C.; Yeo, W.-H. 2020. Printed, wireless, soft bioelectronics and deep learning algorithm for smart human–machine interfaces. *ACS Applied Materials & Interfaces* 12, 49398–49406.

26. Kaushik, A.K.; Dhau, J.S.; Gohel, H.; Mishra, Y.K.; Kateb, B.; Kim, N.-Y.; Goswami, D.Y. Electrochemical SARS-CoV-2 Sensing at Point-of-Care and Artificial Intelligence for Intelligent COVID-19.

27. Uddin, S.; Haque, I.; Lu, H.; Moni, M.A.; Gide, E. 2022. Comparative performance analysis of k-nearest neighbour (KNN) algorithm and its different variants for disease prediction. *Scientific Reports* 12, 6256.

28. Singh, A.K.; Anand, A.; Lv, Z.; Ko, H.; Mohan, A. 2021. A survey on healthcare data: A security perspective. *ACM Transactions on Multimedia Computing Communications, and Applications* 17(25):1–26.

29. Jabeen, T.; Ashraf, H.; Ullah, A. 2021. A survey on healthcare data security in wireless body area networks. *Journal of Ambient Intelligence and Humanized Computing* 12(10):9841–9854.

30. AbuKhousa, E.; Mohamed, N.; Al-Jaroodi, J. 2012. e-Health cloud: Opportunities and challenges. *Future Internet* 4(4):621–645.

31. Arora, S. IoMT (Internet of Medical Things): Reducing cost while improving patient care.

32. Gope, P.; Hwang, T. 2015. BSN-care: A secure IoT-based modern healthcare system using body sensor network. *IEEE Sensors Journal* 16(5), 1368–1376.

33. Allied Health Workforce Innovations for the 21st Century Projects. 1999. The Hidden Health Care Workforce: Recognizing, Understanding and Improving the Allied and Auxiliary Workforce. Available at http://futurehealth.ucsf.edu/AHexecsum.html.

34. Karthick, R.; Ramkumar, R.; Akram, M.; Kumar, M.V. 2021. Overcome the challenges in bio-medical instruments using IoT: A review. *Materials Today. Proceedings* 45, 1614–1619.

35. Khan, R.; Khan, S.U.; Zaheer, R.; Khan, S. 2012. Future internet: The Internet of Things architecture, possible applications and key challenges. In Proceedings of the 2012 10th International Conference on Frontiers of Information Technology, Islamabad, Pakistan, 17–19 December.

36. Li, C.; Zhang, S.; Zhang, H.; Pang, L.; Lam, K.; Hui, C.; Zhang, S. 2012. Using the k-nearest neighbor algorithm for the classification of lymph node metastasis in gastric cancer. *Computational and Mathematical Methods in Medicine* 2012, 876545.

IoT-driven machine learning mechanisms for healthcare applications

Gopalakrishnan Karuppaiah,
Karthikeyan Velayuthapandian,
and Sridhar Raj Sankara Vadivel

20.1 INTRODUCTION: BACKGROUND AND DRIVING FORCES

The healthcare industry has traditionally relied on manual processes and subjective decision-making, resulting in inefficiencies, errors, and suboptimal patient outcomes. However, with the rapid modernization of technologies, particularly the proliferation of the Internet of Things (IoT) and machine learning (ML), the clinical care landscape is undergoing a profound transformation. This convergence of IoT and ML is ushering in a new era of data-driven, personalized healthcare applications that hold immense promise for revolutionizing patient care. Integrating a wide collection of corporeal and ordinal "things" with the burgeoning extensible and sensors, IoT and ML have recently generated additional worldwide perspective on inventiveness in statistics to construct a robust global framework [1].

The phrase "Internet of Things" eventually came into practice in several sensors, such as processors, GPS apps, as well as mobile phones, to incorporate an extensive variety of "things" [2]. A variety of exploratory issues, including system architecture and information analysis with deployments, have been brought about by continual incorporation across an Internet-related phase and the supplementary infrastructure that includes such sensors. Nowadays, IoT innovation has made rapid strides in a variety of technical and automatic controls, most notably in the health facilities [3]. The outcome is the growth of IoT technology, and ML has impacted medical care by bringing routine medical testing and other health services into people's homes and making it easier for both doctors and patients to use medical equipment. It would streamline medical care for individuals, particularly in urgent situations. In addition, hospitals might lessen their workload by fluctuating simple and doable responsibilities to patients' homes. One of the key rewards is a decrease in costs, as patients may evade paying clinic fees when they saw a doctor. The limitations of the existing network architecture, which prevent it from supporting real-time, IoT-based applications, are another challenge; hence, Software Defined Networking is anticipated to be an appropriate network setup for these applications [4, 5]. Therefore, it will be necessary in

DOI: 10.1201/9781003487647-20

the foreseeable future to introduce recent advances in the healthcare sector to produce cutting-edge medical technology and easily track patients from afar. The patient's physical condition and medication history are recorded and analyzed as part of the monitoring process [6]. The proliferation of IoT has led to a rise in the use of embedded sensors, labeling, etc. With the use of IoT, portable sensors can be used to collect more precise information. It is possible to improve the device's usability with the help of a pharmaceutical container and an Android app. When properly timed, the deployment of numerous advancements such as IoT will drastically alter several given area of the clinical sector [7]. The standard of living could be raised, thanks to IoT. Multiple good changes might be made to information interpreting, regulated communications, and digital management of data solutions with the use of integrated technologies [8–10]. Many wearable healthcare technologies and applications are still in development [11]. Using IoT and ML, this chapter will highlight the most crucial aspects of patient-centered healthcare. Showcase some existing investigation on IoT and ML for individualized medical care, highlighting relevant concerns and limitations.

In healthcare, IoT devices range from wearable's and implantable medical devices to remote monitoring systems, smart hospital equipment, and even smart home-based healthcare systems. These devices generate a vast amount of real-time data about patient health, vital signs, activities, and environmental conditions.

On the other hand, a specific type of computational intelligence known as ML permits machines to acquire knowledge through information and formulate judgments or recommendations with no the use of explicit code. ML algorithms can process and analyze large datasets to identify patterns, trends, and correlations, allowing for more accurate predictions and decision-making.

The IoT-driven ML processes used in medical applications are depicted in Figure 20.1. Biosignal sensors, which are easily extracted from the human body by means of wearable electronics, provide the data needed for healthcare

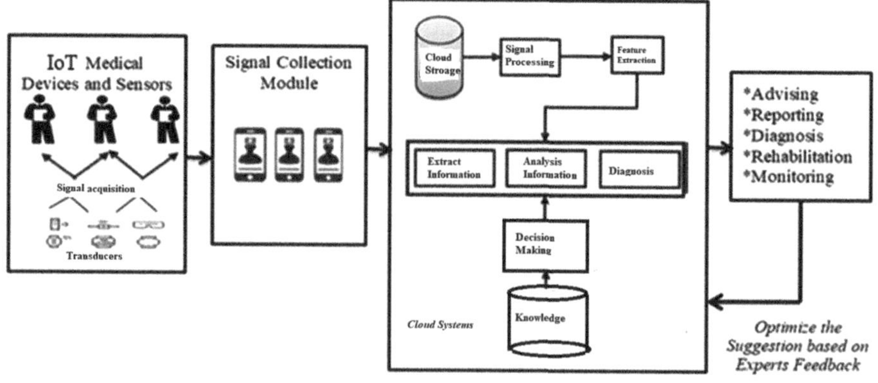

Figure 20.1 Basic block diagram for IoT-driven ML mechanisms for healthcare applications.

analysis. Using IoT, these records are put to use in areas like identification and medical care. Wearable or flexible electronics has grown rapidly as a field of study in recent decades because of its inherent flexibility and cheap weight. It has several potential applications, including but not limited to motion tracking, rehabilitation, human–machine interface (HMI), illness diagnostics, etc. Data from sensors is gathered and prepared for use by signal collecting modules, which are then sent into a data storage media. The decision-making system then takes what it has learned from this processing and offers the sought-after facts. This data is sent to those in positions of authority. Cloud-based authority feedback and iterative processing lead to increasingly precise outcomes.

20.2 DRIVING FORCES FOR IoT-DRIVEN ML MECHANISMS IN HEALTHCARE APPLICATIONS

Some of the driving forces for IoT-driven ML mechanisms in healthcare applications are as follows:

- *Real-time Patient Monitoring*: IoT-enabled medical devices provide continuous and real-time monitoring of health indicators for clients, including heartbeat, arterial pressure, blood sugar levels, and more. ML algorithms can analyze this data in real time, alerting healthcare providers to any deviations from normal values and enabling early intervention for critical conditions.
- *Personalized Medicine:* The combination of IoT-generated data and ML algorithms empowers medical professionals to cultivate personalized individualized therapy programs for patients. By considering a patient's unique health data, medical history, and genetic information, ML can recommend tailored therapies and interventions, leading to more effective treatments and improved patient outcomes.
- *Remote Patient Care:* IoT devices facilitate remote patient monitoring, lowering the requirement for repeated hospital appointments and enabling clinical care providers to monitor patients from a distance. ML-powered analytics can detect trends and patterns in the data, allowing for timely adjustments to treatment plans and reducing the burden on healthcare facilities.
- *Predictive Analytics:* ML algorithms excel at analyzing large and complex datasets, making them valuable tools for predicting disease outbreaks, identifying at-risk patient populations, and optimizing resource allocation. By leveraging historical data, ML models can forecast potential health issues and assist in proactive planning and preventive measures.
- *Drug Discovery and Development:* In pharmaceutical research, ML techniques are being employed to analyze vast datasets, including genetic

information, molecular structures, and clinical trial results. This accelerates drug development through the selection of possible drug candidates along with the prediction of their effective and safe characteristics.

- *Health System Efficiency:* The integration of IoT devices and ML algorithms streamlines healthcare processes and enhances operational efficiency. ML-powered predictive maintenance can ensure that medical equipment functions optimally, reducing downtime and enhancing patient care.
- *Improved Patient Engagement:* IoT devices and ML-powered applications can facilitate better patient engagement through personalized health insights and feedback. By empowering patients to monitor their health and make informed decisions, they become active participants in their care.

20.3 METHOD OF PROVIDING MEDICAL TREATMENT

Preventative medicine, identification, diagnostic, and therapy are the four fundamental stages of the medical care practice (see Figures 20.2–20.4).

Preventative Medicine: Everybody is familiar with the adage "prevention is better than cure," so the goal of that initial phase in the process of medical care is to maintain individuals health. This stage encompasses things like sleeping with nets to avoid infectious diseases, being physically active to avoid obesity, having a healthy diet along with access to pure drinking water, or quitting smoking to prevent lung disease [12].

Identification: Both patients and the general public need to be aware of their own physical state, routinely monitor their blood pressure and glucose levels, and seek medical attention right away if any odd health issues arise [13].

Diagnostics: Examinations must be performed whenever strange signs are found. In order to find a therapy that is effective, data needs to be obtained, combined, and properly analyzed. The individual may be examined, a medical examination may be carried out, diagnostic procedures may be carried out, or clinicians might talk to clarify any ambiguity in order to make identification [14]. An accurate evaluation can guarantee that an individual's medical condition can be appropriately comprehended, allowing for the taking of suitable actions to attain a satisfied health result.

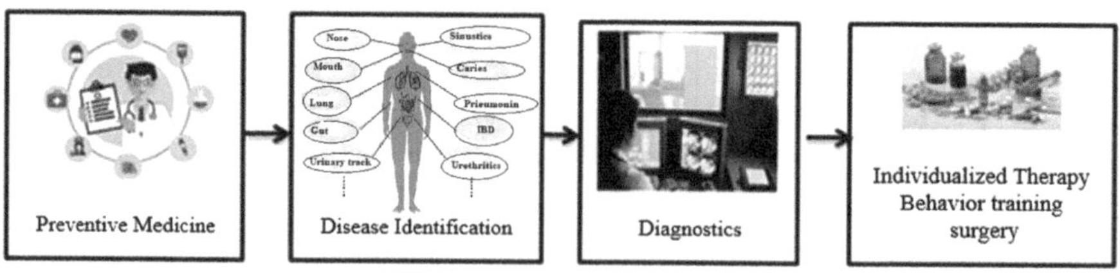

Figure 20.2 Healthcare process.

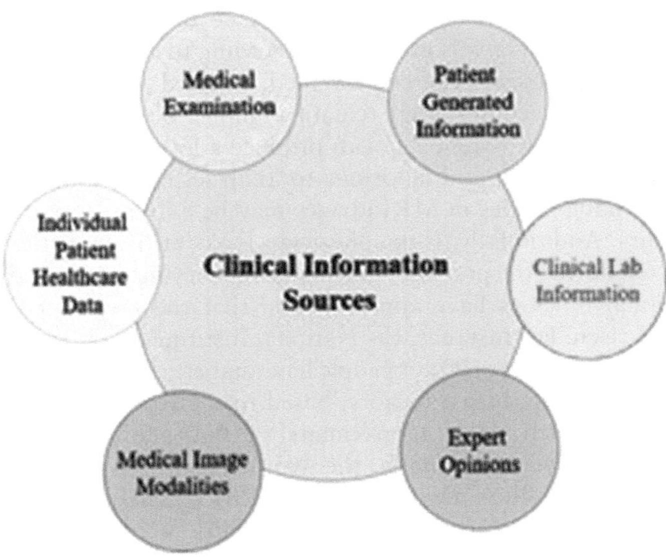

Figure 20.3 Healthcare data collection sources.

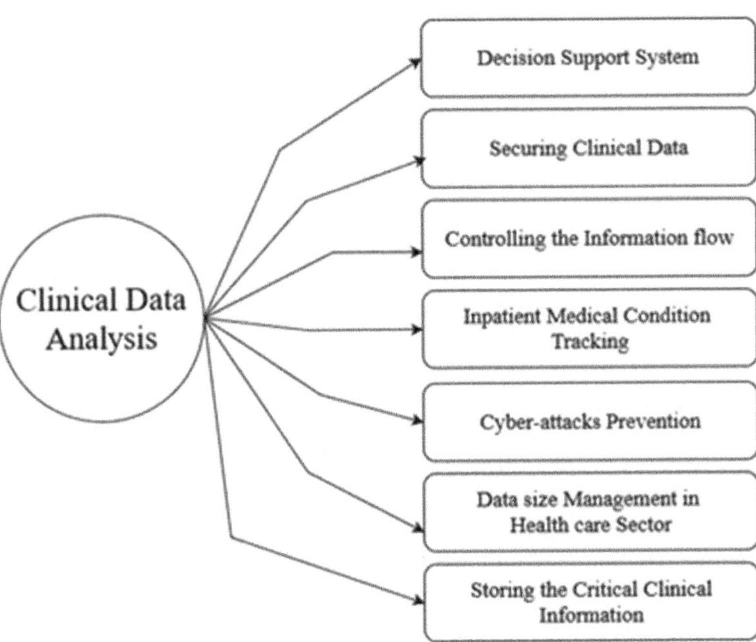

Figure 20.4 Reasons for clinical data analysis.

Therapy: To offer, collaborate with, or regulate an individual's medical condition, a successful therapy is prescribed according to each diagnostic. Despite the fact that a few illnesses can be prevented, detected, diagnosed, and treated through medical procedures, there remain a number of downsides [15, 16].

The problem is that diagnosing can produce a lot of information, thereby rendering it challenging and laborious to analyze. For instance, identifying preliminary malignancies in MRI images may be extremely challenging and require hours. Additionally, if the physician looks at the statistical information collected during the previous consultations, they may deduce that numerous additional illnesses have appeared and that the prevalence of various illnesses has risen. For instance, the National Institute of Nutrition and Food Technology estimate that 19% of people have diabetes. Nearly 30% of females have been affected by breast tumors, based to the Regional Administration of Healthcare, which states approximately 2,600 additional instances are discovered annually. Additionally, the World Health Organization reports that out of the 8.8 million deaths globally in 2015, malignancy remained the nation's second leading cause of mortality [14, 16].

Although medical professionals are making great efforts to enhance medical care, there remains room for improvement to produce enhanced results as well as preserve numerous lives. ML was therefore developed to assist and advance the healthcare sector in many different ways.

20.3.1 Healthcare information

In the modern age of massive information, there are many various forms of healthcare information, like disease prediction, healthcare documentation, personally identifiable information, and diagnostic imaging [17]. Additionally, by evaluating this information and applying it to the right uses, the healthcare sector may undergo a major improvement. The efficient application of health-related information may "raise the United States of America healthcare business to the amount of $350 trillion and so reduce the cost of medical care approximately 7%," according to Chen [18]. Because of how it was gathered or its nature, medical data is complex. There are many parameters and factors which make it complicated and extremely multidimensional and represent a class disparity [19]. Information about patients went missing as a consequence of improper healthcare information gathering [17].

There are ML mechanisms established that are explicitly tailored for clinical information mining, allowing them to lessen the impact of the previously mentioned limitations [20, 21]. It can assist with identifying unlabeled data, retrieving significant details in unorganized data, simplifying it to a standardized format, and interacting with datasets that have a wide range of information types. Furthermore, addressing these difficulties, ML algorithms offer a wide range of uses in the evaluation of healthcare information, particularly in areas such as medical diagnosis, including therapy, implementations for general healthcare studies, and the administration of populations [22].

20.4 OVERVIEW OF ML TECHNIQUES IN HEALTHCARE

Identifying the proper attributes (descriptors) regarding the information in order to anticipate the right categorization (label) corresponds to one of the most important jobs for ML in the healthcare sector. For instance, in the past, highly competent doctors, along with additional clinical and wellness professionals, were able to analyze clinical images. Based on their extensive expertise in the field, they were going to develop useful identifiers that correspond to particular labeled outputs on a health-related database [23]. But because so much data is produced on a daily basis, ML approaches can produce predictions that are virtually identical to those made by subject-matter specialists [23]. In order to assist physicians in identifying early signs during the course of treatment of malignancy, ML algorithms have demonstrated the ability to precisely harvest appropriate characteristics from medical CT palettes [24]. Medical utilization of ML can also benefit doctors. Physicians' duties, including prediction, assessment, image analysis, and therapy, can be aided by predictions made using ML approaches [25].

20.4.1 Support vector machines (SVMs)

SVM is a supervised ML approach that is applied to problems associated with binary classification in many different domains, particularly in the discipline of healthcare. The informational elements from a conventional SVM framework are mapped onto a higher-dimensional space, whereby a decision plane is used to divide the dualistic categories having the least amount of overlap [26, 27]. With no prior understanding regarding the tracking, a SVM employs dot function products within the feature domain of the map, which are identified as kernels, to determine the best possible hyperplane separator, as shown in Eq. (20.1), where w^T is the vector that holds the weight for the input vector x with the bias b. Increasing the separation among both classes using a linearly distinct hyperplane is a mathematical issue:

$$w^T x + b = 0 \tag{20.1}$$

SVMs were initially developed for regular, discrete categorizations. It can also create dynamic approaches, though. To categorize the information, the kernel's operations might add additional characteristics at a subsequent level [28]. SVMs are frequently employed in the discipline of healthcare for uses such as health forecasting and detection since they employ a driven-by-data computational strategy and perform best on databases that contain fewer observations proportional to the parameters (Figure 20.5) [29].

SVMs have been employed in binary classification experiments in Alzheimer's prognostic studies [29] to determine whether individuals who have moderate cognitive impairment have dementia. SVMs are additionally used for forecasting infections of the bladder [30], detecting hypertension of

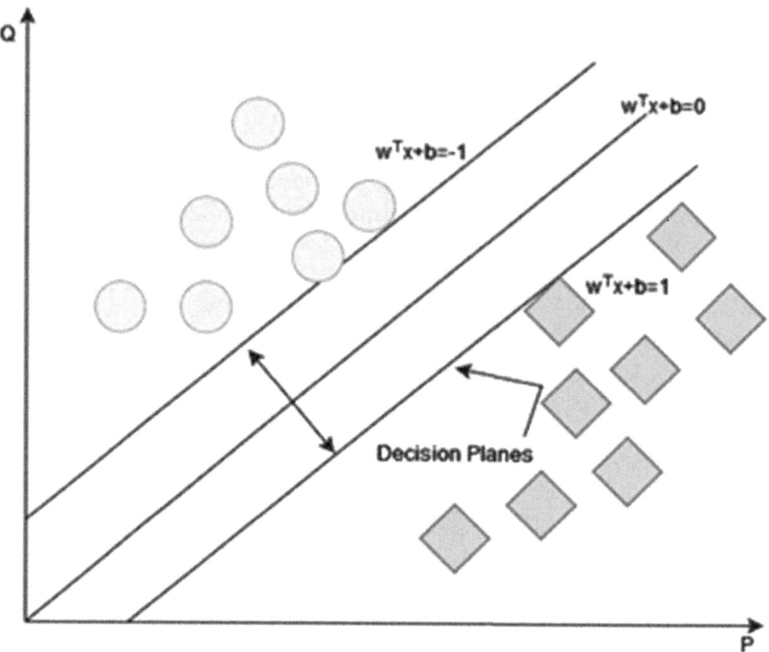

Figure 20.5 Decision plane of SVM.

the lungs [31], and determining the best treatment option [32], among other healthcare categorization issues. SVMs are widely utilized in tumor genomics studies, according to Huang et al. [28], resulting in the identification of novel tumor biomarkers, therapeutic desired outcomes, and improved understanding about tumor driving mutations [33]. SVMs are advantageous for particularly upcoming malignancy genome uses because of their adaptability in binary classification challenges as well as the freedom to select the correct settings unique to healthcare information.

20.4.2 Clustering

Recognizing communes and trends among a collection of information and grouping them together into groups is known as clustering [34]. The technique of clustering divides the unlabeled information into logical groupings with no tags to ensure that identical information can be grouped into distinct clusters [35]. Random as well as unlabeled medicinal and scientific information, such as gene manifestations and enzyme fields, is frequently categorized using clustering methodologies like k-means [36]. A more compact form of the k-means scheme called C-means grouping has produced promising outcomes for categorizing malignancies such as breast cancer as well as liver illnesses in UCI healthcare datasets [37,38]. In this section, a preclassifier is implemented to organize the information when the categories are employed, using the fuzzy C-means segmentation approach, in which an individual point might belong to multiple groups. Similar steps are taken in the C-means aggregating approach reminiscent of k-means, but a set of possible groupings is used. Class-based clustering classifier (CBCC), an approach for categorizing healthcare information into groups for nine standard datasets, including the Australian, Cleveland, Ecoli, German, Hepatitis, Wine, Iris, Pima, and Wisconsin [39], was suggested by Yelipe et al. (2018) [33]. It focuses on determining the distance between Euclidean points using fuzzy measurements. Similar to k-means, clustering may yield greater outcomes if additional expertise is made accessible as a supplement to the unprocessed information [40].

20.4.3 Decision trees (DTs)

Through the use of conditional logic, DT calculates learned information gathered from a collection of data into a tree [29]. By computing every branch's knowledge acquisition and entropy, the instructional parameter corresponding to every node in the tree iteratively assesses how effectively every node can categorize the tagged input.

$$\text{Entropy}(D) = -\sum_{k=1}^{d} p_k \log_2 p_k \tag{20.2}$$

p_k in Eq. (20.2) stands for the likelihood that a feature in class k will be represented. The entropy and estimation of the information's dependability or instability is calculated using this method. Entropy aids in determining how the knowledge needs to be divided to achieve an even distribution of categories, or an ideal categorization, combined with a knowledge gain (G).

$$G(D,B) = \text{Entropy}(D) - \text{Entropy}(D\,/\,B) \tag{20.3}$$

To calculate the amount by which the overall entropy of database D has decreased with more knowledge regarding characteristic B, the entropy measurement in database D provided by characteristic B is deducted from the total entropy of database D prior to any potential modifications. DTs are employed in the discipline of medicine, particularly for diagnostic research [29], illness prognosis [41, 42], forecasting hypertension [31], forecasting the consequences of critical care [32], as well as predictions of coronary artery disease [43].

20.4.4 Random forest (RF)

RF structures comprise a group of DT structures that collectively decide on the categorization problem; the majority of these "votes" select the appropriate

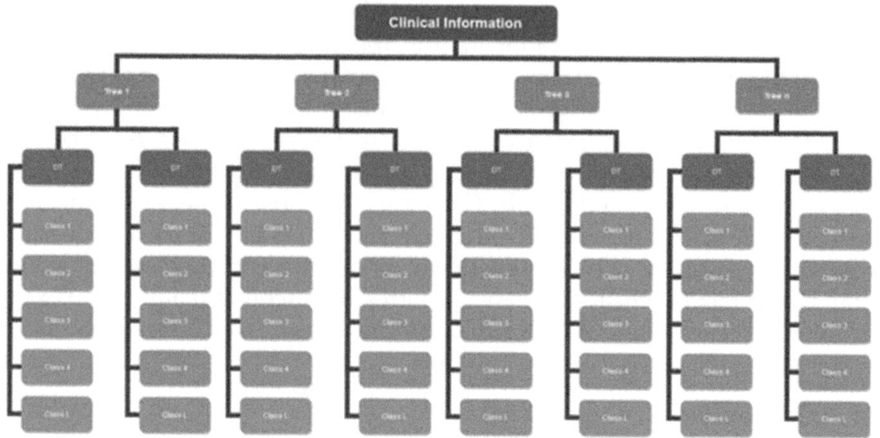

Figure 20.6 DT formation in RF.

class for the previously unidentified information source [44, 45]. The variation (overfitting) issue involving one particular DT is thus addressed because RFs have multiple DTs (Figure 20.6). In cases of extreme class disparity, the voting rules may be altered [46].

$$\hat{z} = \frac{1}{n} \sum_{k=1}^{p} \sum_{j=1}^{q} X_k(y_j, y') \tag{20.4}$$

Zhu et al. [47] suggested a weighted polling RF framework to address the issue of large-scale class unbalance whenever utilizing RFs, whereby every predictor's (DT's) voting gets multiplied with a load to increase the validity of that classification. In order to prevent excessive fitting in the forecasting of healthcare costs for people with recognized mellitus in the United States, Wang and Shi [48] employed RF models that included many DTs with little relationship with one another.

20.4.5 K-nearest neighbors (KNNs)

A different categorization method is KNN, which operates on the principle of labeling the unregulated point of information that corresponds closest to a classified information source (Figure 20.7) [49].

Unlike every other segmentation method, KNN primarily uses the measure of Manhattan distance (M_D) (Eq. (20.6)) or Euclidean distance (E_D) (Eq. (20.5)) measurements to determine the separation among the information's elements. Whenever the information points have the characteristics corresponding to continuous factors, these metrics are employed; nevertheless, for categorical parameters, the Hamming distance (H_D) measurement

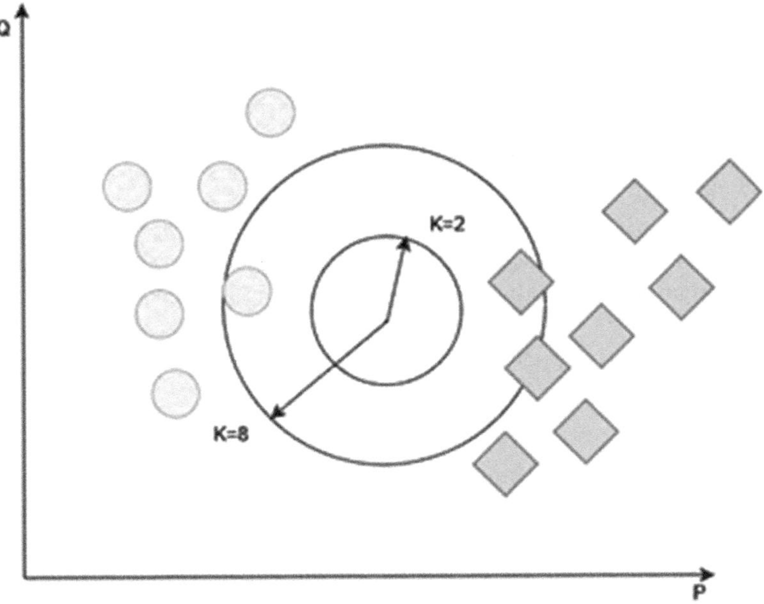

Figure 20.7 Sample KNN representation.

is utilized (Eq. (20.7), where H_D is larger compared to 0 if $p \neq q$ and equals zero if $p = q$).

$$M_D = \left(\sum_{j=1}^{l} \left(p_j - q_j \right)^2 \right)^{1/2} \tag{20.5}$$

$$E_D = \sum_{j=1}^{l} \left| p_j - q_j \right| \tag{20.6}$$

$$H_D = \sum_{j=1}^{l} \left| \left(p_j - q_j \right)^2 \right| \tag{20.7}$$

By addressing the issue of each recognized specimen being accorded the identical precedence when choosing the group classification for an unidentified or unstructured information point, the fuzzy KNN method was developed by Keller et al. [50].

The relevance of correctly organizing healthcare information for an algorithm like KNN is demonstrated mathematically by Zhang [51]. The effectiveness of the KNN algorithm's diagnostic capabilities might be confirmed by establishing hyperparameters unique to healthcare information using the appropriate value of K. The researchers assert that in 30% of the instances when KNN was employed to the clinical databases examined in Reference [52], KNN produced the highest accuracy outcomes.

20.4.6 Naive Bayes (NB)

With the help of a collection of characteristics that describe a particular instance and the knowledge of additional instances, the NB information categorization approach predicts a category utilizing a single case.

$$p(d \mid y) = \frac{p(y \mid d)p(d)}{p(y)} \tag{20.8}$$

$p(y \mid d)$ represents the conditional likelihood of occurrence d in Eq. (20.8), depending on the knowledge of y. By computing every feature's likelihood according to the knowledge acquired from additional characteristics, we can increase the autonomous nature of the attributes, which means that they do not collaborate until they are mutually dependent, influencing likelihood [43].

NB is a crucial method for improving the precision of classification by removing irrelevant characteristics [43]. Therefore, NB may be employed to pick characteristics successfully [53]. It has produced significant outcomes for text categorization in the healthcare sector, serving as a potent preliminary processing activity that enhances the written content classifier's adaptability and effectiveness [53]. Utilizing healthcare databases, NB demonstrates that it is incredibly easy and successful because of its susceptibility to the selection of features. Domain-specific selection of features is incredibly important to healthcare professionals and is therefore beneficial. NB demonstrated the greatest performance when analyzed alongside KNN as well as other classifications in Shen et al.'s [54] analysis regarding the prediction of recuperation from femoral neck displacement.

20.4.7 Neural networks (NNs)

The majority of the models used in deep learning are built on NNs. Cells make up NNs, and everyone has its own activation function, weight, and bias variables. The weight and bias of the cells are used to determine the values supplied proportionately. Whether an operation is straightforward or complicated, NNs are capable of solving it [55]. To reduce the error rate of predictions on formerly unobserved points of information, aggregates of equivalent artificial NNs might be used [56].

$$z = \alpha(w^T y + c) \tag{20.9}$$

A skillfully designed NN is put out in Reference [57] that forecast the vertebral trabecular bone's strength under compression (CS) in individuals with advanced rheumatism. This NN also utilizes a back propagation approach employing a mean-square error expense function to determine the discrepancy among the predicted CS readings and the genuine CS parameters. It employs a tanh function of activation for the layers that are hidden and a linear activation function for the results. An excellent, powerful multi-instance artificial NN for healthcare diagnosis tasks involving classification was constructed by Wang et al. [58], and it was especially built on low-quality and fragmented databases of postoperative data. Both databases were from medical practice for the recognition of schizophrenic exacerbation and traditional Chinese Medicine for the diagnostic of acupuncture obstruction. They collected inter-instance characteristics employing multi-instance NN and subsequently separated the key characteristics for training and employing them for the ultimate categorization in the framework they developed. For this objective related to healthcare evaluation, particularly when considering partial and inferior information, their innovative approach outperformed existing ML algorithms. Additionally, Le [38] suggested an integration of NNs and the k-means clustering technique to increase the precision of diagnosis, which has been investigated on samples derived from the UCI 2016 categorization of liver disorders and breast tumors [37].

20.5 HEALTHCARE APPLICATION OF ML

20.5.1 Forecasting and diagnosis of conditions using ML techniques

Different ML techniques have been employed to forecast or identify diseases in their earliest stages, making treatment easier and increasing the likelihood that the individual receiving treatment will recover. These methods have allowed for the detection of several diseases, although with varying degrees of effectiveness according to the technique, characteristic collection, learning a database, and other variables. Cancer cells with specific traits might be subsequently refined via principal component analysis (PCA) to produce more accurate predictions [59], recognizing benign and malignant tumors in breast cancer. Following that, categorization is used to extract image attributes, including consistency, dimension, and smoothness [60].

Due to the striking similarity between small-cell lung cancer (SCLC) and carcinoma with no distinguishing features, the detection of SCLC in people is a significant challenge. In order to identify SCLC, deep learning methodologies created on convolutional neural networks (CNNs) and other algorithms that utilize ML may be applied. The forecasting of type 2 diabetics has been rendered conceivable through the utilization of predictive ML computational methods like the Gaussian naive Bayes algorithm

(GNB), LR, KNN, CART, RFA, and SVM in conjunction with parameters in digital health information like serum–glucose 1 and serum–glucose 2 levels, a person's body mass index, racial or ethnic background, sex, creatinine amount, and so on [61].

20.5.2 Diagnostic imaging using ML

Research in imaging for clinical purposes is expanding quickly since it is frequently necessary for determining disorders. While examining the ML process for producing recommendations from imagery, several processes may be distinguished. An image will be broken into many pieces after being provided as a feed in order to focus on the desired location. Attributes are able to be drawn out of these locations using data acquisition strategies. The necessary characteristics are picked out of them, plus the disruption is eliminated. After classifying the retrieved information, the ML algorithm will next generate recommendations depending on the categorization.

Currently, an extensive number of imaging techniques for medical purposes have been employed for various evaluations, including biopsy specimens, tumor reconstruction, seizures, blood vessel circumstances, and more [62]. These include electromagnetic resonance imaging (MRI), computed tomography (CT), ultrasound, single-photon release CT, and fluoroscopy. The interpretation of healthcare images is constantly changing as a result of technological advancement. The development of 3D virtual models also contributes to this goal by enhancing comprehension of complicated anatomical structures and by offering efficient instruments for surgical scheduling and postoperative guidance. These days, medical care is increasingly utilizing fetal MRI and 3D ultrasound images [63].

The effective method of histogram equalization (HE) could potentially be applied to enhance contrast. HE has undergone a number of different modifications that have been in place to enhance the technique's effectiveness. A number of ML methods are utilized to analyze clinical images, including linear discriminant analysis, SVM, as well as RF. ML techniques are being utilized to build low binary structure descriptions that might be utilized for medical imagery. In order to analyze the specifics of an illness, clinical images are examined using a NN approach. Specialist systems focused on medicine may utilize ML to assist in clinical imaging [64].

20.5.3 ML in biomedical science

Databases on gene activity include evaluations of a group of chromosomes' varying degrees of translation. Gene expression assessments are often made using specimens of tissue or individuals over a period or interval, and the results are displayed as numerical matrices. Each of the nodes in the structure of interactions between proteins stands for biological molecules, and the boundaries signify interconnections. Since it might be challenging for individuals to provide accurate numbers, it remains preferable to utilize a minimal amount of input from users throughout the segmentation process. If the aforementioned user contributions are inaccurate, the precision of the algorithm might be impacted [65].

Statistics must be analyzed, understood, and used to take appropriate action before they can be helpful. To carry out the previously mentioned operations with databases, computations are necessary. As a result, modern medical practice requires the use of cutting-edge analytical instruments in the ML sector. In a qualitative database, ML is unable to resolve the basic difficulties with inference about causality. It should be stated that while the model is effective for forecasting consequences, these variables do not correspond to cause and effect [66].

20.5.4 Retrieval of medical events using ML

Disease–drug interactions, disease–gene interactions, drug–drug interactions, and protein–protein interactions are all examples of biological processes with intricate architectures. The volume of unorganized and partially structured medical information is continually expanding, making clinical data mining technologies essential for effectively and reliably extracting these biological occurrences.

With the use of SVM, it is feasible to divide the process of extracting occurrences into various categorization assignments, with every assignment focusing on identifying the trigger phrases that define activities and the supporting data that specifies what proteins or enzymes participate in these occurrences. This depends on algorithms for supervised learning as well as labeled information. Although these might be taken into account while utilizing a semi-supervised ML strategy for clinical occurrence in the extraction process, sparse characteristics that have been processed by supervised ML methods might be employed to improve the efficiency of the framework [67]. Enzyme sequencing information might be used to extrapolate the effective, fundamental, and developmental properties of the enzyme. Protein categorization aims at precisely gathering this data, and only the use of ML techniques has made this achievable. Figure 20.8 illustrates the basic medical events combined with IoT mechanism for the smart healthcare mechanism.

20.5.5 ML toward polypharmacology

The goal of polypharmacology is to create drugs that may activate various receptors. Despite the fact that a medicine might be intended to address one or more targets, its effectiveness and hazard are a consequence of numerous interconnections involving pharmacodynamic, pharmacokinetic, epigenetic, biological, and contextual variables. In order to facilitate the forecasting and evaluation of experimental and animal drug–response characteristics, ML-related computational strategies are needed [68].

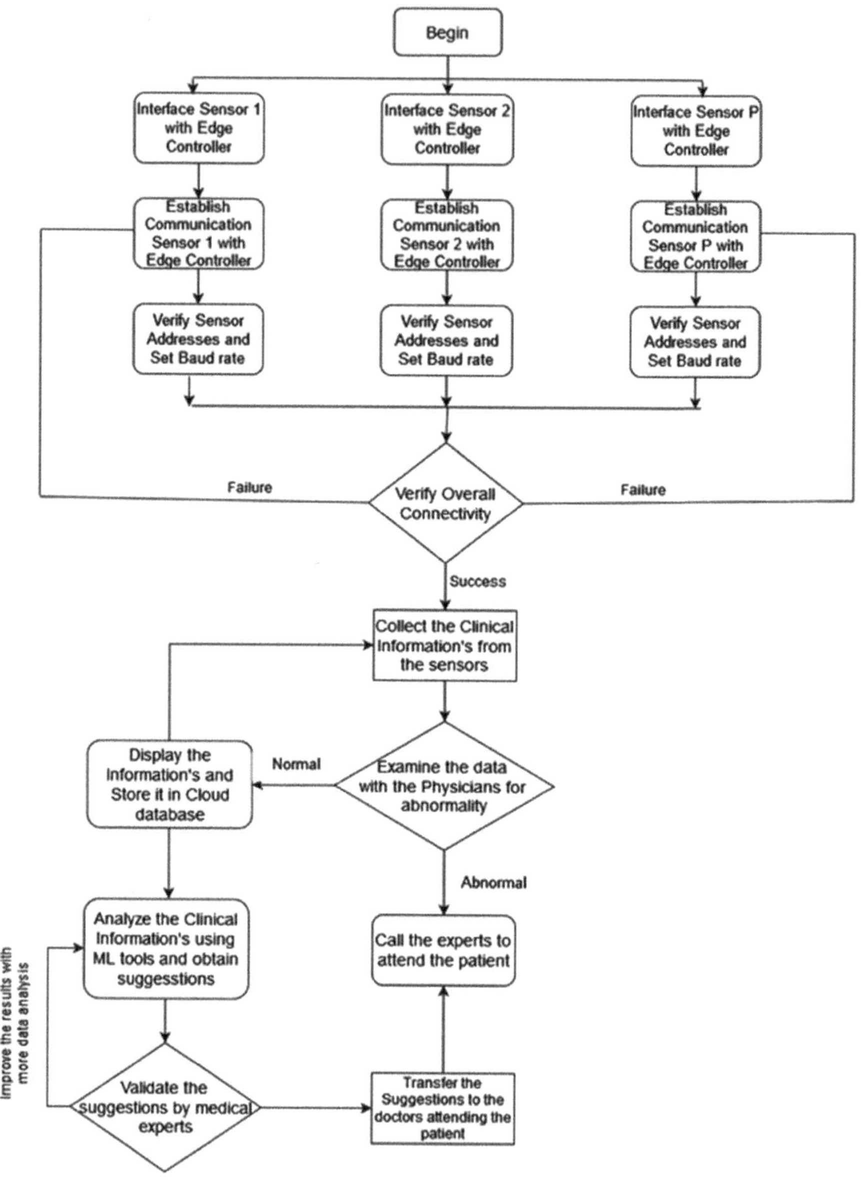

Figure 20.8 Retrieval of medical events using ML.

Recommendations are made using ML techniques using historical information. The Google flu serves as a reminder of the potential issues with the forecasting of time series when using information from just one quarter. Possessing a lot of knowledge from previous periods has less value. In order to make more precise inferences, it is often discovered during studies on decision-making systems that it seems preferable to employ information gathered in the most recent year rather than historical information from a number of years. While assessing forecasting techniques, the primary emphasis is on the reliability of the systems' capacity to anticipate patterns in the future rather than their capacity to replicate previous patterns [68]. It is evident that by employing complicated and unpredictable information, ML approaches may enhance the precision of forecasts using traditional regression techniques.

20.5.6 Integrative bioscience and ML towards drug recycling

During the initial stages of clinical research, over 90% of medications failed for reasons like undesirable responses, adverse effects, or ineffectiveness. Reusing drugs was recently discussed as a solution to such problems. The understanding of disease-related genetic material, pharmaceutical targets, signaling systems, and gene–gene communications is combined to create a drug disease network (DDN) that encompasses every one of the associations among pharmaceutical targets and genomes associated with a particular illness outlined in KEGG signaling channels. The Pearson correlation coefficient among the genome disruption characteristics of the drug–disease combinations, which can range from 1 to –1, is used to determine the recycling ratings of the drug–disease combinations. If the result is highly favorable, it means that the medicine and the medical condition affect the immune system in a comparable manner, and if it is extremely adverse, it means that the two exhibit contradictory characteristics of genome disruption. A drug's potential as an intervention for a specific condition can be assessed by utilizing this number [69].

20.6 INNOVATIONS AND TECHNIQUES IN THE TREATMENT OF THE ELDERLY

In a study by Alex et al. [70], they discussed an innovative Medicine Box integrated with a wireless-enabled smart home system and an Android application (Health-IoT). This setup facilitates enhanced communication between patients and doctors. The Medicine Box, a key component of the system, serves as a reminder for patients to take their medications punctually. Through wireless connectivity, the box ensures timely notifications about prescribed medicines, which are synchronized with the client's smart device through the Android app. The system proactively alerts patients, ensuring accurate medication adherence. Additionally, the system is equipped to send SMS notifications to a preconfigured guardian in case of critical health indicators. In a related study, Kinthada et al. [71] proposed a framework for monitoring patients' medication consumption. This approach encompasses the distribution of prescribed drugs and the tracking of prescription histories. The system advises patients through warnings and assists in locating missed injections, which healthcare professionals can rectify. This advanced system, compared to traditional devices, is smaller, more affordable, precise, lightweight, and operationally simplified. The recommended system holds potential to aid elderly patients, particularly those who might struggle with literacy, in adhering to their medication schedules. Furthermore, Pinto et al. [72] highlighted the growing elderly population globally and the need for comprehensive support. They emphasized that the IoT could revolutionize healthcare by providing personalized, preventive, and collaborative care. The study introduced an IoT solution targeting elderly individuals, enabling them to keep track of and document important data while offering alert warning capabilities [72]. Their research proposed a cost-effective wireless networking solution involving a cloud-connected bracelet for elderly patient support. This innovation signifies a promising direction for contemporary healthcare.

20.7 ML AND BIG DATA TECHNIQUES IN CLINICAL CARE

In a study conducted by Hosseini et al. [73], the focus was on exploring the characteristics of a brain–machine interface by means of various sensors, including electroencephalography. The study aimed to extract information from epileptic brains through techniques such as diffusion tensor imaging and imagery [73]. The proposed method incorporated advanced computation to deliver an instantaneous context-aware approach, employing both invasive and noninvasive techniques to monitor and analyze brain activity. The primary objective was to predict the onset of seizures ("ictal start") in a timely manner, contributing to effective epilepsy management. Addressing the requirements of healthcare systems, which demand a network structure capable of supporting Quality of Service (QoS) for video and real-time applications, is crucial.

Akhil et al. [74] discussed the utilization of ML in the healthcare sector, anticipating a transformative impact in the coming years. ML and artificial intelligence (AI)-driven decision support systems (DSS) are expected to offer predictive solutions for both patients and medical practitioners [74]. Leading companies like Enclitic, MedAware, and Google have introduced substantial efforts to improve AI-based healthcare systems. This technological advancement is projected to enhance efficiency, precision, and accessibility in healthcare delivery, leading to improved patient outcomes while minimizing costs.

Yadav and Jadhav [3] primarily focused on dual significant statistics skills, namely, medical data mining and the IoT. The integration of big data analytics (BDA) with IoT offers a comprehensive framework for managing and sharing vast volumes of structured as well as unstructured information. BDA is instrumental in handling extensive datasets that are commonly encountered in business contexts [3]. On the other hand, IoT facilitates the seamless exchange of information among various physical, electronic, and sensor-based devices that are interconnected within a network.

Healthcare providers are now collecting more data than ever before, from electronic health records (EHRs) to wearable devices. This data can be used to track patients' health over time, identify patterns, and make predictions about future diseases. However, the sheer volume of data can make it difficult to process and analyze manually. ML algorithms can be employed to automate the analysis of healthcare data. These algorithms can identify patterns and make predictions that would be difficult or unmanageable for physicians to confirm themselves. ML algorithms can also be utilized to classify patients into different risk groups, which can help healthcare providers target interventions more effectively. AI-powered healthcare data analysis can lead to improved diagnoses, treatments, and patient results. As an instance, AI algorithms have the potential to detect individuals at risk of specific illnesses, prior to any visible symptoms. This information can be used to intervene early and prevent the disease from developing. AI algorithms can also be used to develop new treatments for diseases that are currently incurable.

There are various AI technologies that can be used for healthcare data analysis, including classification, regression, clustering, and association. Classification algorithms can be used to identify patients into different groups based on their characteristics. Regression algorithms can be utilized for forecasting upcoming results by relying on historical data. Clustering algorithms can be used to group patients together based on their similarities. Association algorithms can be employed to recognize trends within datasets. AI-powered healthcare data analysis can help healthcare providers make better decisions about patient care. For instance, based on a patient's particular condition, AI algorithms may be able to recommend the best course of treatment. They can also identify people who may need hospital readmissions. The application of AI has been thoroughly studied in the healthcare industry.

Professionals specializing in data within the healthcare sector leverage large datasets for a range of purposes, spanning from enhancing patient satisfaction to developing intricate ML algorithms with the capability to diagnose medical ailments through X-ray imagery. In achieving these accomplishments, these experts harness analytics to efficiently handle and scrutinize substantial datasets, ultimately generating valuable insights, pinpointing trends, and facilitating informed decision-making processes.

In summary, these research endeavors contribute to the advancement of biomedical technology, healthcare management, and data analytics. They underscore the potential of innovative techniques like BMI, ML, and IoT in revolutionizing medical practices and improving patient care while addressing the complex challenges of prediction, real-time monitoring, and data management.

20.8 BIG DATA APPLICATIONS

Professionals within the healthcare domain harness the potential of big data across an expansive spectrum of objectives, encompassing tasks like unraveling insights in biomedical exploration and tailoring medical solutions to individual patients. Several illustrative applications of big data within healthcare encompass the following:

- Crafting predictive analytics to construct ML frameworks with the capacity to forecast the probability of a patient potentially developing a specific ailment.
- Facilitating real-time notifications to medical personnel through ongoing monitoring of patients' conditions within a medical establishment.
- Elevating security measures concerning the handling of delicate medical information, including aspects like insurance claims and medical histories.

This section provides an in-depth exploration of a healthcare system empowered by ML through IoT integration. The impact of IoT on healthcare is highly beneficial, positively impacting the lives of countless individuals. It thoroughly assesses the healthcare landscape, effectively diagnosing ailments and offering personalized care for the betterment of patients. IoT technologies offer a wide array of data, encompassing appointment reminders, exercise monitoring, calorie tracking, blood pressure, disease status, heart health, body temperature, and body positioning. The proposed healthcare system's design is illustrated in Figure 20.9.

IoT facilitates the connection of machinery, tools, and medical apparatus, creating intelligent information systems tailored to each patient's specific needs. Integrating IoT technologies significantly benefits advanced medical devices catering to individualized solutions. These technologies enable the capture,

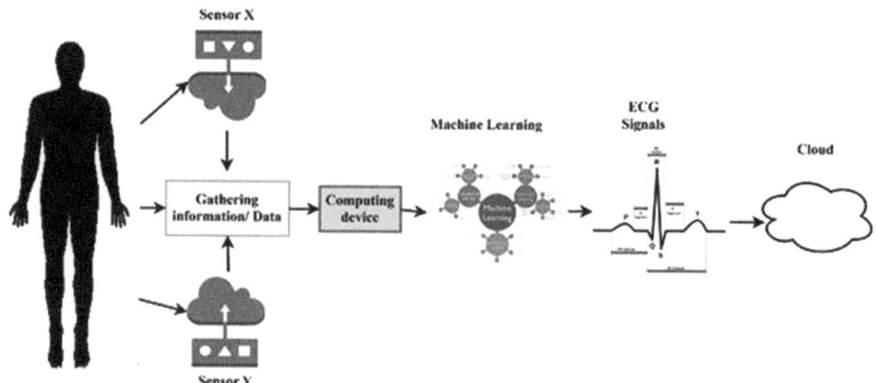

Figure 20.9 The structure of a healthcare system enabled by ML and IoT.

storage, and analysis of digital medical information. All medical records are maintained digitally, with internet resources enabling seamless transfer of patient data during emergencies, ultimately enhancing doctors' efficiency.

The medical IoT framework merges the advantages of big data, ML, and IoT technology within the medical domain. Moreover, it delineates the procedures for relaying patient data from diverse sensors and medical tools to a dedicated medical network. The configuration of distinct IoT healthcare system components harmoniously integrated to cater to clinical care needs is called an IoT healthcare topology.

A variety of sensors, including pulse sensors, blood pressure (BP) sensors, temperature sensors, and tilt sensors, are utilized to gather medical information from patients. This information encompasses blood pressure, heart rate, temperature, oxygen saturation, ECG (electrocardiogram) readings, body postures, and more. A wearable sensor-based IoT system is employed to track important signs such as pulse, body temperature, and BP, offering the potential for critical health monitoring. Sensors play a crucial role in perceiving, collecting, and transmitting essential data related to patient health and illnesses. Within this context, all physical objects are interconnected through the Internet, enabling real-time process monitoring via devices. Specific medical practitioners receive pertinent patient data tailored to their requirements. Regular measurements are taken, and if any of these indicators deviate from established healthy ranges, the central hub can transmit the data to the cloud for immediate notification of emergency services.

The ECG provides a sequence of sinus rhythms that depict the heart's condition. Among the widely employed tests for identifying cardiac disorders, the ECG stands out due to its affordability and effectiveness in pinpointing specific conditions. The model developed to predict outcomes for various illnesses and differentiate between normal and pathological ECG readings can also be applied to forecast the progression of other conditions lacking prior analysis. The primary objective is to determine which algorithm yields optimal results for disease prognosis. This study employs four distinct ML algorithms, which are discussed as follows.

The DT, a supervised learning technique, is commonly utilized for solving categorization problems. It functions with categorical or continuous input and output variables. The model learns straightforward decision rules based on data characteristics when predicting the target variable's value. In essence, the population or sample is segregated into two or more uniform clusters using the most prominent differentiation in input parameters.

In the KNN method, instances of training data are stored and label estimation is performed using the training samples closest to the new data point. This instance-based learning technique employs an instance-based training set. NB employs multivariate Bernoulli distributions for data distribution, serving as a training and categorization algorithm suitable for linear classification. It assumes binary values for each feature, requiring decision rules and sample representation as binary-valued feature vectors.

The supervised learning technique SVM is engaged for outlier detection, regression, and classification. Given labeled training information, the scheme generates a finest decision plane for classifying different cases. Categorization is performed by creating a hyperplane in a multidimensional space, dividing instances of different label classes. A typical heart maintains a steady sinus rhythm with a heartbeat between 60 and 100 beats per minute (specifically 82 bpm). Minor alterations in the PQRST (P-wave, QRS-Complex, T-Wave) segment can indicate various cardiac diseases.

The P wave, QRS complex, T wave, and U wave constituting a typical ECG tracing of a cardiac cycle are usually detectable in 50–75% of ECGs. The section of the ECG trace follows the T wave, or in certain cases the U wave, before the subsequent P wave represents the baseline (flat segments). In a healthy, normally functioning heart, the baseline is nearly isoelectric. Based on the ECG report and symptoms, this system determines whether an individual has heart disease. If heart disease is detected, it is further classified as coronary artery disease or myocardial infarction.

To ensure optimal care and diagnosis in the future, all records are securely stored in the cloud. Secure preservation of patient-provided medical information is essential for continuous use. Combining IoT and ML algorithms enhances the performance of doctors and surgeons in heart disease prediction and classification, thus achieving accuracy and reliability in therapy.

20.9 FUTURE TRENDS FOR ML WITH IoT IN MEDICAL SERVICES: CRITICAL RESEARCH CHALLENGES

Despite the numerous advantages, the implementation of IoT-driven ML mechanisms in healthcare also faces challenges. Data security, privacy concerns, interoperability, and the need for regulatory compliance are critical factors that need to be addressed to ensure the responsible and widespread adoption of these technologies. However, as the capabilities of IoT and ML continue to expand, their integration in healthcare applications holds immense potential to transform the industry and ultimately improve the lives of patients worldwide. ML and the IoT are playing a crucial role in revolutionizing healthcare by enabling data-driven decision-making, personalized treatments, and remote patient monitoring. However, several research issues and future directions remain to be addressed to fully unlock the potential of ML and IoT in healthcare. Some key areas are provided in Table 20.1.

Overall, addressing these research issues and focusing on the future directions outlined above will be pivotal in fully leveraging the potential of ML and IoT in healthcare, ultimately resulting in improved results for patients and improved efficiency in medical systems. The solution to these problems involves cooperation between clinical professionals, data scientists, policymakers, and technology experts. Research and development efforts must focus on creating robust and secure ML algorithms, developing standardized

Table 20.1 Future trends of ML with IoT in medical services

Ref. No.	Medical services	Applications of ML with IoT in respective fields
[75]	Remote patient monitoring	ML algorithms process IoT-generated patient data for real-time monitoring of vital signs and health conditions remotely, enabling early anomaly detection and proactive healthcare interventions
[76]	Predictive analytics	ML models analyze historical patient data from IoT devices to predict disease progression, medication adherence, hospital readmissions, and overall health outcomes, optimizing treatment plans
[77]	Personalized medicine	ML algorithms utilize IoT-collected data to tailor treatment plans and medications based on individual patient characteristics, enhancing treatment efficacy and minimizing side effects
[11]	Health wearables and devices	ML integrated with IoT enhances accuracy and interpretation of data from wearable devices, providing insights into an individual's health and lifestyle patterns for early intervention and recommendations
[78]	Data security and privacy	ML-powered algorithms enhance data security and privacy for healthcare IoT devices, detecting anomalies and potential security breaches to ensure compliance with privacy regulations
[77]	Drug development and research	ML algorithms process vast amounts of IoT-collected data to expedite drug discovery, clinical trials, and research, leading to faster development of new treatments and therapies
[79]	Telemedicine optimization	ML optimizes telemedicine services by leveraging IoT data to improve diagnostic accuracy, treatment recommendations, and patient–doctor interactions, enhancing the efficiency and accessibility of services
[77]	Healthcare resource management	ML algorithms integrated with IoT optimize resource allocation in healthcare settings, predicting patient admissions, optimizing staff schedules, and managing medical inventory more efficiently

interfaces, addressing biases in data and models, and ensuring compliance with ethical and regulatory standards. Additionally, educating healthcare stakeholders about the benefits and limitations of ML and IoT in medical care is essential for successful integration and adoption.

20.10 CONCLUSION

In conclusion, the fusion of IoT and ML has ushered in a transformative era for healthcare applications. This synergy has empowered the healthcare industry to harness the power of data-driven insights, real-time monitoring, and predictive analytics to enhance patient care, streamline operations, and drive medical advancements. IoT-driven ML mechanisms offer numerous benefits across various healthcare domains. Remote patient monitoring has become more comprehensive and personalized, allowing healthcare professionals to detect anomalies, predict deteriorations, and intervene proactively. Chronic disease management has been revolutionized, enabling patients to take an active role in their health through continuous data collection and personalized treatment plans. Furthermore, the integration of IoT sensors and devices with ML algorithms has optimized hospital operations, improving resource allocation, patient flow, and staff management. Predictive maintenance of medical equipment ensures uninterrupted services and minimizes downtime, enhancing the overall efficiency of healthcare facilities. However, this convergence also presents challenges that must be addressed. Data security and patient privacy are paramount concerns, necessitating robust cybersecurity measures and adherence to regulatory standards such as HIPAA. The interoperability of diverse IoT devices and platforms remains an ongoing technical challenge, requiring standardized protocols and seamless integration. As we look ahead, the trajectory of IoT-driven ML in healthcare appears promising. Continued advancements in sensor technology, data analytics, and algorithm development will likely lead to more accurate diagnoses, personalized treatments, and better health outcomes. Collaborations between healthcare professionals, data scientists, and technologists will play a pivotal role in shaping the future of healthcare, ensuring that innovations are not only technologically sound but also ethically responsible and patient-centric. In essence, IoT-driven ML mechanisms are a cornerstone of the modern healthcare landscape, enabling a paradigm shift from reactive to proactive, patient-centered care. By leveraging the vast potential of data and intelligent algorithms, healthcare stands poised to achieve new heights of precision, accessibility, and effectiveness, ultimately leading to healthier populations and improved quality of life.

REFERENCES

1. Hamad, Z. J., & Shavan, A. (2021). Machine learning powered IoT for smart applications. International journal of science and business, 5(3), 92–100.
2. Qi, J., Yang, P., Min, G., Amft, O., Dong, F., & Xu, L. (2017). Advanced internet of things for personalised healthcare systems: A survey. Pervasive and mobile computing, 41, 132–149.
3. Yadav, S., & Jadhav, S. (2019). Machine learning algorithms for disease prediction using IoT environment. International journal of engineering and advanced technology, 8, 4303–4307. doi:10.35940/ijeat.F8914.088619.
4. Askar, S. (2016). Adaptive load balancing scheme for data center networks using software defined network. Journal of university of Zakho, 4(A)(2), 275–286.
5. Askar, S. (2017). SDN-based load balancing scheme for fat-tree data center networks. Al-Nahrain journal for engineering sciences (NJES), 20(5), 1047–1056.
6. Keti, F., & Askar, S. (2015). Emulation of Software Defined Networks Using Mininet in Different Simulation Environments. 6th International Conference on Intelligent Systems, Modelling and Simulation, Kuala Lumpur, 2015, pp. 205–210. doi: 10.1109/ISMS.2015.46

7. Reena, J. K., & Parameswari, R. (2019). A Smart Health Care Monitor System in IoT Based Human Activities of Daily Living: A Review. 2019 International Conference on Machine Learning, Big Data, Cloud and Parallel Computing (COMITCon).

8. Shailaja, K., Seetharamulu, B., & Jabbar, M. (2018). Machine Learning in Healthcare: A Review. 2018 Second International Conference on Electronics, Communication and Aerospace Technology (ICECA).

9. Aziz, M. N., & Islam, A. (2020). Reviewing data mining as an enabling technology for BI. International journal of science and business, 4(7), 46–51.

10. Atiqur, R., Liton, A., & Wu, G. (2020). Content caching strategy at small base station in 5G networks with mobile edge computing. International journal of science and business, 4(4), 104–112.

11. Rakhmatulin, I. (2020). Review of EEG feature selection by neural networks. International journal of science and business, 4(9), 101–112.

12. McGowan, B., Gibb, M., Cullen, K., & Craig, C. (2019). Non-cognitive symptoms of dementia (NCSD): Guidance on non-pharmacological interventions for healthcare and social care practitioners.

13. Mathew, T. K., & Zubair, M., & Tadi, P. (2024). Blood Ducrose Control. StatPearls Publishing.

14. Garg, A., & Mago, V. (2021). Role of machine learning in medical research: A survey. Computer science review, 40, 100370.

15. Kaplan, R. M. (2003). The significance of quality of life in health care. Quality of life research, 12, 3–16.

16. Smiti, A. (2020). When machine learning meets medical world: Current status and future challenges. Computer science review, 37, 100280.

17. Smiti, A., & Elouedi, Z. (2012). DBSCAN-GM: An improved clustering method based on gaussian means and DBSCAN techniques. In 2012 IEEE 16th international conference on intelligent engineering systems (INES) (pp. 573–578). IEEE.

18. Chen, C. H. (2014). A hybrid intelligent model of analyzing clinical breast cancer data using clustering techniques with feature selection. Applied soft computing, 20, 4–14.

19. Cox, D. R. (1958). The regression analysis of binary sequences. Journal of the Royal Statistical Society series b: Statistical methodology, 20(2), 215–232.

20. Lavrač, N. (1999). Machine learning for data mining in medicine. In Joint European Conference on Artificial Intelligence in Medicine and Medical Decision Making (pp. 47–62). Berlin, Heidelberg: Springer.

21. Dinov, I. D. (2016). Methodological challenges and analytic opportunities for modeling and interpreting big healthcare data. Gigascience, 5(1), s13742-016.

22. Rumsfeld, J. S., Joynt, K. E., & Maddox, T. M. (2016). Big data analytics to improve cardiovascular care: Promise and challenges. Nature reviews cardiology, 13(6), 350–359.

23. Shen, D., Wu, G., & Suk, H. I. (2017). Deep learning in medical image analysis. Annual review of biomedical engineering, 19, 221–248.

24. Zhou, M., Scott, J., Chaudhury, B., Hall, L., Goldgof, D., Yeom, K. W., & Gatenby, R. (2018). Radiomics in brain tumor: Image assessment, quantitative feature descriptors, and machine-learning approaches. American Journal of neuroradiology, 39(2), 208–216.

25. Chen, J. H., & Asch, S. M. (2017). Machine learning and prediction in medicine: Beyond the peak of inflated expectations. The new England journal of medicine, 376(26), 2507.

26. Suykens, J. A., & Vandewalle, J. (1999). Least squares support vector machine classifiers. Neural processing letters, 9, 293–300.

27. Lin, C. F., & Wang, S. D. (2002). Fuzzy support vector machines. IEEE transactions on neural networks, 13(2), 464–471.
28. Huang, S., Cai, N., Pacheco, P. P., Narrandes, S., Wang, Y., & Xu, W. (2018). Applications of support vector machine (SVM) learning in cancer genomics. Cancer genomics & proteomics, 15(1), 41–51.
29. Dallora, A. L., Eivazzadeh, S., Mendes, E., Berglund, J., & Anderberg, P. (2017). Machine learning and microsimulation techniques on the prognosis of dementia: A systematic literature review. *PLoS one*, 12(6), e0179804.
30. Taylor, R. A., Moore, C. L., Cheung, K. H., & Brandt, C. (2018). Predicting urinary tract infections in the emergency department with machine learning. *PLoS one*, 13(3), e0194085.
31. Leha, A., Hellenkamp, K., Unsöld, B., Mushemi-Blake, S., Shah, A. M., Hasenfuß, G., & Seidler, T. (2019). A machine learning approach for the prediction of pulmonary hypertension. PLoS one, 14(10), e0224453.
32. Meiring, C., Dixit, A., Harris, S., MacCallum, N. S., Brealey, D. A., Watkinson, P. J., & Ercole, A. (2018). Optimal intensive care outcome prediction over time using machine learning. PLoS one, 13(11), e0206862.
33. Yelipe, U., Porika, S., & Golla, M. (2018). An efficient approach for imputation and classification of medical data values using class-based clustering of medical records. Computers & electrical engineering, 66, 487–504.
34. Jain, A. K., Murty, M. N., & Flynn, P. J. (1999). Data clustering: A review. ACM computing surveys (CSUR), 31(3), 264–323.
35. Xu, R., & Wunsch, D. (2008). Clustering. John Wiley & Sons, Inc.
36. Wiwie, C., Baumbach, J., & Röttger, R. (2015). Comparing the performance of biomedical clustering methods. *Nature methods*, 12(11), 1033–1038.
37. UCI datasets (1995). https://archive.ics.uci.edu/ml/datasets.php
38. Le, T. L. (2019). Fuzzy c-means clustering interval type-2 cerebellar model articulation neural network for medical data classification. IEEE access, 7, 20967–20973.
39. KEEL datasets (2011). https://sci2s.ugr.es/keel/datasets.php#sub1
40. Wagstaff, K., Cardie, C., Rogers, S., & Schrödl, S. (2001). Constrained k-means clustering with background knowledge. ICML, 1, 577–584.
41. Chen, M., Hao, Y., Hwang, K., Wang, L., & Wang, L. (2017). Disease prediction by machine learning over big data from healthcare communities. IEEE access, 5, 8869–8879.
42. Nilashi, M., bin Ibrahim, O., Ahmadi, H., & Shahmoradi, L. (2017). An analytical method for diseases prediction using machine learning techniques. Computers & chemical engineering, 106, 212–223.
43. Ramalingam, V. V., Dandapath, A., & Raja, M. K. (2018). Heart disease prediction using machine learning techniques: A survey. International journal of engineering & technology, 7(2.8), 684–687.
44. Breiman, L. (2001). Random forests. Machine learning, 45, 5–32.
45. Erickson, B. J., Korfiatis, P., Akkus, Z., & Kline, T. L. (2017). Machine learning for medical imaging. *Radiographics*, 37(2), 505–515.
46. Liaw, A., & Wiener, M. (2002). Classification and regression by random forest. R news, 2(3), 18–22.
47. Zhu, M., Xia, J., Jin, X., Yan, M., Cai, G., Yan, J., & Ning, G. (2018). Class weights random forest algorithm for processing class imbalanced medical data. IEEE access, 6, 4641–4652.
48. Wang, J., & Shi, L. (2020). Prediction of medical expenditures of diagnosed diabetics and the assessment of its related factors using a random forest model, MEPS 2000–2015. International journal for quality in health care, 32(2), 99–112.
49. Cover, T., & Hart, P. (1967). Nearest neighbor pattern classification. *IEEE transactions on information theory*, 13(1), 21–27.

50. Keller, J. M., Gray, M. R., & Givens, J. A. (1985). A fuzzy k-nearest neighbor algorithm. *IEEE transactions on systems, man, and cybernetics*, 4, 580–585.
51. Zhang, Z. (2016). Introduction to machine learning: k-nearest neighbors. Annals of translational medicine, 4(11).
52. Uddin, S., Khan, A., Hossain, M. E., & Moni, M. A. (2019). Comparing different supervised machine learning algorithms for disease prediction. BMC medical informatics and decision making, 19(1), 1–16.
53. D'souza, K. J., & Ansari, Z. (2018, November). Big data science in building medical data classifier using naïve Bayes model. 2018 IEEE International Conference on Cloud Computing in Emerging Markets (CCEM) (pp. 76–80). IEEE.
54. Shen, L., Chen, H., Yu, Z., Kang, W., Zhang, B., Li, H., & Liu, D. (2016). Evolving support vector machines using fruit fly optimization for medical data classification. Knowledge-based systems, 96, 61–75.
55. Nielsen, M. A. (2015). Neural Networks and Deep Learning (vol. 25, pp. 15–24). San Francisco, CA: Determination press.
56. Hansen, L. K., & Salamon, P. (1990). Neural network ensembles. *IEEE transactions on pattern analysis and machine intelligence*, 12(10), 993–1001.
57. Shaikhina, T., & Khovanova, N. A. (2017). Handling limited datasets with neural networks in medical applications: A small-data approach. Artificial intelligence in medicine, 75, 51–63.
58. Wang, Z., Poon, J., Sun, S., & Poon, S. (2019, July). Attention-based multi-instance neural network for medical diagnosis from incomplete and low quality data. 2019 International Joint Conference on Neural Networks (IJCNN) (pp. 1–8). IEEE.
59. Mishra, V., Singh, Y., & Rath, S. K. (2019). Breast cancer detection from thermograms using feature extraction and machine learning techniques. 2019 IEEE 5th International Conference for Convergence in Technology (I2CT) (pp. 1–5). IEEE.
60. Dhahri, H., Al Maghayreh, E., Mahmood, A., Elkilani, W., & Faisal Nagi, M. (2019). Automated breast cancer diagnosis based on machine learning algorithms. Journal of healthcare engineering, 2019, 4253641.
61. Mani, S., Chen, Y., Elasy, T., Clayton, W., & Denny, J. (2012). Type 2 diabetes risk forecasting from EMR data using machine learning. AMIA Annual Symposium Proceedings (vol. 2012, p. 606). American Medical Informatics Association.
62. Miner, R. C. (2017). Image-guided neurosurgery. *Journal of medical imaging and radiation sciences*, 48(4), 328–335.
63. Pratt, R., Deprest, J., Vercauteren, T., Ourselin, S., & David, A. L. (2015). Computer-assisted surgical planning and intraoperative guidance in fetal surgery: A systematic review. Prenatal diagnosis, 35(12), 1159–1166.
64. Murtza, I., Saadia, A., Basri, R., Imran, A., Almuhaimeed, A., & Alzahrani, A. (2022). Forex investment optimization using instantaneous stochastic gradient ascent: Formulation of an adaptive machine learning approach. Sustainability, 14(22), 15328.
65. Andreopoulos, B., An, A., Wang, X., & Schroeder, M. (2009). A roadmap of clustering algorithms: Finding a match for a biomedical application. Briefings in bioinformatics, 10(3), 297–314.
66. Obermeyer, Z., & Emanuel, E. J. (2016). Predicting the future: big data, machine learning, and clinical medicine. The new England journal of medicine, 375(13), 1216.
67 Wang, J., Xu, Q., Lin, H., Yang, Z., & Li, Y. (2013). Semi-supervised method for biomedical event extraction. Proteome science, 11(1), 1–10.
68. Xie, L., Xie, L., Kinnings, S. L., & Bourne, P. E. (2012). Novel computational approaches to polypharmacology as a means to define responses to individual drugs. Annual review of pharmacology and toxicology, 52, 361–379.

69. Peyvandipour, A., Saberian, N., Shafi, A., Donato, M., & Draghici, S. (2018). A novel computational approach for drug repurposing using systems biology. Bioinformatics, 34(16), 2817–2825.
70. Alex, G., Varghese, B., Jose, J. G., & Abraham, A. M. (2016). A modern health care system using IoT and Android. Journal for Research, 8(4).
71. Kinthada, M. R., Bodda, S., & Mande, S. B. K. (2016). eMedicare: MHealth solution for patient medication guidance and assistance. 2016 International Conference on Signal Processing, Communication, Power and Embedded System (SCOPES).
72. Pinto, S., Cabral, J., & Gomes, T. (2017). We-care: An IoT-based health care system for elderly people. 2017 IEEE International Conference on Industrial Technology (ICIT).
73. Hosseini, M.-P., Tran, T. X., Pompili, D., Elisevich, K., & Soltanian-Zadeh, H. (2017). Deep learning with edge computing for localization of epileptogenicity using multimodal rs-fMRI and EEG big data. 2017 IEEE International Conference on Autonomic Computing (ICAC).
74. Akhil, J., Samreen, S., & Aluvalu, R. (2018). The future of health care: Machine learning. International journal of engineering and technology (UAE), 7, 23–25. doi:10.14419/ijet.v7i4.6.20226
75. Waleed, M., Kamal, T., Um, T. W., Hafeez, A., Habib, B., & Skouby, K. E. (2023). Unlocking insights in IoT-based patient monitoring: Methods for encompassing large-data challenges. Sensors, 23(15), 6760.
76. Shastry, K. A., & Shastry, A. (2023). An integrated deep learning and natural language processing approach for continuous remote monitoring in digital health. Decision analytics journal, 8, 100301.
77. Javaid, M., Haleem, A., Singh, R. P., Rab, S., Haq, M., & Raina, I. U. (2022). Internet of things in the global healthcare sector: Significance, applications, and barriers. International journal of intelligent networks, 3, 165–175.
78. Dash, K. (2023). Machine Learning Applications for Detecting Anomalies and Ensuring Data Integrity in Clinical Trials.
79. Amjad, A., Kordel, P., & Fernandes, G. (2023). A review on innovation in healthcare sector (Telehealth) through artificial intelligence. Sustainability, 15(8), 6655.

Index

A

ABAC (attribute-based access control), 244
Access control list (ACL), 104
Adaptive spatial kernel separation measure based fuzzy c-means (ASKFCM), 193
Advanced Encryption Standard (AES), 312
Advanced imaging tools like CT scanners, 28
Age-related macular degeneration (ARMD), 188
Albumin (Heller's test), 121, 125
Alexnet, 147
AMQP (Advanced Message Queuing Protocol), 308
Amwell, 233
Arrhythmia detection, 88
Artificial Intelligence (AI), 132
Artificial kidney, 116
Artificial limbs, 32–33
Artificial neural networks (ANNS), 48
Asthma, 93

B

Bayes, support vector machine (SVM), 3
Big data, 2–4
Big data applications, 398
Bile salt (Smith's Test), 121, 126
Biomedical applications, 323
Black hole attack, 279
BLE security (Bluetooth low-energy security), 309
Blockchain, 101
Blood pressure (BP), 343

Blood pressure monitors track cardiovascular health, 28
Blood tests, 106
Bluetooth low energy (BLE), 50
Body sensor networks (BSNs), 45–48
Brain tumor, 145
Breast cancer diagnosis, 78
Brute force attack, 280

C

CA-125, 99
Cardiac care, 93
Cardiovascular diseases, 86
ChatGPT, 202
Chromosome, 58
Chromosome data augmentation (CDA), 60
Chronic kidney disease, 192
Clinical data analysis, 383
Clinical decision support system (CDSS), 197
Cloud IOT, 273
Clustering, 386
COAP (Constrained Application Protocol), 258, 307
COCO (common objects in context) annotator, 64
Cognitive behavioural therapy (CBT), 169
Complex event processing (CEP), 119
Composite peak signal to-noise ratio (CPSNR), 134
Computerized tomography (CT), 79
Convolutional neural networks (CNNs), 3, 58
Coordinate reference frame (CRF), 81
CouchDB, 104

Cranial surgery, 81
Cross-site request forgery (CSRF), 242
Cross-site scripting (XSS), 243
Cybersecurity, 229
Cybersecurity threats, 303

D

DASS (depression anxiety stress scale), 167, 173
Data security, 369
Datagram transport layer security (DTLS), 307
Data-level/sensor-level fusion, 30
Decision trees (DTs), 52, 387
Decision-level fusion, 30
Deep learning, 102
Denial of service (DOS), 277
Dental, 131
Detectron2, 67
Diabetes mellitus (DM), 190
Diabetic retinopathy (DR), 188
Dipstick test, 120
Distributed cloud computing, 250
DPWsim, 206
DRCN (deeply recursive convolutional network), 69
DRRN (deep recursive residual network), 69
Drug discovery, 19, 77
Drug recycling, 395
DTI, 150

E

Early disease detection, 33
Early sepsis detection, 264
ECG analysis, 84
ECG sensors monitor heart activity, 28
Edge computing, 248
Edge gateway deployment, 254
e-health clouds, 236
e-healthcare, 222
Electrocardiogram (ECG) analysis, 12, 77
Electroencephalogram (EEG), 12
Electronic health, 300
Electronic health record (EHR), 196, 300, 356
Electronic medical records (EMRS), 356
Elliptic curve cryptography (ECC), 281
End-stage renal disease (ESRD), 117
ENT surgery, 81

Epidemiological surveillance, 94
Event processing language (EPL), 119
Extremal regions (ER), 62

F

Facebook artificial intelligence research (FAIR), 67
Fast R-CNN, 67
Feature-level fusion, 30
Federated learning (FL), 16–18
Fedhealth, 18
Fog computing, 251
FSRCNN (fast SR convolutional neural network), 69
Functional magnetic resonance imaging (FMRI), 92
Fuzzy decision method, 134

G

Gated recurrent unit (GRU), 3–4
Gaussian naive Bayes algorithm (GNB), 392
General-purpose input and output system (GPIO), 47
Github, 49

H

Health Insurance Portability and Accountability Act (HIPAA), 223, 225
Healthcare technologies, 345
Hearing aids, 32
Hemodialysis (HD), 116
Hippocampal subregions, 92
Histogram equalization (HE), 392
HITRUST (health information trust alliance), 262
HLF blockchain, 103
Hospital management system (HMS), 351
Hybrid cloud–edge data management strategies, 257
Hypertext markup language (HTML), 204
Hypertext transfer protocol (HTTP), 204

I

Image-guided surgery (IGS), 77, 80
Implantable devices, 31

Industrial IoT (IIOT), 321
Industry 4.0, 345
Information and communication technology (ICT), 341
Integrated development environment (IDE), 210
International System for Human Cytogenetic Nomenclature, 64
Internet of medical things (IoMT), 188
IOT architecture, 25
IPSec (Internet Protocol Security), 308

J

Jamming attack, 278

K

Karyotyping, 58
K-nearest neighbour (KNN), 172, 388

L

Laplacian pyramidal superresolution network (LaPSRN), 58
LaPSRN model, 68
Layers of IOT architecture, 26
LDR, 123
Ledger, 106
Lightweight cryptography, 280
Long short-term memory (LSTM), 3–4
Low-power wide-area networks (LPWAN), 1

M

Magnetic resonance imaging (MRI), 79
Mammography, 107
Medical identity theft (MIDT), 243
Medical image analysis, 188
Medical use, 41
Membership service provider (MSP), 105
Mental health, 167
Mineral bone disease (MBD), 117
ML algorithm, 13, 26–28
ML-enabled IoT, 327
Mobile edge computing (MEC), 251
Model-agnostic meta-learning (MAML), 15–16
Model-to-model (M2M), 51
Monitoring tools, 313
MQTT (message queuing telemetry transport), 84, 307

MRI, 145
Multi-distributed generated advertising network (MD-GAN), 62
Multifactor authentication (MFA), 234

N

Naive Bayes (NB), 390
Naive Bayes (NBs) algorithm, 79
Natural language processing (NLP) techniques, 209
Nature biotechnology, 46
Network intrusion detection systems (NIDS), 314
Neural networks (NNS), 390
Neural pathways, 93

O

OpenCV, 68
Optical coherence tomography (OCT), 193
Ovarian cancer, 98

P

Pacemakers, 8
Peak signal-to-noise ratio (PSNR), 134
Personal healthcare (PH), 9
Personalized medicine, 36–37
Phenotype representation learning (PRL), 79
Plushcare, 233
Polypharmacology, 393
Population health management, 33
Positron emission tomography (PET), 92
Practical Byzantine fault tolerance (PBFT), 104
Prioritized colored petri net (PCPN) model, 119
Privacy, 222
Private cloud, 240
Public cloud, 238
Public healthcare records (PHRs), 356
Pulse oximeters measure blood oxygen levels, 28

R

Random forest (RF), 387
Ransome attack, 280
RBAC (role-based access control), 244, 261

Real-time location system (RTLS), 49
RECIST (response evaluation criteria in solid tumors), 79
Recurrent neural networks (RNNS), 3
Reinforcement learning, 102
Relay, 124
Remote patient monitoring, 262
Remote patient monitoring (RPM) system, 224
Remote patient monitoring systems (RPMS), 225
Renal replacement therapy (RRT), 116
Residual convolutional recurrent attention neural network (Res-CRANN), 61
ResNet50 Model, 145
Resource description framework (RDF), 7–8
Retinal diseases, 190
Robot-assisted surgery, 77
Robotic process automation (RPA), 276

S

Secure sockets layer (SSL), 261
Security, 222
Security information and event management (SIEM), 315
Skin temperature, 12
Small-cell lung cancer (SCLC), 391
Smart health management system, 351
Smart healthcare system, 344
Smart therapist, 167
Software defined networking (SDN), 43
Spine surgery, 81
Special International Commission on Illumination (S-CIELAB), 134
SRCNN (SR convolutional neural network), 69
Structural similarity index (SSIM), 134
Structural similarity sugar (Benedict test), 121
Supervised learning, 102
Support vector machine (SVM), 52, 78, 128, 385
Surgical robots, 31
Surgical workflows, 264
Sybil attack, 279
Synaptic plasticity, 93
Synthetic minority oversampling technique (SMOTE), 137

T

Teladoc, 233
Telehealth solutions, 262
Telemedicine, 231
Threat intelligence feeds, 314
Transport layer security (TLS), 306
Tumor proportional scoring (TPS), 79

U

Ultrasound, 107
Ultrasound transducers, 32
U-Net, 150
Uniform resource finder (URF), 204
Unsupervised learning, 102
Urea (hypobromite test), 121, 126

V

VDSR (very deep SR), 69
Virtual network function (VNF), 207
Visual studio code (Vscode), 210
VITA master, 132

W

Wearable biosensors, 46
Wearable devices, 29
Web of things (WoT), 202
Web ontology language (OWL), 7–8
Websockets with SSL, 310
Wireless body area network (WBAN), 43, 48
Wireless sensor networks (WSNs), 320
Word sense disambiguation (WSD), 283
Wormhole attack, 279

X

X-ray machines aid, 28

Y

Yottabyte mark, 44
You Only Look Once (YOLO), 67

Z

Zigbee security, 309